AWHONN
Association of Women's Health, Obstetric and Neonatal Nurses

Fetal Heart Monitoring Principles and Practices

Third Edition

Editors

Nancy Feinstein, PhD, RNC
Keiko L. Torgersen, BSN, MS, RNC
Jana Atterbury, MS, RNC

Contributors

Donna Adelsperger, RN, MEd
Jana Atterbury, MS, RNC
Rebecca L. Cypher, PNNP, MSN(c)
Gay L. Goss, PhD, RNC, WHNP, CNS
Nancy Feinstein, PhD, RNC
G. Eric Knox, MD
Kathleen Mahoney, APN, C
Patricia Robin McCartney, PhD, RNC, FAAN

Gina M. Mikkelsen, RNC, MSN
Faith Wight Moffatt, BN, MS(N), RN
Anne Santa-Donato, RNC, MSN
Judy V. Schmidt, EdD, RNC
Kathleen Rice Simpson, PhD, RNC, FAAN
Keiko L. Torgersen, BSN, MS, RNC
Vickie J. Waymire, RNC, MSN

KENDALL/HUNT PUBLISHING COMPANY
4050 Westmark Drive   Dubuque, Iowa 52002

Any procedure or practice described in this book should be applied by the health care practitioner under appropriate supervision in accordance with professional guidelines used with regard to the specific circumstances of each practice situation. The information contained in this book does not define a standard of care, nor is it intended to dictate an exclusive course of management. It presents general methods and techniques of practice that are currently acceptable, based on current research and used by recognized authorities. Proper care of individual patients may depend on many individual factors as well as professional judgment. The information presented here is not designed to define standards of practice for employment, licensure, discipline, legal or other purposes. Variations and innovations that are consistent with law and that demonstrably improve the quality of patient care should be encouraged. Care has been taken to confirm the accuracy of information presented and to describe generally accepted practices. However, the authors, editors, and publisher cannot accept any responsibility for error or omissions or for any consequences resulting from the application of the information in this book and make no warranty, express or implied, with respect to the contents of the book.

The authors and publisher have exerted every effort to ensure that drug selection and dosage set forth in this text are in accordance with current recommendations and practice at the time of publication. However, in view of ongoing changes in government regulations, and the constant flow of information relating to drug therapy and drug reactions, the reader is urged to check the package insert for each drug for any changes in indications and dosage and for added warnings and precautions. This is particularly important when the recommended agent is a new or infrequently used drug. It is the responsibility of the health care provider to ascertain the FDA status of drugs or devices planned for use in their clinical practice.

Electronic Fetal Heart Rate Monitoring: Research Guidelines developed by the National Institute of Child Health and Human Development (NICHD) Research Planning workshop was published in 1997.* This document contains a proposed nomenclature system for electronic fetal monitoring interpretation. Many health care facilities have adopted the NICHD nomenclature for the purposes of conducting research. As future trends in bedside practice evolve based on research about these guidelines, AWHONN will update its programs accordingly.

*The NICHD report was published concurrently in the November/December 1997 issues of AWHONN's *Journal of Obstetric, Gynecologic, and Neonatal Nurses (JOGNN)* and in the *American Journal of Obstetrics and Gynecology.*

Second printing July 2003. The second printing of this edition includes updated information about the use of Nellcor® fetal pulse oximetry technology (the OxiFirst® Fetal Pulse Oximetry System including the N-400 monitor and fetal sensor) as an adjunct to electronic fetal monitoring. This update is based on revisions to the clinical management protocol disseminated by Nellcor Puritan Bennett, Inc, Pleasanton, California in a letter of February 3, 2003 from David Swedlow, MD and Madeleine Bolling. The full text of the letter can be downloaded from *www.fda.gov/cdrh/psn/show16-Nellcor.html.* The new information is presented in Chapter 8 on pages 185 and 186.

Acknowledgements

This book is dedicated to the memory of Jana L. Atterbury, RNC, MSN, a former member of the AWHONN Board of Directors and contributor to the development and publication of this text. Jana's dedication and years of service to AWHONN are greatly appreciated and will be missed.

First edition Authors of *Fetal Heart Monitoring Principles and Practices*:

Donna Adelsperger, RNC, MEd
Julie Carr, RN, MSN
Deborah Davis, RNC, BSN
Nancy Feinstein, RNC, MSN
Judy Schmidt, RNC, EdD, Chair

Our most sincere appreciation goes to the original authors, who also served on the Fetal Heart Monitoring Education Program Steering Committee (1990–1995), for providing us with a quality product as the foundation for this revision. We also thank the editors and contributors to the 2nd edition of the *Fetal Heart Monitoring Principles and Practices* (FHMPP) textbook. The 3rd edition of *FHMPP* is built upon the framework and content of the 1st and 2nd editions. The contributions of the content reviewers for the 1st, 2nd, and 3rd editions also are acknowledged and appreciated.

3rd Edition Task Force Members:

Donna Adelsperger, RN, MEd, Chair
Rebecca L. Cypher, PNNP, MSN(c)
Kathleen Mahoney, APN, C
Faith Wight Moffatt, BN, MS(N), RN
Vickie J. Waymire, RNC, MSN

3rd Edition Editors:

Nancy Feinstein, PhD, RNC
Keiko L. Torgersen, BSN, MS, RNC
Jana L. Atterbury, RNC, MSN

3rd Edition Content Reviewers:

Donna Adelsperger, RN, MEd
Jennifer Bradle, MSN, RN, CNS
Rebecca L. Cypher, PNNP, MSN(c)
Lisa A. Dreyer, MSN, RNC, CNS
Carol Harvey, RNC, MS
Gail Heathcote, MSN, CNM
Ashley Hodges-Segars, MSN, CRNP, MA
Sylvia Hong, RN, MSN
Reneé Jones, RNC, MSN, WHNP
Audrey Lyndon, RNC, MS, CNS
Kathleen Mahoney, APN, C

2nd Edition Editors:

Nancy Feinstein, RNC, MSN
Patricia McCartney, RNC, PhD

2nd Edition Contributors:

Nancy Feinstein, RNC, MSN
Susan Gilson, RNC
Tracey Kasnic, RNC, BSN
Patricia McCartney, PhD, RNC, Revision Task
   Force Chair
Keiko L. Torgersen, BSN, MS, RNC
Catherine Weiser, RN, MS, FNP

2nd Edition Content Reviewers:

Donna Adelsperger, RNC, MEd
Julie Carr, RN, MSN
Janet Cunningham, RNC, BSN, MS
Deborah Davis, RNC, BSN
Michelle Murray, RNC, PhD
Anna Romig Nickels, RNC, BSN
Julian T. Parer, MD, PhD
Jeffrey P. Phelan, MD, JD
Judith Poole, RNC, MN
Judy Schmidt, RNC, EdD

Elizabeth McIntire, BSN, RNC
Patricia Robin McCartney, PhD, RNC, FAAN
Faith Wight Moffatt, BN, MS(N), RN
Nancy O'Brien-Abel, MN, RNC
Kathleen O'Connell, MN, RN
Patricia Purfield, RNC, MSN
Shirley Scott, RN, MS
Ann Sprague, RNC, BN, MEd
Elizabeth Rouleau MSN, RNC, WHNP
Marie-Josée Trépanier, RN, BScN, Med
Vickie J. Waymire, RNC, MSN

Marie-Josée Trépanier, RNC, MEd
Joyce Vogler, RN, Dr.PH, MS
Faith Wight Moffatt, BN, MS(N), RN

1st Edition Content Reviewers:

Anne T. Barrett, RNC, MSN
Micki Cabaniss, MD
Catherine Driscoll, RN, BSN
Timothy R. B. Johnson, MD
Julian T. Parer, MD, PhD
Catherine C. Rommal, RNC, BS
Kent Ueland, MD

A special thanks is extended to Patricia Wagner, RNC, MSN, innovator, contributor, member and Chair of the Fetal Heart Monitoring Education Program Steering Committee form 1990 to 1991.

A special thanks is also extended to all of the AWHONN Fetal Heart Monitoring Principles and Practices Instructor Trainers and Instructors for their continuing support and participation. A special thanks is also extended to the AWHONN staff for their assistance in the production of the book and materials that accompany the FHMPP program.

Auscultation Station:
A special thanks is extended to Marilyn R. Lapidus, RNC, BSN, Director, Clinical and Scientific Affairs, at Corometrics for her help in developing audiotaped materials used in this skill station.

Instrumentation Station:
A special thanks is extended to Utah Medical for sponsoring the original video edition for "Spiral Electrode and Intrauterine Pressure Catheter Placement" video.

Contents

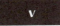

SECTION THREE

Maternal-Fetal Assessment: Development of the Nursing Database

SECTION FOUR

Fetal Monitoring: Nursing Diagnosis and Intervention

Rebecca L. Cypher, PNNP, MSN(c)
Donna Adelsperger, RN, MEd
Keiko L. Torgersen, BSN, MS, RNC

CHAPTER 8:   *Assessment of Fetal Oxygenation and Acid-Base Status*

Rebecca L. Cypher, PNNP, MSN(c)
Donna Adelsperger, RN, MEd

SECTION FIVE

Application of Fetal Heart Monitoring Data

Rebecca L. Cypher, PNNP, MSN(c)

SECTION SIX

Advanced Fetal Heart Monitoring Principles and Practices

Jana L. Atterbury, RNC, MSN
Gina M. Mikkelsen, RNC, MSN
Anne Santa-Donato, RNC, MSN

Keiko L. Torgersen, BSN, MS, RNC

Preface

The Fetal Heart Monitoring Principles and Practices Workshop (FHMPP) is a 2-day workshop (18.3 contact hours) focusing on the application of essential fetal heart monitoring (FHM) knowledge and skills in nursing practice. The workshop is a method of validating a nurse's knowledge and skills to determine competence. The didactic session is an analysis of case studies that requires the synthesis of key principles pertinent to the physiologic basis of fetal heart monitoring technology, tracing interpretation, nursing intervention, and verbal and written communication skills. The skill sessions focus on demonstration and practice of skills including auscultation, Leopold's maneuvers, placing an intrauterine pressure catheter and spiral electrode, interpreting tracings, identifying indicated nursing interventions, and communication and documentation. Each section of the workshop builds upon principles addressed in the previous section. Successful completion of written examinations and performance evaluations is a requirement for competence validation and earning continuing education credit. Participants attending the entire program who do not successfully complete the written examinations and skills performance evaluations may earn continuing education credits only.

The FHMPP workshop is based on nursing and educational theory. The instructional design incorporates critical thinking and decision making and is targeted toward professional nurses with previous FHM experience. Participants analyze multiple realistic case studies of increasing complexity and difficulty. Workshop participants are expected to have prior education and experience with both auscultation and EFM. Although the content of the workshop is comprehensive, specific nursing responsibilities vary according to institution, state, province, or region. Nurses who take the course are advised to be familiar with institutional policies and their state, provincial, or regional nurse practice act. Each institution should identify practice responsibilities as well as competence criteria and measurement.

Purpose: To validate the knowledge and skills of experienced nurses in a standardized FHM course.

Goal: To improve the assessment, promotion, and evaluation of fetal well being through dissemination of a standard course designed to validate the knowledge and skills of nurses whose practice includes FHR monitoring.

Objectives: Upon successful completion of the workshop, the participant will be able to:

- ◆ Demonstrate the decision-making process necessary for the proper selection and verification of FHM techniques
- ◆ Analyze fetal heart rate patterns, uterine activity and their implications for fetal well-being
- ◆ Correlate indicated clinical interventions with related maternal-fetal physiology
- ◆ Describe the role and responsibility of the professional nurse in the use of FHM in intrapartum care
- ◆ Simulate the psychomotor skills used in FHM
- ◆ Communicate verbal and written data about patient status and verify accountability.

Content: The workshop applies principles of fetal heart monitoring to practice. The instructional methodology includes the FHMPP textbook, the didactic presentation, and the skill sessions.

     1. *Manual:* The participant's FHMPP textbook reviews basic knowledge and skills used in FHM and is the companion text for the workshop. Text chapters address the content areas pertinent to the didactic case-study session topics and the nursing process (assess-

ment, interpretation, intervention, evaluation, and communication). Each chapter presents principles specific to topic areas covered. The chapters review important areas of knowledge and skill and build upon the nurse's prior knowledge. Content includes a physiologic framework for decision making, contemporary technology, and complementary labor care. Professional guidelines for practice and clinical research are included with the discussion of practice principles.

New with this 3rd Edition are chapters covering antenatal tesing, fetal dysrythmias and advanced case study exercises. A chapter about maternal-fetal assessment has also been added. The 3rd Edition *Fetal Heart Monitoring Principles and Practices* textbook is intended primarily to support the workshop objectives, but may also be a useful resource for perinatal health care professionals.

2. *Didactic:* Didactic sessions present cognitive principles through case studies and include audiovisual and discussion methods. Actual case studies are used to provide practice-based discussion. Each case illustrates one or more specific principles or issues. Each section of the didactic portion builds upon the principles addressed in the previous section. Cases become successively more complex. The didactic discussion format allows participants to ask or respond to questions that help:

   ◆ Extract key information
   ◆ Identify the problem
   ◆ Define the issues involved
   ◆ Make decisions regarding appropriate nursing interventions
   ◆ Evaluate outcome of interventions
   ◆ Communicate and document the entire process
   ◆ Formulate principles for handling future cases

3. *Skill Sessions:* The hands-on skill sessions combine cognitive problem-solving simulations and psychomotor skills. The sessions include mechanisms for hands-on practice and validation of knowledge and skills using audiovisual and simulation models developed exclusively for the workshop. The skill sessions include:

   ◆ Demonstration, practice, and testing of auscultation, Leopold's maneuvers, placement of intrauterine pressure catheter and spiral electrode skills
   ◆ Interpretation of tracings
   ◆ Identification of indicated nursing interventions
   ◆ Identification of appropriate communication and documentation methods.

Instruction and Administration:

For information regarding the AWHONN FHMPP workshop or other AWHONN workshop resources, please visit our website at *http://www.awhonn.org* and the Fetal Heart Monitoring Principles and Practices pages, or telephone headquarters at (800) 673-8499 if calling from the United States and (800) 245-0231 if calling from Canada.

Workshops scheduling and preparation of instructors is conducted through this office. Workshop fees support administrative expenses, including staff support, design and production of course materials, distribution of materials, and committee activity.

SECTION ONE

Theoretical Basis for Fetal Heart Monitoring

CHAPTER 1

Intrapartum Fetal Monitoring: A Historical Perspective

Patricia Robin McCartney
Judy V. Schmidt

☞ INTRODUCTION

This introduction to fetal heart monitoring (FHM) education includes an overview of the history of fetal heart rate (FHR) assessment, a summary of the evidence supporting practice, the development of professional guidelines, the evolution of FHM education and the use of the nursing process as a framework for applying FHM education to practice. These elements provide the historical context and an understanding of the state of the science as a basis for the Fetal Heart Monitoring Principles and Practices (FHMPP) workshop.

☞ HISTORY OF INTRAPARTUM FETAL SURVEILLANCE

The history of fetal surveillance provides the background for understanding the role of FHM in professional perinatal practice. Assessment of the FHR is an important indirect measure of fetal oxygenation in antepartum and intrapartum care.

This overview highlights the development of techniques to assess the FHR and uterine activity (UA), along with adjunct assessment techniques such as ultrasonography, fetal scalp blood sampling, fetal scalp stimulation, acoustical stimulation, pulse oximetry and computer analysis. A more comprehensive historical review may be found elsewhere (Goodlin, 1979; Schmidt & McCartney, 2000; Wulf, 1985). Notable historical events are summarized in Table 1-1.

Clinicians and researchers seeking ways to prevent fetal death (mortality) and neurological damage (morbidity) shaped the evolution of FHM techniques. Clinical assessment of the FHR and UA began with unassisted auscultation (examiner's ear on the maternal abdomen) and palpation (examiner's hands on the abdomen) and expanded with the addition of mechanical devices and electronic technology. Contemporary practice is the result of more than a century of research and development by practitioners dedicated to promoting optimal birth outcomes by identifying best practices for fetal heart assessment, interpretation and intervention.

TABLE 1-1

A Chronology of Major Fetal Heart Monitoring Developments*

DATE	DEVELOPMENT
1818	Mayor listens to FHR with ear on woman's abdomen.
1821	Kergaradec obtains FHR by stethoscope and relates FHR to fetal life and well-being.
1833	Kennedy publishes text describing FHR and Kergaradec's technique.
1849	Kilian proposes using FHR to identify fetal distress and need for intervention.
1893	Winckel publishes text with specific auscultation criteria for diagnosing fetal distress.
1906	Cremer uses abdominal and intravaginal leads for fetal ECG.
1917	Hillis describes the head fetoscope.
1947	Reynolds measures uterine tension with a multichannel tocodynamometer.
1952	Williams and Stallworthy place polyethylene catheter in cervix to measure intrauterine pressure.
1958	Hon reports preliminary EFM research.
1961	Saling measures fetal scalp pH.
1964	Callagan adapts Doppler ultrasonography to detect FHR.
1967	Fifth World Congress of Gynecology and Obstetrics agrees on EFM deceleration patterns.
1968	Hammacher and Hewlett-Packard market commercial EFM.
1971	International conference approves EFM pattern terminology.
1972	Hon develops the spiral fetal scalp electrode.
1976	Haverkamp reports results of the Dublin Trial comparing EFM and auscultation.
1977	Read uses acoustical stimulation to assess fetal well-being.
1982	Clark uses scalp stimulation to assess fetal well-being.
1985	Manning reports findings on the biophysical profile.
1986	Paine publishes the auscultation acceleration test.
1992	AWHONN introduces a standardized FHR monitoring course (FHMPP).
1996	PISUG forms to address educational needs related to computer information systems for FHM.
1997	NICHD panel recommends standardized EFM definitions.
2000	FDA approves the fetal pulse oximeter.

Abbreviations: AWHONN, Association of Women's Health, Obstetric and Neonatal Nurses; ECG, electrocardiogram; EFM, electronic fetal monitoring; FDA, U.S. Food and Drug Administration; FHMPP, Fetal Heart Monitoring Principles and Practices; FHR, fetal heart rate; NICHD, National Institute of Child Health and Human Development; PISUG, Perinatal Information System Users Group.

FHR

Clinical assessment of the FHR began almost 200 years ago, when both the Swiss surgeon Mayor in 1818 and the French physician and nobleman Kergaradec (Jean-Alexandre Le Jumeau, Vitcomte de Kergaradec) in 1821 reported the presence of fetal heart sounds obtained by auscultation (Goodlin, 1979). Mayor used the ear-to-abdomen method, but Kergaradec used a wooden stethoscope and is credited as the first practitioner to recommend assessing fetal heart sounds for diagnostic purposes. In 1833, Evory Kennedy in Dublin wrote a comprehensive monograph, *Observations on Obstetric Auscultation,* intended to convince doubting colleagues to use Kergaradec's auscultation technique (Goodlin, 1979). Kennedy's textbook described the slowness of the FHR return when a contraction "is passing on," and the effects of fetal head compression and funic compression on the FHR.

During the mid-1800s, a number of investigations using auscultation were reported, including identifying the normal FHR range and correlating FHR with other clinical findings such as maternal fever, gestational age, fetal weight, fetal sex and fetal movement. Clinicians debated methods of auscultation (stethoscope vs. ear-to-abdomen), the ideal positioning of the patient (standing vs. supine) and the necessity of exposing the pregnant woman's abdomen during the procedure. Clinicians also investigated physiologic causes for changes in the FHR. In Germany in 1858, Schwartz wrote in a text that the FHR be counted during labor, both between and during contractions, as a method of assessing fetal well-being (Goodlin, 1979). Schwartz related fetal bradycardia to both compression of the fetal head and decreased placental function caused by the reduction in blood flow during uterine contractions. He is also credited as the first to investigate fetal breathing activity. In 1885, Schatz described umbilical cord compression; in 1903, Seitz claimed FHR decelerations were indicators of fetal oxygenation and described head compression (Wulf, 1985).

In 1849 in America, Kilian proposed that FHR findings of rates less than 100 beats per minute (bpm) or greater than 180 bpm could identify fetal distress that required forceps intervention (Goodlin,

1979). Von Winckel in Germany in 1893 formulated specific criteria to identify fetal distress, as determined by auscultation: tachycardia greater than 160 bpm, bradycardia less than 120 bpm, or irregularity of the FHR (Goodlin, 1979). Von Winckel's criteria and auscultation guidelines were followed for the next 75 years (Wulf, 1985).

In the early 1900s, the fetoscope replaced auscultation with the ear or binaural or monaural stethoscope. The head fetoscope was first described in the literature by Hillis (1917) as a metal band over the head attached to a common binaural stethoscope. The original purpose for the device was to enable the obstetrician to listen to second-stage fetal heart tones without using his hands, thus remaining "surgically prepared" for the delivery. However, additional benefits were improved assessment from bone conduction and the ability to press the bell of the stethoscope firmly against the abdomen. This device came to be known as the DeLee-Hillis fetoscope to acknowledge both obstetrician inventors.

As the practice of FHR auscultation grew, researchers began to study the measurement accuracy of clinicians (reliability) and the relationship between FHR findings and neonatal outcomes (validity). In 1958, Hon observed obstetricians counting a FHR from an audiotape and found their rates varied widely (Hon, 1958). He concluded human auditory interpretation of the FHR had poor reliability. In 1968, a federally funded, multi-center trial referred to as the Collaborative Project compared intrapartum auscultated FHR findings based on Von Winckel's criteria with neonatal outcomes (Benson, Shubeck, Deutschberger, Weiss & Berendes, 1968). The authors' conclusions suggested auscultated FHR findings had poor validity. These two studies are commonly cited as catalysts for the rejection of auscultation in favor of newer electronic monitoring methods.

The use of technologic devices to assess the FHR began about 100 years ago with indirect measurement using abdominal devices and direct measurement using fetal devices. Pestalozza in 1891 and Hofbauer and Weiss in 1908 reported their endeavors with phonocardiography, a mechanical process using a microphone-like apparatus that amplified and continuously recorded the FHR through the maternal abdomen (Goodlin, 1979; Wulf, 1985). Many years later Hammacher in 1962 improved the clarity of the phonocardiographic signal and connected the FHR with the recording of uterine contractions. Also about 100 years ago (in 1906), the cardiologist Cremer applied both abdominal and vaginal electrodes to obtain a fetal electrocardiogram (ECG) as a demonstration project on a woman who was not in labor (Wulf, 1985).

In the 1950s, three pioneers of electronic fetal monitoring (EFM)—Hon in America, Caldeyro-Barcia in Uruguay and Hammacher in Germany—began reporting success with electronic monitors that could continuously record indirect abdominal phonocardiography and electrocardiography. One of the earliest reports was by Hon in 1958 described using silver electrodes inside light plastic shells on the mother's abdomen and thigh (Hon, 1958). Hon compared the FHR and patterns of FHR changes with labor variables and neonatal outcomes; at this time he did not find the actual configuration of the fetal ECG complex to be useful. Because of poor signal quality of the early abdominal fetal ECG, clinicians experimented with multiple devices to record the FHR directly from the fetus. Hon developed a disposable fetal scalp electrode in 1972 that successfully obtained a direct fetal ECG and remains the basis for the devices used today (Goodlin, 1979). In 1964, Callagan adapted Doppler ultrasound technology to indirectly assess fetal heart motion through the maternal abdomen (Goodlin, 1979). This external measurement technique became widespread in both antepartum and intrapartum settings, with progressive engineering improvement in the signal quality and accuracy.

Uterine Activity

Clinical assessment of uterine activity with technologic devices actually began a little earlier than FHR technology. In 1872, Schatz reported measuring uterine activity by placing balloons within the uterus to record intrauterine pressures on a graph called a "pain tracing" (Goodlin, 1979). Two decades later, Schaeffer measured uterine activity externally by placing a hood with a tube connected to a spirometer over the pregnant woman's abdomen (Goodlin, 1979). These early investigators examined normal uterine activity and uterine response to anesthetics and drugs such as epinephrine, ether and morphine. By 1947, an external device, the tocodynamometer, was designed to detect, and eventually to continuously record, tension changes in the abdomen resulting from uterine contractions. This device provided a visual wave displaying the frequency, duration and relative strength of uterine contractions.

The first internal assessment of uterine activity was reported by Williams and Stallworthy in 1952; they inserted a polyethylene catheter through the cervix of a woman in labor (Goodlin, 1979). However, Williams and Stallworthy concluded, "No instrument was as discerning as the experienced hand in assessing the quality of uterine contractions." Also in 1952, Caldeyro-Barcia reported inserting catheters into the uterus directly through an amniocentesis needle in the abdominal wall. Caldeyro-Barcia coined the term "Montevideo units" as a quantifiable measure of intrauterine pressure. Eventually, a commercial intrauterine pressure catheter (IUPC) was developed that could be inserted into the uterus through the cervix and attached to an external strain gauge transducer to record pressure changes. With advances in microchip computers, a small, solid-state transducer that could detect pressure changes was placed at the distal end of the IUPC, replacing the strain gauge transducer.

EFM

The simultaneous measurement of FHR and uterine contractions came to be called cardiotocography (CTG) or simply EFM. Hammacher and Hewlett-Packard developed the first commercially available electronic FHR monitor in 1968, initially using external microphone phonocardiography and later adding external ultrasound and internal fetal ECG devices (Freeman, Garite & Nageotte, 1991). Today, the term phonocardiography refers to the sound signal from ultrasound technology (National Library of Medicine, 2002). The computerized sampling of the raw ultrasound signal, the mathematical calculation of rate and the visual representation all progressively improved. As ultrasound FHR signal sampling and calculation were improved through engineering, the devices came to be called "second-generation monitors." Wireless transmission of the ultrasound signal later enabled ambulatory telemetry.

An important result of this electronic technology was the conversion of an auditory signal into a visual waveform and the creation of a continuous visual pattern of the FHR, permanently recorded on paper. Thus, FHR assessment changed from unassisted auscultation using auditory skills to automated auscultation using visual skills. The development of EFM dramatically altered obstetric practice. In many settings, EFM became the primary technique for FHR monitoring, while intermittent auscultation became a screening or secondary technique. In some settings, auscultation remained the primary technique for FHM.

Adjunct Surveillance Methods

A number of adjunct methods were developed to complement the assessment of the FHR, not only during labor but in the late antepartum period as well. These innovations enhanced FHM techniques, provided additional information about fetal oxygenation status or improved FHM information management. More tools for fetal assessment in late pregnancy introduced a new field of care: antepartum fetal surveillance. Expansion of fetal evaluation led to the development of specialized antepartum testing centers (Afriat, 1981).

A reassuring EFM tracing identifies an oxygenated and neurologically intact fetus with a high level of sensitivity (ability to identify only a healthy fetus as healthy) and has few false-negative results (when an assessment falsely identifies a compromised fetus as healthy). When a tracing is reassuring, clinicians usually agree the fetus is healthy. However, a nonreassuring EFM tracing has a low level of specificity (ability to identify only a compromised fetus as compromised) and many false-positive results (when an assessment falsely identifies a healthy fetus as compromised). With a nonreassuring tracing, clinicians need more information to assess oxygenation and avoid unnecessary intervention. There

is less clinician agreement with a nonreassuring tracing. Adjunct surveillance methods were developed to provide more information.

In the 1960s, clinicians observed that late decelerations during labor were associated with an increased risk of metabolic acidosis. In the 1970s, physicians began using low dose oxytocin in antepartum testing, and the term "oxytocin challenge test" (OCT) was introduced (Freeman, 1975). Clinicians observed that the fetal heart rate response to mild induced contractions could predict the FHR response to the stress of labor. The technique was broadened to become the "contraction stress test" (CST) using either oxytocin or stimulation of the breast or nipple (breast stimulation test: BST). The CST has been controversial from the beginning primarily because of its high false-positive rates (falsely identifying a healthy fetus as being at risk).

During the 1970s, Schifrin and colleagues adopted observation by Hammacher and Kubli to test and introduce the nonstress test (NST) (Rochard et al., 1976). The NST would identify FHR accelerations without inducing contractions and serve as a useful, noninvasive predictor of fetal well-being. However, when it was introduced, the NST required the use of electronic monitors generally only available at fetal testing centers. Manufacturers progressively developed more portable monitors specifically suited for antepartum testing in clinicians' offices and in homes. In 1986, Paine and colleagues described an auscultated acceleration test using a fetoscope to auscultate and graph FHR accelerations (Paine, Zandari, Johnson, Rorie & Barger, 2001). This "low-tech" approach to fetal evaluation has been internationally tested and recommended for settings where more advanced technology is not accessible.

Ultrasound was first used in the late 1950s to measure fetal biparietal diameter. By the 1970s, ultrasound had become widely used to identify fetal and placental structure and position. Real-time scanning technology was added, and evaluation of the fetal heart became possible. The biophysical profile was pioneered in the 1970s (Manning, Platt & Silos, 1980), and it became a standard fetal assessment test during the 1980s. Early work with ultrasound technology projected its potential use for assessing uterine and umbilical blood flow (Goodlin, 1979). Ultrasonography, or Doppler velocimetry (Doppler flow), is now used to measure blood flow in the uterine artery, umbilical arteries and fetal middle cerebral artery as indicators of vascular status and fetal compensatory responses.

Saling reported a technique to measure fetal acidosis through scalp blood pH sampling in 1961, long before continuous EFM was widely used in labor (Goodlin, 1979). The analysis of fetal capillary blood correlated with subsequent umbilical cord blood samples taken at birth, and together these biochemical assessments of pH were viewed as the "gold standard" for measures of fetal status. Scalp sampling later fell into disfavor because the technique was invasive and technically challenging, often requiring a prolonged maternal supine position, and resulting pH measures were found to have poor specificity (ability to identify only a compromised fetus as compromised) (Clark & Paul, 1985).

Several investigators identified methods to stimulate a FHR acceleration that is now known to be associated with a nonacidotic fetus. Clark and colleagues reported that a FHR acceleration following the stimulation of the scalp during a fetal blood sampling procedure (puncture) was associated with a nonacidotic fetus (Clark, Gimovsky, & Miller, 1982). These same researchers found that a FHR acceleration following fetal scalp stimulation with pinching and pressure was also associated with a nonacidotic fetus (Clark, Gimovsky, & Miller, 1984). Prior to Clark's work, Read and Miller (1977) reported that a FHR acceleration in response to abdominal acoustic stimulation correlated with OCT outcomes and fetal well-being. This association was later tested using an artificial larynx for intrapartum acoustic stimulation (or vibroacoustical stimulation) and fetal scalp pH levels for measures of fetal well-being (Smith, Ngyguen, Phelan, & Paul, 1986). A FHR acceleration was proven to be associated with the absence of acidosis. Both scalp stimulation and acoustical stimulation are now recognized as effective tests of fetal well-being.

The initial efforts to directly assess fetal oxgenation attempted to measure scalp oxygen tension

and peripheral pulse oxygen saturation (Goodlin, 1979). Adult pulse oxygen saturation technology (pulse oximetry) was adapted for fetal use with a single, thin, fetal sensor that both emits and receives light. Fetal pulse oximetry was developed, researched and commercially available in Europe in the 1990s but was not approved for use in the United States until 2000 (Simpson & Porter, 2000). Measurement of fetal oxygen saturation (FS_PO_2) is currently used in some settings to assess oxygen status when the EFM tracing is nonreassuring or uninterpretable. ACOG (2001) and SOGC (2002) do not recommend fetal pulse oximetry as a standard of care at this time.

Because human visual analysis is subjective and limited by human sensory capacities, even the earliest electronic monitors used computer technology to aid human pattern recognition. Computer analysis (CA) of the FHR uses artificial intelligence (AI) to objectively analyze the auditory signal according to predetermined criteria, alert care providers, interpret patterns and even offer management options. Automated analysis has provided objective, standardized and reproducible data for research on FHR responses in the antepartum and intrapartum setting. There are a number of published studies on automated methods of fetal assessment in North American (McCartney, 2000). Several investigators have compared computer analysis to visual analysis and generally found similar or better performance with computer analysis in assessing FHR characteristics (McCartney, 2000). One early device had flashing yellow and red lights for detection of "ominous FHR patterns" (Yeh, Jilek & Hon, 1974). In 1978 in England, Dawes and colleagues began developing software and rules (Dawes-Redman criteria), now available in the commercial Sonicaid monitor (Sonicaid monitor, Oxford Medical Ltd., United Kingdom), which have been used for CTG analysis in numerous studies around the world. In the United States, Devoe also has researched and published widely on automated methods of fetal assessment (McCartney, 2000).

Obstetric clinical information systems, also known as perinatal information systems, became commercially available for patient care in the 1990s. Although originally perceived as "central monitoring," these powerful computer systems are capable of more than simultaneous displays of EFM results. Information systems interface with EFM devices and can be used to enter, display, document, transmit, store, query, analyze and retrieve FHR data and generate reports in both hospital and ambulatory settings (Kelly, 1999). Perinatal systems have great potential for influencing practice and research on FHR assessment.

The Effect of Technology on Intrapartal Nursing Practice

With the introduction of technological advances, nurses had to make EFM fit into their clinical practice. Nurses who experienced the introduction of EFM in their clinical settings were challenged to reconcile the conflict between the use of technology for biomedical objectivity and personalized, natural childbirth (Sandelowski, 2000). The field of nursing has had to work to ensure that constant attention to the glamour of new technology does not overshadow the fundamental practices of labor support.

⌨ EVIDENCE FOR FHR ASSESSMENT

When clinicians first experimented with FHM techniques, they recorded their observations as evidence for practice. This kind of reporting gradually evolved into the present expectations for rigorous clinical trials to produce evidence for practice. Key research issues, debates, and historical studies are summarized here.

The initial purpose of EFM was to identify unfavorable or nonreassuring FHR characteristics that indicate a fetus at risk for asphyxia, thus enabling intervention to prevent fetal death and neonatal morbidity. Years of research and practice with FHM have produced considerable information about both favorable and unfavorable FHR characteristics and implications. The purpose of FHM now is to identify the FHR characteristics indicating fetal well-being as well as those that suggest the fetus might be at risk. Information on favorable or reassuring FHR characteristics is equally helpful in clinical care.

Research on the reliability, validity and efficacy of both auscultated and electronic FHR assessment has been controversial. Each method was incorporated into clinical practice without confirming research evidence. Frequently cited studies on the ability of humans to accurately auscultate FHR or interpret EFM patterns and the relationship of auscultated FHR or EFM patterns to fetal outcomes are summarized here. A more complete review of the research is available elsewhere (Feinstein, 2000; Feinstein, Sprague & Trepanier, 2000; Haggerty, 1999; Thacker & Stroup, 1999; Thacker, Stroup & Peterson, 1995).

Auscultation vs. EFM

Two early studies on auscultation skill and outcomes have been widely cited in the literature, despite concerns raised about their methodologies. The earliest report on auscultation skill was mentioned in Hon's 1958 paper. In a short introductory background paragraph, a study was mentioned without original sources (Hon, 1958). Hon believed periodic auscultatory sampling between contractions was inaccurate, so he engaged 15 obstetricians to "count" eight rates recorded on a magnetic tape (ranging from 75–204 bpm). Hon found the counted values varied within a range of 6–68 bpm of the true recorded FHR and subsequently concluded electronic techniques prevented this human error. However, Hon's report did not describe the counting method, the nature of the recording or the obstetricians' experience with auscultation.

A report was published in 1968 on the findings of a government funded, multicenter, prospective observational study on auscultated FHR related to fetal distress, titled the "Collaborative Study of Cerebral Palsy, Mental Retardation, and Other Neurological Diseases and Blindness" (Benson et al., 1968). In this study, the FHR was auscultated by observers that were specially trained (qualifications were not identified) every 15 minutes during the first stage of labor. The short report states that four auscultated FHR measures were related to fetal distress based on the computer analysis of the data; however, the author could not identify one auscultatory FHR that was a reliable indicator of fetal distress except for bracycardia which the authors call "save in extreme degree." The authors (Benson et al., 1968) acknowledged the study was limited by the absence of a definition of fetal distress that was acceptable. However, in this study, the FHR was not obtained during a contraction or for 30 seconds following a contraction, and FHRs obtained during the second stage of labor were not used in the final analysis.

A number of subsequent studies have examined individuals' skill in assessing FHR, rhythm and accelerations; compared auscultatory devices such as Doppler and Pinard devices (Mahomed, Nyoni, Mulambo, Kasale & Jacobus, 1994) and evaluated the cost-effectiveness of auscultation in labor (Feinstein, 2000; Feinstein et al., 2000; Miller, Pearse & Paul, 1984). Further information about auscultation can be found in Chapter 5.

On the other side of the debate, clinicians and consumers pointed to the invasive nature and high equipment costs associated with EFM and questioned the widespread application of an unproven technology. The evidence for reliability—or the accuracy of clinicians' measurements—with EFM patterns is inconsistent. Some studies show clinicians differ in their interpretations of an EFM pattern (interrater or interobserver reliability) and that the same clinician may give different interpretations of the same EFM pattern when reviewed at different times (intrarater or intraobserver reliability). There is some evidence to support validity—or the relationship of EFM patterns to neonatal outcomes such as cerebral palsy. However, as predictors, these associations have unacceptably high false-positive rates (Nelson, Dambrosia, Ting & Grether, 1996).

In 1976, Haverkamp and colleagues reported the first prospective, randomized clinical trial (RCT) comparing intrapartum EFM and auscultation, known as the Dublin Trial (Haverkamp, Thompson, McFee & Cetrulo, 1976). The findings demonstrated no benefit in fetal or neonatal health with EFM over auscultation. Critics and supporters of EFM debated the methodology of the study and the implications; however, later investigations also did not find any fetal or neonatal benefits with EFM over auscultation. Collectively, the findings from 12 RCTs published between 1976 and 1994 and subsequent meta-analyses of these RCTs

demonstrated no benefit with EFM compared with auscultation (Thacker & Stroup, 1999; Thacker et al., 1995). The RCTs compared the safety and efficacy of EFM with intermittent auscultation in low-risk and high-risk pregnancies. (Staffing was not a consideration in these studies.) Although neonatal outcomes did not differ with respect to the method of monitoring, the use of EFM did increase the likelihood of cesarean delivery and operative vaginal delivery.

Professionals and consumers agree that more research with sound methodology is needed on FHM. Yet, practice variations demonstrate that even the existing research has not been fully implemented (Haggerty, 1999).

☞ STANDARDIZATION AND PROFESSIONAL GUIDELINES

Practice differences have existed throughout the history of FHR assessment. In 1999, the Institute of Medicine (IOM) released a report on measures to reduce the incidence of health care errors (Institute of Medicine, 1999). Measures that improve safety include standardized language and both standardization and simulation in training. The IOM report specifically directs professional organizations to facilitate patient safety by developing and promoting practice guidelines and by standardizing technology and education. The Association of Women's Health, Obstetric and Neonatal Nurses (AWHONN) responded by reiterating its commitment to solutions that ensure patient safety, including the FHMPP workshop (AWHONN, 2000b). Several important efforts toward consensus and standardization in FHM are summarized here, although disagreement continues.

Standardized Language, Controversy and Consensus

Uniform FHR terminology and interpretation are necessary to facilitate meaningful communication, legally defensible documentation, functional information databases and sound research. A standardized approach to both auscultation and electronic monitoring requires criteria that are quantifiable, objectively measurable, unambiguous, reproducible and generally accepted. Clinicians and researchers have often disagreed about FHR assessment, interpretation and intervention. Lively controversy and debate continues about which method of monitoring is appropriate; how FHR characteristics are defined, named and measured; which characteristics and changes are assessed and when; what constitutes "normal" and which interventions are indicated.

Physicians began to describe slight variations in baseline FHRs as early as the 1950s, using different terminology (Goodlin, 1979). Present FHR pattern definitions originated from the pioneering work of Hon, Hammacher and Caldeyro-Barcia and colleagues during the 1950s and 1960s. These physicians agreed on descriptions of similar patterns but used different terms and classifications (see Table 1-2). They described baseline rates, oscillations from the baseline rate (called accelerations and decelerations) and fluctuations of the baseline rate referred to as variability (classified by the amplitude of the FHR changes and the number of cycles of change per minute) (Freeman et al., 1991). Some international agreement on deceleration patterns was achieved at the Fifth World

Congress of Gynecology and Obstetrics in 1967 (Goodlin, 1979).

An international conference panel on fetal monitoring convened in 1971 in the United States and again in 1972 in Amsterdam to develop consensus on terminology and measurement (Freeman et al., 1991). The panel agreed upon the terminology of baseline "variability," and "early, late and variable" decelerations. Hon's pattern descriptions formed the basis for deceleration pattern definitions. No agreement was reached on a monitor paper scale or speed, nor on the categorization of variability. Consequently, discrepant terminology (e.g., oscillations, variability, beat-to-beat variability, variation) and categorizations of variability evolved (see Table 1-3). There has never been consensus on categorization of variability.

Some automated analysis systems, such as the Sonicaid system and the SisPorto project (SisPorto, Oporto University, Portugal) do apply standard criteria for computer analysis. The SisPorto project is an Internet-accessible program and database for an international multicenter study using automated analysis of antepartum and intrapartum cardiotocography. The SisPorto FHR analysis uses standardized and agreed-upon criteria developed

TABLE 1-2

Historical Classifications of Fetal Heart Rate Characteristics

HON (1963)	CALDYERO-BARCIA, MENDEZ-BAUER & POSIER (1966)	HAMMACHER (1969)
Baseline irregularity	Bradycardia	Type 0 oscillation silent
Bradycardia	Tachycardia	Type 1 oscillation narrow undulatory
Tachycardia	Type I dip	Type 2 oscillation undulatory
Early deceleration	Type II dip	Type 3 oscillation saltatory
Late deceleration	Baseline rapid fluctuation	Type 0 dip
Variable deceleration	Transient ascents of FHR	Type 1 dip
	Long term variability	Type 2 dip
	Short term variability	

TABLE 1-3

*Categories of Fetal Heart Rate Variability**

RANGE OF FETAL HEART RATE CHANGES IN BEATS PER MINUTE (bpm)	5 CATEGORIES	4 CATEGORIES	4 CATEGORIES OF NICHD	3 CATEGORIES	2 CATEGORIES
Undetectable	Absent	Absent	Absent	Decreased	Absent
0–2			Minimal		
3–5	Minimal	Minimal			
6–15	Average	Average	Moderate	Average	Present
15–25	Moderate				
> 25	Marked	Marked	Marked	Increased	

* Adapted from Chez & Harvey, 1994.

by the International Federation of Gynecology and Obstetrics (FIGO) (Ayres-de Campos, Bernardes, Garrido, Marques-de-Sa & Pereira-Leite, 2000). Commercial perinatal information systems may apply standardized criteria in alerting functions or allow the individual users to define their own parameters for EFM pattern recognition and alerts.

In the 1970s, nurses began to work on a standardized language or classification system for nursing practice that could be used in a computerized database and would help nurses document their contribution to patient care, including intrapartum care (Eganhouse, McCloskey & Bulechek, 1996). The Nursing Intervention Classification (NIC) system includes the intervention "6772: Electronic Fetal Monitoring: Intrapartum Intervention," which is comprised of standardized procedures and actions and cites the FHMPP workshop as a reference (McCloskey & Bulechek, 2000).

Standardized nomenclature is necessary for many other aspects of clinical practice, such as documentation, reimbursement and bibliographic databases. Many experts have expressed concern about the continued use of imprecise terms such as "fetal distress" and "birth asphyxia." In 1998, the American College of Obstetricians and Gyne-

cologists (ACOG) recommended the term "fetal distress" be replaced with "nonreassuring fetal status," followed by a further description of the assessment findings (ACOG, 1998). In 1998, the perinatal International Classification of Disease (ICD) code removed all inclusion terms for fetal distress except metabolic acidosis (ACOG, 1998). The National Library of Medicine (NLM) Medical Subject Headings (MeSH) identifies the terms "fetal heart rate," "fetal monitoring," "cardiotocography," and "phonocardiography" for searching the literature database on FHR assessment (National Library of Medicine, 2002).

Professional Guidelines

Professional organizations have issued a number of guidelines to promote standardization and competence in fetal heart assessment (Table 1-4). These resources are periodically revised on the basis of new research findings, technological developments and practice changes. Some resources focus on a specific assessment technique while others are comprehensive. Some resources are interdisciplinary or international in scope.

TABLE 1-4

Chronology of Professional Standards and Guidelines for Fetal Heart Monitoring

SOURCE	YEAR	TITLE
NAACOG	1980	*The Nurse's Role in Electronic Fetal Monitoring* (Technical bulletin)
NAACOG	1986	*Electronic Fetal Monitoring: Joint ACOG/NAACOG Statement* (Position statement)
NAACOG	1986	*Electronic Fetal Monitoring: Nursing Practice Competencies and Educational Guidelines* (Guidelines)
NAACOG	1988	*Nursing Responsibilities in Implementing Fetal Heart Rate Monitoring* (Position statement)
NAACOG	1990	*Fetal Heart Rate Auscultation* (OGN nursing practice resource)
NAACOG	1991a	*Nursing Practice Competencies and Educational Guidelines: Antepartum Fetal Surveillance and Intrapartum Fetal Heart Monitoring* (2nd ed.) (Guidelines)
NAACOG	1991b	*NAACOG Standards for the Nursing Care of Women and Newborns* (4th ed.) (Standards)
NAACOG	1991c	*Appropriate Use of Technology in Nursing Care* (Committee opinion)
ACNM	1991	*Appropriate Use of Technology in Childbirth* (Position statement)
NAACOG	1992	*Nursing Responsibilities in Implementing Fetal Heart Rate Monitoring* (Position statement)
AWHONN	1993	*Didactic Content and Clinical Skills Verification for Professional Nurse Providers of Basic, High Risk and Critical Care Intrapartum Nursing* (Guidelines)
SOGC	1995*	*Fetal Health Surveillance in Labor* (Policy statement)
ACOG	1995*	*Fetal Heart Rate Patterns: Monitoring, Interpretation, and Management* (Technical bulletin)
AWHONN	1998a*	*Standards and Guidelines for Professional Nursing Practice in the Care of Women and Newborns* (Standards and guidelines)
AAP and ACOG	1997	*Antepartum and Intrapartum Care Guidelines for Perinatal Care* (4th ed.) (Guidelines)
AWHONN	1998b*	*Clinical Competencies and Educational Guide: Antepartum and Intrapartum Fetal Heart Rate Monitoring* (Guidelines)
ACOG	1998*	*Inappropriate Use of the Terms Fetal Distress and Birth Asphyxia* (Committee opinion)
AWHONN	1999*	*Basic, High-Risk and Critical Care Intrapartum Nursing: Clinical Competencies and Education Guide*

(table continues)

	TABLE 1-4 (cont.)	
	Chronology of Professional Standards and Guidelines for Fetal Heart Monitoring	
SOURCE	**YEAR**	**TITLE**
AWHONN	2000a*	*Fetal Assessment* (Position statement)
AAP and ACOG	2002*	*Guidelines for Perinatal Care* (5th ed.) (Guidelines)
SOGC	2002*	*Fetal Health Surveillance in Labour* (Part I and Part II) (Clinical Practice Guideline, Number 112)

Abbreviations: AAP, American Academy of Pediatrics; ACNM, American College of Nurse Midwives; ACOG, American College of Obstetricians and Gynecologists; AWHONN, Association of Women's Health, Obstetric and Neonatal Nurses (formerly NAACOG); NAACOG, Nurses Association of the American College of Obstetricians and Gynecologists; SOGC, Society of Obstetricians and Gynaecologists of Canada.

* Current publications. Professional standards, guidelines and position statements are reviewed and revised or withdrawn in an ongoing basis.

Several guidelines address the choice of FHM method. No professional association of providers involved in childbirth has ever authored a guideline recommending EFM over intermittent auscultation for low-risk births. Because clinical trials have demonstrated that auscultation is as effective as EFM, recent guidelines address the option of intermittent auscultation for low-risk births. For example, AWHONN "supports the use of fetal auscultation" as well as the "judicious, appropriate application of intrapartum EFM" and does not support the use of EFM as a substitute for appropriate professional nursing care (AWHONN, 2000b). Further, AWHONN recommends each facility develop a policy regarding appropriate use of each FHR monitoring method. In 1995, ACOG stated, "Current data indicate that FHR monitoring is equally effective whether done electronically or by auscultation," and outlined factors to consider in the choice of technique (ACOG, 1995). The Society of Obstetricians and Gynaecologists of Canada stated that intermittent auscultation is the recommended method of FHR surveillance for women at low risk during labor (SOGC, 1995). Professional guidelines have been useful for establishing consistency in the frequency of FHR assess-

ment in labor (AAP & ACOG, 1997; ACOG, 1995; SOGC, 1995). Despite the many guidelines available, practices differ, and professionals continue to work toward consensus.

In 1995, the U.S. National Institute of Child Health and Human Development (NICHD) convened an international panel of researchers and clinicians who developed standardized, quantitative definitions for EFM to be used for both visual and computer interpretation (Table 1-5). These operational definitions were published simultaneously in nursing and medical specialty journals; they were recommended to improve the reliability of pattern interpretation in studies and to better compare findings among studies. To date, little research has been reported on the use of the new nomenclature or on the reliability of FHR pattern interpretation, the validity of interpretation, correlation of patterns with fetal outcomes or the development of computer applications. One study compared the analyses of clinicians using the NICHD definitions with the analyses of a computerized fetal monitor alerting system and found the NICHD definitions did not reduce human interobserver differences in pattern interpretation (Devoe et al., 2000).

TABLE 1-5	
National Institute for Child Health and Human Development Definitions for Electronic Fetal Monitoring (NICHD, 1997)	
TERM	**DEFINITION**
Baseline Rate	110–160 beats per minute (bpm) Mean fetal heart rate (FHR) from a 10-minute segment of recording rounded to nearest 5 bpm interval
Baseline Variability	Fluctuations in baseline FHR > 2 cycles per minute (peak to trough); irregular in amplitude and frequency Absent = amplitude undetectable Minimal = 5 bpm or fewer Moderate = 6–25 bpm Marked = 25 bpm or more
Accelerations	Abrupt = Acceleration to peak level in < 30 seconds, at least 15 bpm and 15 seconds in duration, but < 2 minutes in duration (For fetus < 32 weeks of gestation, acceleration of at least 10 bpm and 10 seconds in duration) Prolonged acceleration = Acceleration for ≥ 2 minutes but < 10 minutes in duration
Decelerations	Late = Gradual decrease ≥ 30 seconds to nadir, nadir delayed, after Uterine Contraction (UC) peak Early = Gradual decrease ≥ 30 seconds to nadir, nadir coincident with UC peak Variable = Abrupt decrease < 30 seconds to nadir, ≥ 15 bpm and ≥ 15 seconds in duration but < 2 minutes; if associated with UC, timing varies Prolonged deceleration = 15 bpm or more below baseline for > 2 minutes but < 10 minutes in duration
Changes/Trends	Baseline change = Acceleration or deceleration of 10 minutes or more in duration Sinusoidal = No variability, regular amplitude and frequency, excluded from definition of variability

☛ FETAL MONITORING EDUCATION

The implementation of continuous EFM required skilled personnel at the bedside to interpret patterns throughout labor; understandably, this responsibility became part of nurses' work. Nurses quickly found themselves in need of new knowledge and skills to use this tool. Collectively and diligently, nurses initially addressed their immediate needs for education and later emerged as the leaders in fetal monitoring education. Although the term "fetal monitoring" is often used to refer to electronic methods, it applies to both manual and electronic methods. Professional fetal monitoring education should include the knowledge and skills for both auscultation and electronic fetal heart assessment.

Early EFM Education

When EFM was introduced in the 1960s, little formal education existed beyond that provided by manufacturers' consumer services divisions. Most nurses learned the basic skills through on-the-job-training. Independent clinicians gradually began to develop and teach EFM education programs throughout the United States. These independent educators were instrumental in early EFM instruction and continue to be primary providers of basic and advanced instruction today. Some educators went on to develop "train the trainer" programs that prepared others with the knowledge and skills necessary to teach basic EFM (Adelsperger, 1990; Traber, Leppein & Billmaier, 1993).

Continuing Education Needs

In the 1970s, nurses encountered new technology and few learning resources. Textbooks and journals were only beginning to include basic instruction on EFM. Even today, new nurses generally do not have basic skills in either auscultation or EFM because of limitations in both theory and clinical practice. By the early 1980s, the content, style and emphasis in education programs had become quite diverse. Clinicians recognized a need for resources that would 1) identify a standard core of FHM knowledge and skills and 2) establish mechanisms for validating knowledge and skills. Nurses turned to professional organizations such as NAACOG, now known as AWHONN, and ACOG for resources to meet these needs.

Guidelines

In 1980, NAACOG released a technical bulletin on EFM, followed by a joint position statement with ACOG in 1985 and educational guidelines in 1986. These resources were followed in the years to come with numerous other position statements, standards, guidelines and educational resources on EFM and FHM for nurses (Table 1-4). The

AWHONN web site includes a list of current guidelines (www.awhonn.org); AWHONN remains the recognized authority for nursing practice guidelines in FHM.

Resources

Late in the 1970s, ACOG released a slide-tape module on the basics of EFM that was widely used for education in hospital inservice programs; NAACOG followed with a textbook, videos and manuals. To date, AWHONN continually revises and diversifies FHM education resources. Information on current educational resources is available on AWHONN's web site (www.awhonn.org).

Today, many continuing education resources for FHM offer didactic knowledge and some measure skill proficiency. A variety of providers offer continuing education activities, such as professional organizations, nurse entrepreneurs, commercial companies and health care institutions. Activities that validate participant completion include traditional conferences, hands-on skills workshops, case studies, independent or home self-study assessment modules, journals, computer-assisted or computer simulation programs and audio, video and satellite conferencing. These resources as well as many other publications and audiovisual programs also enable individuals or institutions to continue learning without formal participant validation.

In 1995, nurses and vendors working with clinical information systems began to raise questions and share strategies through the Perinatal Nursing Internet Discussion List; in 1996, this group organized to form the Perinatal Information System Users Group (PISUG). A nonprofit professional organization, PISUG sponsors annual conferences for networking, education and product demonstration. This organization has become an important educational resource for nurses using computer information systems in fetal heart monitoring.

Instruction Methods

Competence in fetal monitoring requires didactic knowledge as well as critical-thinking, decision-making and psychomotor skills. Most standards and guidelines for FHM education include content outlines and suggested evaluation methods. The AWHONN guidelines outline both core (basic) and ongoing (experienced) instructional programs. A core program includes essential knowledge and skills to achieve minimal competence, while an ongoing program includes additional knowledge and skills to maintain competence. Programs for novices emphasize the rules and structure (core) for basic assessment and intervention and focus on factual information. Programs for experienced clinicians provide opportunities for ongoing consideration and problem-solving through case studies, discussion and reflection. Both basic education and experience are necessary to achieve skill in clinical judgment (Benner, 1984).

Instruction and evaluation methods may include examination, case-study analysis, tracing interpretation, role-playing, policy debate, documentation discussion and skill demonstration. Mahley, Witt and Beckmann (1999) developed and evaluated an EFM teaching tool for undergraduate students based on the nursing process which could also be used by intrapartum nurses.

Competence Validation and Certification

Competence validation is the process of documenting that an individual has received instruction and evaluating the individual's knowledge and skills. A variety of instruction and performance evaluation tools can be used for competence validation (Simpson & Creehan, 1998). Certification is recognition awarded by an accredited credentialing agency to an individual who completes predetermined criteria, usually limited to didactic knowledge, demonstrated by means of a psychometrically sound exam. The advantages and disadvantages of subspecialty certification in didactic EFM knowledge have been debated (Afriat, Simpson, Chez & Miller, 1994; McCartney, 1999; Murray, 1999).

Research

Although a variety of educational resources for learning and validating competence in FHR

assessment exist, research on their effectiveness is limited. The few reported investigations include studies on educational content and methods (Kinnick, 1989, 1990; Murray & Higgins, 1996; Sauer, 1993; Trepanier et al., 1996) and studies on assessment of skill (Chez et al., 1990; Haggerty, 1996; Haggerty & Nuttall, 2000; McCartney, 1995; Morrison et al., 1993). Haggerty (1996) found expert intrapartal nurses identified four clinical parameters to assess the severity of fetal stress: duration of stress, fetal reserve status, reversibility and specific signs of stress. Later, Haggerty and Nuttall (2000) reported that the most important clinical factors experienced nurses considered in determining fetal risk were scalp pH, maternal parity, amniotic fluid color and long-term FHR variability.

🖳 DEVELOPMENT OF THE FHMPP PROGRAM

In 1990, NAACOG initiated the development of a standardized fetal monitoring course to validate the cognitive knowledge and psychomotor skills of the experienced nurse in comprehensive fetal heart monitoring (both auscultation and EFM). The AWHONN FHMPP workshop complements existing AWHONN resources and institutional programs on basic fetal heart monitoring. Because of increasing interest in the auscultation method and prevailing continuing education philosophy emphasizing skills verification, the course validates didactic knowledge as well as skill in auscultation, EFM and abdominal palpation. The FHMPP workshop was designed to be part of an overall plan for competence validation in specialty practice for the individual or institution. Many institutions identify the FHMPP as a component of the nurse's core competencies for institutional accreditation purposes.

Throughout the development of the FHMPP, the goal was to create a course that would emphasize the physiologic basis of assessment and intervention and help nurses apply these concepts to practice through the use of small group exercises, case studies, decision-making activities and hands-on skill practice. Fetal monitoring is taught within the nursing model, as a component of overall nursing knowledge and skills, and not as an isolated technical skill. Case studies are presented in segments, and students work in small groups to systematically assess, analyze and interpret problem cues and discuss intervention. Students are expected to build on prior knowledge, and faculty are expected to guide, stimulate and foster critical-thinking skills as well as present structured, advanced information. Learning through case studies requires integrating fetal heart monitoring data, including both technologically generated data and manually assessed data, into a broader clinical assessment.

The NAACOG Committee on Education appointed a National Steering Committee of six member experts in fetal monitoring education from geographically diverse areas. This volunteer committee met regularly for 2 years and created the 2-day course along with a workshop manual, audiovisual materials and skill models (Schmidt, 2000). The course plan included training qualified NAACOG members as instructors to teach the course and as instructor-trainers to prepare additional instructors; it was piloted in 1992. An Instructor Enhancement Course was added in 1994 for training course instructors. In 1997, the newsletter *The Beat Goes On* was initiated to communicate workshop information to instructors and instructor-trainers. An Advanced FHMPP course was added in 1998.

Ten years later, in 2002, there were more than 1,700 FHMPP instructors throughout the United States and abroad. More than 4,000 FHMPP workshops have been conducted since 1993, including more than 38,000 participants in the United States, Canada, Germany, Italy, Spain and Turkey.

A complete description of the FHMPP workshop and information is included in the Preface.

◘ THE NURSING PROCESS AND THE FHMPP EDUCATION PROGRAM

The nursing process model—assessment, interpretation, intervention and evaluation—provides the theoretical framework for the content of this book and the didactic components of the FHMPP workshop. The process of FHM decision-making is based on the critical-thinking skills of analysis, synthesis and evaluation that are central to the nursing process (Figure 1-1).

◘ RECOMMENDATIONS FOR FURTHER RESEARCH

Fetal heart monitoring is a pervasive assessment tool in perinatal care today. The goal of FHM is secondary prevention, or screening (early detection) for signs of fetal compromise to enable prompt intervention and prevent an unfavorable outcome. However, regardless of how important the target condition is, "Clinicians should be selective in providing preventive services" (Department of Health and Human Services, 1998). The use of FHM in nursing practice should be based on research findings and not on tradition or practices favored by an influential clinician. Gennaro, Hodnett and Kearney (2001) offer nurses a guide for incorporating existing research into practice.

Areas for further research include assessment, interpretation and intervention practices. Assessment research needs include examining observer skill, observer reliability, comparisons of monitoring methods including computer analysis, monitoring frequency, identification of who is at risk and other methods of measuring fetal oxygenation. Interpretation research needs include describing the relationship of FHR characteristics and neonatal outcomes. Intervention research needs include testing interventions in relationship to neonatal outcomes and in an effort to validate FHM as a secondary prevention screening tool. Further research should capitalize on the opportunity to collect data using perinatal information systems. Education also should be based on research findings, including nurses' cognitive and skill development, novice/expert differences and efficacy of instruction and evaluation methods.

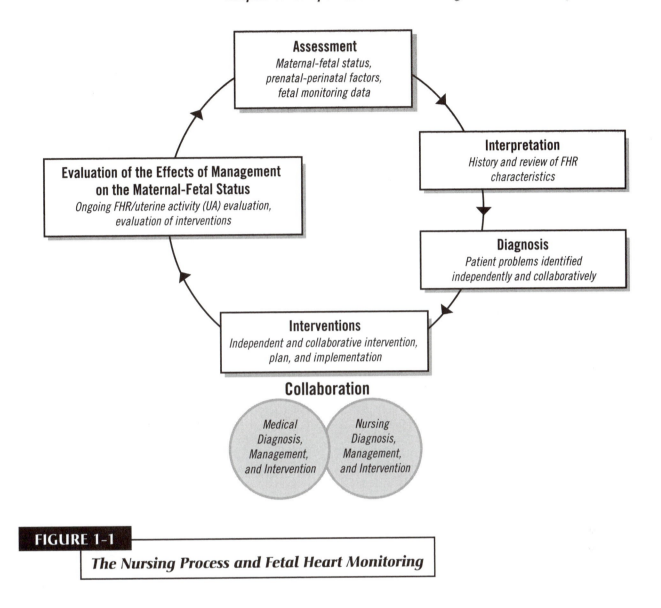

FIGURE 1-1

The Nursing Process and Fetal Heart Monitoring

🖙 REFERENCES

Adelsperger, D. (1990). *Train the trainer program.* (Continuing Education Program). Washington, D.C.: AWHONN.

Afriat, C. L. (1981). The evolution of an antepartum testing program. *Journal of Obstetric, Gynecologic and Neonatal Nursing, 10*(2), 110–112.

Afriat, C. L., Simpson, K. R., Chez, B. F., & Miller, L. A. (1994). Electronic fetal monitoring competency—to validate or not to validate: The opinions of experts. *Journal of Perinatal and Neonatal Nursing, 8*(3), 1–16.

American Academy of Pediatrics, American College of Obstetricians and Gynecologists. (1997). *Guidelines for perinatal care* (4th ed.). Elk Grove Village, IL, and Washington, D.C.: Authors.

American Academy of Pediatrics, American College of Obstetricians and Gynecologists. (2002). *Guidelines for perinatal care* (5th ed.). Elk Grove Village, IL, and Washington, D.C.: Authors.

American College of Nurse Midwives. (1991). *Appropriate use of technology in childbirth* (Position Statement). Washington, D.C.: Author.

American College of Obstetricians and Gynecologists. (1995). *Fetal heart rate patterns: Monitoring, interpretation, and management* (ACOG Technical Bulletin No. 207). Washington, D.C.: Author.

American College of Obstetricians and Gynecologists. (1998). *Inappropriate use of the terms fetal distress and birth asphyxia* (ACOG Committee Opinion No. 197). Washington, D.C.: Author.

American College of Obstetricians and Gynecologists. (2001, September). *Fetal pulse oximetry* (Committee Opinion No. 258). Washington, D.C.: Author.

Association of Women's Health, Obstetric and Neonatal Nurses. (1993). *Didactic content and clinical skills verification for professional nurse providers of basic, high risk, and critical care intrapartum nursing* (withdrawn). Washington, D.C.: Author.

Association of Women's Health, Obstetric and Neonatal Nurses. (1998a). *AWHONN standards and guidelines for professional nursing practice in the care of women and newborns* (5th ed.). Washington, D.C.: Author.

Association of Women's Health, Obstetric and Neonatal Nurses. (1998b). *Clinical competencies and educational guide: Antepartum and Intrapartum fetal heart rate monitoring.* Washington, D.C.: Author.

Association of Women's Health, Obstetric and Neonatal Nurses. (1999). *Basic, high-risk and critical care intrapartum nursing: Clinical competencies and education guide.* Washington, D.C.: Author.

Association of Women's Health, Obstetric and Neonatal Nurses. (2000a). *Fetal assessment* (Position Statement). Washington, D.C.: Author.

Association of Women's Health, Obstetric and Neonatal Nurses. (2000b). *Written statement of AWHONN to Subcommittee on Health, Committee on Ways and Means on the Institute of Medicine Report on Medical Errors* [On-line]. Retrieved March 31, 2000: http://www.awhonn.org/advocacy/iomstatement.htm

Ayres-de Campos, D., Bernardes, J., Garrido, A., Marques-de-Sa, J., & Pereira-Leite, L. (2000). SisPorto 2.0: A program for automated analysis of cardiotocograms. *Journal of Maternal-Fetal Medicine, 9*(5), 311–318.

Benner, P. (1984). *From novice to expert: Excellence and power in clinical nursing practice.* Menlo Park, CA: Addison-Wesley.

Benson, R. C., Shubeck, F., Deutschberger, J., Weiss, W., & Berendes, H. (1968). Fetal heart rate as a predictor of fetal distress: A report from the Collaborative Project. *Obstetrics and Gynecology, 32*(2), 259–266.

Caldeyro-Barcia, R., Mendez-Bauer, E., & Poseiro, J. (1966). Control of human fetal heart rate during labor. In D. E. Cassels (Ed.), *The heart and circulation in the newborn and infant.* New York: Grune and Stratton.

Chez, B. F., & Harvey, C. (1994). *Essentials of electronic fetal heart monitoring* (2nd ed.). (Videotape series, Association of Women's Health, Obstetric and Neonatal Nurses). Baltimore, MD: Williams & Wilkins.

Chez, B. F., Skurnick, J. H., Chez, R. A., Verklan, M. T., Biggs, S., & Hage, M. L. (1990). Interpretations of nonstress tests by obstetric nurses. *Journal of Obstetric, Gynecologic, and Neonatal Nursing 19*(3), 227–232.

Clark, S. L., Gimvosky, M. L., & Miller, F. C. (1982). Fetal heart rate response to scalp blood sampling. *American Journal of Obstetrics and Gynecology, 144*(6), 706–708.

Clark, S. L., Gimvosky, M. L., & Miller, F. C. (1984). The scalp stimulation test: A clinical alternative to fetal scalp blood sampling. *American Journal of Obstetrics and Gynecology, 148*(3), 274–277.

Clark, S. L., & Paul, R. H. (1985). Intrapartum fetal surveillance: The role of fetal scalp blood sampling. *American Journal of Obstetrics and Gynecology, 153*(7), 717–720.

Devoe, L., Golde, S., Kilman, Y., Morton, D., Shea, K., & Waller, J. (2000). A comparison of visual analyses of intrapartum fetal heart rate tracings according to the new National Institute of Child Health and Human Development guidelines with computer analyses by an automated fetal heart monitoring system. *American Journal of Obstetrics and Gynecology, 183*(2), 361–66.

Eganhouse, D. J., McCloskey, J. C., & Bulechek, G. M. (1996). How NIC describes MCH nursing. *MCN, The American Journal of Maternal/Child Nursing, 21*(5), 247–252.

Feinstein, N. F. (2000). Fetal heart rate auscultation: Current and future practice. *Journal of Obstetric, Gynecologic, and Neonatal Nursing, 29*(3), 306–315.

Feinstein, N. F., Sprague, A., & Trepanier, M. J. (2000). *Fetal heart rate auscultation.* Washington, D.C.: AWHONN.

Freeman, R. K. (1975). The use of the oxytocin challenge test for antepartum clinical evaluation of uteroplacental respiratory function. *American Journal of Obstetrics and Gynecology, 121*(4), 481–489.

Freeman, R. K., Garite, T. J., & Nageotte, M. P. (1991). *Fetal heart rate monitoring* (2nd ed.). Baltimore, MD: Williams & Wilkins.

Gennaro, S., Hodnett, E., & Kearney, M. (2001). Making evidenced-based practice a reality in your institution. *MCN, The American Journal of Maternal/Child Nursing, 26*(5), 236–244.

Goodlin, R. C. (1979). History of fetal monitoring. *American Journal of Obstetrics and Gynecology, 133*(3), 323–352.

Haggerty, L. A. (1996). Assessment parameters and indicators in expert intrapartal nursing decisions. *Journal of Obstetric, Gynecologic, and Neonatal Nursing, 25*(6), 491–499.

Haggerty, L. A. (1999). Continuous electronic fetal heart rate monitoring: Contradictions between practice and research. *Journal of Obstetric, Gynecologic, and Neonatal Nursing, 28*(4), 409–416.

Haggerty, L. A., & Nuttall, R. L. (2000). Experienced obstetric nurses' decision-making in fetal risk situations. *Journal of Obstetric, Gynecologic, and Neonatal Nursing, 29*(5), 480–490.

Hammacher, K. (1969). The clinical significance of cardiotocography. In P. Huntingford, K. Huter, & E. Salez (Eds.), *Perinatal medicine, 1st European Congress, Berlin.* New York: Academic Press.

Haverkamp, A. D., Thompson, H. E., McFee, J. G., & Cetrulo, C. (1976). The evaluation of continuous fetal heart rate monitoring in high-risk pregnancy. *American Journal of Obstetrics and Gynecology, 125*(3), 310–320.

Hillis, D. S. (1917). Attachment for the stethoscope. *Journal of the American Medical Association, 68,* 910.

Hon, E. (1958). The electronic evaluation of the fetal heart rate. *American Journal of Obstetrics & Gynecology, 75*(6), 1215–1230.

Hon, E. (1963). The classification of fetal heart rate: A revised working classification. *Obstetrics and Gynecology, 22,* 137–146.

Institute of Medicine. (1999). *To err is human: Building a safer health system.* Washington, D.C.: National Academy Press.

Kelly, C. S. (1999). Perinatal computerized patient record and archiving systems: Pitfalls and enhancements for implementing a successful computerized medical record. *Journal of Perinatal and Neonatal Nursing, 12*(4), 1–14.

Kinnick, V. G. (1989). A national survey about fetal monitoring skills acquired by nursing students in baccalaureate programs. *Journal of Obstetric, Gynecologic, and Neonatal Nursing, 18*(1), 57–58.

Kinnick, V. G. (1990). The effect of concept teaching in preparing nursing students for clinical practice. *Journal of Nursing Education, 29*(8), 362–366.

Mahley, S., Witt, J., & Beckmann, C. Teaching nursing students to critically evaluate fetal monitor tracings. *Journal of Obstetric, Gynecologic, and Neonatal Nursing, 28*(3), 237–240.

Mahomed, K., Nyoni, R. Mulambo, T., Kasale, J., & Jacobus, E. (1994). Randomized controlled trial of intrapartum fetal heart rate monitoring. *British Medical Journal, 308,* 497–500.

Manning, F., Platt, L., & Sipos, L. (1980). Antepartum fetal evaluation: Development of a fetal biophysical profile. *American Journal of Obstetrics and Gynecology, 136*(6), 787–795.

McCartney, P. R. (1995). Fetal heart rate pattern analysis by expert and novice nurses. *Dissertation Abstracts International, 56-07,* 3677–3944B. Unpublished doctoral dissertation. (University Microfilms No. 9538106).

McCartney, P. R. (1999). Certification in fetal heart monitoring: Is it really worth the additional effort and expense for perinatal nurses? Con position. *MCN, The American Journal of Maternal/Child Nursing, 24*(1), 11.

McCartney, P. R. (2000). Computer analysis of the fetal heart rate. *Journal of Obstetric, Gynecologic, and Neonatal Nursing, 29*(5), 527–536.

McCloskey, J. C., & Bulechek, G. M. (Eds.) (2000). *Nursing interventions classification (NIC)* (3rd ed.). St. Louis: Mosby-Year Book.

Miller, F. C., Pearse, K. E., & Paul, R. H. (1984). Fetal heart pattern recognition by the method of auscultation. *Obstetrics and Gynecology, 64*(3), 332–336.

Morrison, J. C., Chez, B. F., Davis, I. D., Martin, R. W., Roberts, W. E., Martin, J. N., & Floyd, R. C. (1993). Intrapartum fetal heart rate assessment: Monitoring by auscultation or electronic means. *American Journal of Obstetrics and Gynecology, 168*(1), 63–66.

Murray, M. L. (1999). Certification in fetal heart monitoring: Is it really worth the additional effort and expense for perinatal nurses? Pro position. *MCN, The American Journal of Maternal/Child Nursing, 24*(1), 10.

Murray, M. L., & Higgins, P. (1996) Computer versus lecture: Strategies for teaching fetal monitoring. *Journal of Perinatology, 16*(1), 15–19.

National Institute of Child Health and Human Development Research Planning Workshop. (1997). Electronic fetal heart rate monitoring: Research guidelines for interpretation. *Journal of Obstetric, Gynecologic, and Neonatal Nurses, 26*(6), 635–640.

National Library of Medicine. (2002). *Library services* [On-line]. Retrieved January 15, 2002 from http://www.nlm.nih.gov/libserv.html.

Nelson, K. B., Dambrosia, J. M., Ting, T. Y., & Grether, J. K. (1996). Uncertain value of electronic fetal monitoring in predicting cerebral palsy. *New England Journal of Medicine, 334*(10), 613–618.

Nurses Association of the American College of Obstetricians and Gynecologists. (1980). *The nurse's role in electronic fetal monitoring* (Technical Bulletin, withdrawn). Chicago, IL: Author.

Nurses Association of the American College of Obstetricians and Gynecologists. (1986). *Electronic fetal monitoring: Joint ACOG/NAACOG statement* (Position Statement, withdrawn). Washington, D.C.: Author.

Nurses Association of the American College of Obstetricians and Gynecologists. (1986). *Electronic fetal monitoring: Nursing practice competencies and educational guidelines* (withdrawn). Washington, D.C.: Author.

Nurses Association of the American College of Obstetricians and Gynecologists. (1988). *Nursing responsibilities in implementing fetal heart rate monitoring* (Position Statement, withdrawn). Washington, D.C.: Author.

Nurses Association of the American College of Obstetricians and Gynecologists. (1990). *Fetal heart rate auscultation* (OGN Nursing Practice Resource, withdrawn). Washington, D.C.: Author.

Nurses Association of the American College of Obstetricians and Gynecologists. (1991a). *Nursing practice competencies and educational guidelines: Antepartum fetal surveillance and intrapartum fetal heart monitoring* (2nd ed., withdrawn). Washington, D.C.: Author.

Nurses Association of the American College of Obstetricians and Gynecologists. (1991b). *NAACOG standards for the nursing care of women and newborns* (4th ed., withdrawn). Washington, D.C.: Author.

Nurses Association of the American College of Obstetricians and Gynecologists. (1991c). *Appropriate use of technology in nursing care* (Committee Opinion, withdrawn). Washington, D.C.: Author.

Nurses Association of the American College of Obstetricians and Gynecologists. (1992). *Nursing responsibilities in implementing intrapartum fetal heart rate monitoring* (Position Statement, withdrawn). Washington, D.C.: Author.

Paine, L. L., Zandari, L. R., Johnson, T. R., Rorie, J. A., & Barger, M. K. (2001). A comparison of two time intervals for the auscultated acceleration test. *Journal of Midwifery and Women's Health, 46*(2), 98–102.

Read, J. A., & Miller, F. C. (1977). Fetal heart rate acceleration in response to acoustic stimulation as a measure of fetal well-being. *American Journal of Obstetrics & Gynecology, 129*(5), 512–517.

Rochard, F., Schifrin, B. S., Goupil, F., LeGrande, H., Blottiere, J., & Sureau, C. (1976). Nonstressed fetal heart rate monitoring in the antepartum period. *American Journal of Obstetrics & Gynecology, 126*(6), 699–706.

Sandelowski, M. (2000). Retrofitting technology to nursing: The case of electronic fetal monitoring. *Journal of Obstetric, Gynecologic, and Neonatal Nursing, 29*(3), 316–324.

Sauer, P. (1993, June). *Interpretations of fetal heart rate tracings by obstetric nurses: Comparison of test scores with experience and education in electronic fetal heart rate monitoring.* Poster session presented at the annual meeting of the Association of Women's Health, Obstetric and Neonatal Nurses, Reno, NV.

Schmidt, J. V. (2000). The development of AWHONN's Fetal Heart Monitoring Principles and Practices course. *Journal of Obstetric, Gynecologic, and Neonatal Nursing, 29*(5), 509–515.

Schmidt, J. V., & McCartney, P. R. (2000). History and development of fetal heart assessment: A composite. *Journal of Obstetric, Gynecologic, and Neonatal Nursing, 29*(3), 295–305.

Smith, C. V., Nguyen, H. N., Phelan, J. P., & Paul, R. H. (1986). Intrapartum assessment of fetal well-being: A comparison of fetal acoustic stimulation with acid-base determinations. *American Journal of Obstetrics and Gynecology, 155*(4), 726–728.

Simpson, K. R., & Creehan, P. (1998). *Competence validation.* Philadelphia: Lippincott.

Simpson, K. R., & Porter, M. L. (2000). Fetal oxygenation saturation monitoring. *AWHONN Lifelines, 5*(2), 27–33.

Society of Obstetricians and Gynaecologists of Canada. (1995). SOGC Policy Statement: Fetal health surveillance in labour. *Journal of the Society of Obstetricians and Gynaecologists of Canada, 17*(9), 865–901.

Society of Obstetricians, and Gynaecologists of Canada. (2002, April). Fetal health surveillance in labour (SOGC Clinical Practice Guidelines No. 112). Ottawa, Ontario, Canada: Author.

Thacker, S. B., & Stroup, D. F. (1999). Continuous electronic fetal monitoring versus intermittent auscultation for assessment during labor (Cochrane Review). In *Cochrane Library, Volume 2.* Oxford: Update Software.

Thacker, S. B., Stroup, D. F., & Peterson, H. B. (1995). Efficacy and safety of intrapartum electronic fetal monitoring: An update. *Obstetrics and Gynecology, 86*(4), 613–620.

Traber, E., Leppein, M., & Billmaier, K. (1993, June). *Development of a regional EFM train the trainer program.* Poster session presented at the annual meeting of the Association of Women's Health, Obstetric and Neonatal Nurses, Reno, NV.

Trepanier, M. J., Niday, P., Davies, B., Sprague, A., Nimrod, C., Dulberg, C., & Watters, N. (1996). Evaluation of a fetal monitoring education program. *Journal of Obstetric, Gynecologic, and Neonatal Nursing, 25*(2), 137–144.

U.S. Department of Health & Human Services. (1998). *Put prevention into practice: Clinician's handbook of preventive services.* Washington, D.C.: U.S. Government Printing Office.

Wulf, K. H. (1985). History of fetal heart rate monitoring. In W. Kunzel (Ed.), *Fetal heart rate monitoring: Clinical practice and pathophysiology.* New York: Springer-Verlag.

Yeh, S., Jilek, J., & Hon, E. (1974). On-line diagnosis of ominous fetal heart patterns: A warning device. *American Journal of Obstetrics and Gynecology, 118*(4), 559–563.

SECTION TWO

Physiological Basis for Fetal Heart Monitoring

CHAPTER 2

Extrinsic Influences on the Fetal Heart Rate

Gay L. Goss
Keiko L. Torgersen

The fetus depends on the delivery of oxygenated blood to meet metabolic needs and to withstand the stress associated with uterine contractions and labor. Extrinsic influences on the fetal heart rate (FHR) are factors in the fetal environment that affect the availability of oxygen and the ability to transport oxygen to the fetus, thus affecting the FHR. These include maternal physiologic, uteroplacental, uterine activity, and umbilical cord factors. This chapter includes a brief summary of maternal physiological changes during pregnancy, with a discussion of the relationship of the above extrinsic factors to fetal oxygenation and the FHR. Chapter 3 provides a discussion of the fetal intrinsic influences and homeostatic mechanisms that also affect fetal oxygenation.

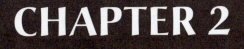 MATERNAL PHYSIOLOGICAL CHANGES DURING PREGNANCY AND IMPLICATIONS FOR FETAL OXYGENATION

Pregnancy is marked by a series of physiologic changes in the maternal reproductive, cardiovascular, hematologic, respiratory, renal, gastroin-testinal, and endocrine systems during the course of pregnancy. These physical and metabolic changes vary with each week of pregnancy and are essential to the growth and well-being of the fetus. Many of the physiologic changes discussed can have a significant impact on the availability of oxygen for transport by the placenta for use by the fetus during growth and development and during labor and delivery.

Reproductive Adaptation

Due to an increase in estrogen and progesterone production during pregnancy, maternal tissues hypertrophy, have hyperplasia and have increased vascularity which contribute to many of the normal discomforts of pregnancy (Bond, 1999; Hunter & Robson, 1992; Torgersen, 2001). The additional vascularity changes the function and size of maternal tissues that is essential to sustain the pregnancy and ensure maternal well-being after delivery. The uterine volume increases from approximately 10 ml in the nonpregnant state to 4–10 liters during pregnancy, a 1,000-fold increase. Additionally, the shape of the uterus changes from an inverted pear to a soft globe and rises out of the pelvis after 12 weeks of gestation.

Contractions may occur as early as the first trimester and continue throughout gestation. Most commonly, contractions noted in early pregnancy are characterized as painless uterine activity. The intensity of these contractions usually measures between 5 and 25 mmHg. Biochemical and physiologic changes occur near term and during parturition, enabling the uterus to contract in a coordinated, efficient manner (Bond, 2000; Caldeyro-Barcia & Poseiro, 1960).

In addition, the uterus undergoes a profound increase in both vasculature and lymphatics. The uterine veins and arteries that interact with the placenta grow larger to meet the increased workload of the fetal-placental unit. Adequate perfusion to the placenta is critical for fetal metabolism, growth and development; and is vital to fetal wellbeing during labor and delivery.

Normal uterine blood flow is determined by the adequacy of maternal arterial blood pressure. The increase in uterine blood flow results in an increase in placental circulation. At term, less than 5% of uterine blood flow goes to the uterine myometrium, 10–15% to the uterine endometrium, and 80–85% to placental circulation (Resnick, 1999). Maternal positions that change maternal blood pressure can also affect uterine blood flow. For example, supine positioning can significantly reduce uterine blood flow by decreasing venous return and uterine arterial blood pressure. Maternal diseases, such as hypertensive disorders and vascular disease, and drugs, such as cocaine, can produce significant vasoconstriction resulting in decreased uterine blood flow, likely secondary to increased sympathetic activity or catecholamine production (Kirkinen, Jouppila, Koivula, Vuori, & Puukka, 1983; Resnick, 1999). Regional analgesia and anesthesia may cause systemic hypotension, which reduces uterine arterial pressure and, therefore, uterine blood flow.

Cardiovascular Adaptation

The cardiovascular system is hyperdynamic and hypervolemic during pregnancy. Pregnancy is considered to be a high flow (high cardiac output) and low resistance (low systemic vascular resistance) state. Physiologic changes in the cardiovascular system include increases in cardiac output, stroke volume, diastolic filling time, and maternal heart rate. Additionally, there are decreases in colloid osmotic pressure, arterial blood pressure, systemic vascular resistance, and pulmonary vascular resistance (Harvey, 1999).

The heart is mechanically displaced to the left and upward due to the growing uterus. The left side of the heart also straightens, increasing the transverse diameter of the heart approximately 1–2 centimeters. In normal pregnancy, the increase in blood volume produces a slight left ventricular hypertrophy yet does not alter left ventricular cardiac function (Harvey, 1999).

Under the influence of progesterone, smooth muscles relax to accommodate the fluid volume increase in pregnancy. Blood volume increases approximately 1,600 ml in a singleton pregnancy and approximately 2,000 ml in a multiple gestation, regardless of the number of fetuses. This increase represents a 50% increase over the nonpregnant state and acts as a protective mechanism against postpartum blood loss.

Maternal cardiac output is a major determinant of placental perfusion and fetal oxygenation. It reflects the overall functional capacity of the left ventricle to maintain satisfactory blood pressure and organ perfusion. Essentially, cardiac output (CO) is heart rate (HR) multiplied by stroke volume (SV) (CO = HR × SV). The mother's cardiac output increases as early as 10 weeks gestation and peaks at 30 weeks gestation at 30–50% above the nonpregnant state. Normal cardiac output in a pregnant woman not in labor and at rest is 6–7 liters per minute (L/min). Pregnant women experiencing increased levels of stress and/or injury can have a cardiac output of 9–11 L/min and women pushing during the second stage of labor can increase their cardiac output to 18 L/min or higher.

During a normal pregnancy, blood volume has increased by 50% at 34 weeks gestation. At term, 6 to 7 L/min of blood is pumped to the uterus. Studies focusing on pregnant women have revealed that cardiac output changes with maternal position, labor, pain, fever, hyperdynamic states, and in the postpartum. One such study reported a 43% increase in cardiac output during pregnancy if mother was in the left lateral recumbent position (Clark et al., 1989). The maternal heart rate also increases throughout pregnancy, approximately 20% (15–20 beats per minute) by the third trimester. As a response to these changes in stroke volume (milliliter of blood pushed out with each heart beat) and heart rate, or maternal cardiac output, 90% of pregnant women will demonstrate one of two types of functional cardiac murmurs. One is a pulmonary systolic murmur, and the second is a supraclavicular systolic murmur (Bond, 1999; Harvey, 1999).

Peripheral circulatory adaptations include a decrease in the systemic vascular resistance (SVR), due in part to the effects of estrogen and progesterone; yet venous pressure remains unchanged. The technical definition for SVR is the measure of tension required for ejection of blood into the circulation. Essentially, this is the resistance the right and left ventricles meet when blood is forced out of the heart or how compliant or tight is the vascular bed. Decreased SVR is responsible for dependent edema in pregnant women, resulting from pooling of blood in the lower extremities. In addition to a decrease in SVR, there is a decrease in uterine vascular resistance, allowing for increased blood flow to the uterus, placenta, and, ultimately, the fetus. Arterial blood pressure decreases in the first weeks of pregnancy but rises to pre-pregnancy values by 20 weeks gestation. Arterial blood pressure is directly related to cardiac output. When arterial blood pressure is decreased, cardiac output is decreased (Mesa et al., 1999). This becomes a concern during labor, when regular progressive uterine activity negatively affects arterial blood pressure (Clark et al., 1989). As a result, if the blood pressure is too low or too high, it can affect the available blood flow to the fetus, thus reducing fetal oxygenation. This decrease in fetal oxygenation can then be reflected in the fetal heart rate.

Hematologic Adaptation

The composition of blood changes as pregnancy advances, and red blood cells (RBC) increase 25–30%, equal to approximately 250 ml/dL due to increased hematopoiesis in the bone marrow and liver. However, plasma volume expands more, to 1,250–1,500 ml, and the increase is not linear to RBC production. This creates a physiologic dilutional anemia, with the most pronounced anemia noticed at 28 weeks gestation. The physiological dilutional anemia, increased hematopoiesis, and associated transfer of approximately 300 mg of maternal iron to the fetus during gestation can create an iron deficit of approximately 800 mg by mid-pregnancy. If maternal anemia is due to iron deficiency or hemoglobinopathies such as thalassemia or sickle-cell disease, or to hemorrhage, the hemoglobin level could be further reduced, limiting available hemoglobin for oxygen transport to the fetus. However, iron supplementation can increase the available RBCs to 400 ml/dL, increasing available hemoglobin for oxygen transport. Normal hemoglobin and hematocrit values in pregnancy are 12–16 gm/dL and 35–45%, respectively.

Pregnancy is a hypercoagulable state, with an increase in clotting factors V, VII, VIII, IX, X, XII, prothrombin, and fibrinogen. The alteration in clotting factors increases the potential for coagulation problems and thrombosis (Bond, 1999; Bonnar, et al., 1969).

White blood cell counts increase by approximately 40 to 50%, tend to increase further during and delivery, and peak in the immediate postpartum.

Pulmonary Adaptation

Anatomical changes in the respiratory system occur in response to the growing uterus and improve gaseous exchange. By 12 weeks gestation, the uterus is no longer contained entirely within the pelvis. Consequently, the level of the diaphragm increases by 4–7 cm, and the subcoastal angle increases 75 to 105 degrees, causing an increase in the anterior/posterior and transverse diameters. The lower ribs flare out to increase space for the lungs. Oxygen consumption increases approximately 20%, with 50% going to the embryo and the fetus. The remaining 50% supports the uterus, breast tissue, and increased respiratory and cardiac demands. Minute ventilation increases by 37% at term due to the growth and development of the fetus, the increased workload of the maternal myocardium, and the growth of the mammary glands (Bond, 1999; Harvey, 1999). In response, ventilation and increased amounts of oxygen result in increased tidal volume (amount of air taken in with each breath) of approximately 39%. Thus, oxygen goes into a smaller residual space, resulting in a more efficient gas exchange, and an increase in alveolar ventilation by 65% or 500 to 700 ml with each exchange. This creates a chronic, compensated, respiratory alkalosis (see Table 2-1) that becomes important during labor, when maternal hyperventilation may exacerbate this alkalotic state. Maternal hyperventilation may increase the maternal pH to the extent that the fetal pH is elevated even in the presence of fetal acidemia, a potentially confounding factor in the interpretation of fetal scalp sampling data.

Baseline maternal arterial oxygen tension is the source for oxygen transported to and used by the fetus. Acute maternal hypoxemia compromises maternal arterial oxygen saturation and tension and decreases oxygen available to the fetus. Acute or chronic maternal respiratory disease such as acute pulmonary edema, chronic asthma, or cystic fibrosis also may reduce oxygen tension and result in compromised fetal or placental growth and development. Maternal smoking results in lowered oxygen saturation despite adequate oxygenation because carbon monoxide molecules displace oxygen on maternal and fetal hemoglobin. Maternal hypoventilation due to breath holding during pushing may transiently decrease oxygen availability.

In response to the increased progesterone, pulmonary resistance stimulates the respiratory center of the brain and increases the pliability of connective tissue. This makes breathing easier for the mother, and she exchanges more air with each breath. However, dyspnea can also occur. The normal respiratory rate for a pregnant woman is approximately 20 breaths per minute.

The respiratory changes create a greater capacity for oxygen transport, increasing the amount of oxygen available to the fetus and to the mother.

Renal Adaptation

Under the influence of progesterone, there is significant dilation of the renal system, especially of the right ureter. Bladder tone is decreased; the bladder is pulled upward, and becomes concave in appearance. These changes predispose the mother to urinary stasis, decreased peristalsis, and subsequent urinary tract infections. In addition, glomerular filtration rates are increased approximately 50%, along with renal clearance. This causes an increase in excreted folate, glucose, urea, sodium and creatinine (Green, 1999).

The renal threshold for glucose is also lowered, which allows for glucose to be spilled into the urine. Urinary tract infection is associated with an increased rate of bladder irritability. Without appropriate treatment, urinary tract infections can lead to coordinated uterine activity. When a urinary tract infection is left untreated, it can cause cervical change, preterm labor, or delivery.

Gastrointestinal Adaptation

Water absorption from the colon increases and causes constipation in the pregnant woman. Gas-

TABLE 2-1

Acid-Base Balance Values

STATUS	PO$_2$	PCO$_2$	pH	BICARB
Pregnant	104–108 mmHg	27–32 mmHg	7.40–7.46	22 mEq/L
Nonpregnant	80–100 mmHg	35–45 mmHg	7.35–7.45	26 mEq/L

(Harvey, 1999)

trointestinal tone and mobility is lowered, increasing gastric emptying time and predisposing the mother to reflux esophagitis, constipation, and nausea. However, gastric secretion of hydrochloric acid and pepsin decrease, which improves peptic ulcer disease and increases the secretory response of histamines (Bond, 1999; Scott, 1999).

Endocrine Adaptation

The thyroid gland increases in size, causing increased iodine metabolism. Thyroid stimulating hormone (TSH) levels decrease, yet thyroxine (T4) levels increase. Additionally, the basal metabolic rate increases 25% by term and is thought to be the cause of maternal palpitations and fatigue during pregnancy. All these changes cause increased perspiration, tachycardia, emotional lability, and heat intolerance. Insulin production increases 30% in the pancreas as a compensatory mechanism for the increase in placental hormones, causing decreased tissue sensitivity to insulin. As a result, women with poor pancreatic function may develop true diabetes during or after pregnancy (Bond, 1999; Harvey, 1999).

Other essential extrinsic factors include the physiology of the utero-placental unit, umbilical cord, and placenta.

☞ PHYSIOLOGY OF THE UTEROPLACENTAL UNIT

Uterine blood flow represents approximately 10% of the maternal cardiac blood flow; however, this number rises progressively throughout pregnancy. About 70–90% of uterine blood flow passes through the intervillous space, and the remainder supplies the myometrium of the uterus. By simple diffusion, oxygen is delivered to the fetus within the placental villi and cotyledons. Major factors affecting the blood flow to the uterus and subsequently the fetus include contractions, maternal positioning, medications, and demands on maternal circulation. Placental considerations include the size and structural integrity of the placenta, and the amount of blood flow to the placenta (Martin & Gingerich, 1976) (see Table 2-2).

The uterine vascular bed is at maximal dilation at rest. Under normal conditions it has little capacity to further dilate and does not respond to changes in respiratory gas tensions.

Uterine contractions decrease uterine blood flow, increase uterine venous pressure, and decrease uterine arterial perfusion pressure (see Figure 2-1). If uterine arterial perfusion pressure is altered without changing the resistance of the uterine vascular bed, there is a direct relationship between uterine blood flow and the uterine pressure. In addition, maternal hyperventilation also may increase catecholamine production, exaggerate the mild compensated respiratory alkalemia of pregnancy, and reduce uterine blood flow. Maternal hyperventilation may increase the maternal pH to the extent that the fetal pH is elevated even in the presence of fetal acidemia, a potentially confounding factor in the interpretation of fetal scalp sampling data.

The placenta is an organ that is often overlooked. The maternal side of placental circulation is comprised of maternal arteries, veins, and spiral arteries. During the nonpregnant state, the spiral arteries are tightly coiled. In the pregnant state, normal physiologic changes in the maternal systems previously discussed cause general vasodilation leading to decreased vascular resistance. The placenta is also affected by these changes. The amount of blood available for transfer to the placental unit is dependent on adequate blood flow to the uterus (King & Parer, 2000) and key to the well-being of the fetus.

The placenta is the organ that bridges the maternal and fetal circulation. The placenta is the fetal organ of respiration, nutrition, and fluid balance and is a major line of defense. It also provides a repository for hormonal function. The placenta is partially formed of villi, which develop early in pregnancy. The villi comprise a direct connection to the maternal spiral arteries.

The intervillous space is an interface between the uterine vasculature and the placenta. Maternal blood circulates within the intervillous space. Surrounded by fetal cotyledons, the intervillous space serves as the major conduit for maternal-

TABLE 2-2

Influences on Uterine Blood Flow

Uterine contractions	Contractions cause < Uterine blood flow > Uterine venous pressure < Uterine arterial perfusion pressure
Maternal positioning	Positioning can cause uterine compression of great vessels, decreased venous return to the heart, decreased blood flow to uterus.
Medications	Sympathetic system involvement from varying medications cause a compensatory hypotension, resulting in decreased blood flow.
Demands on maternal circulation	Demands are caused by metabolism, hydration, activity, and nutrition.
Placental influences	Size, integrity, and blood volume are influences.

Adapted from Bond, 1999; Martin & Gingerich, 1976; Meschia, 1999.

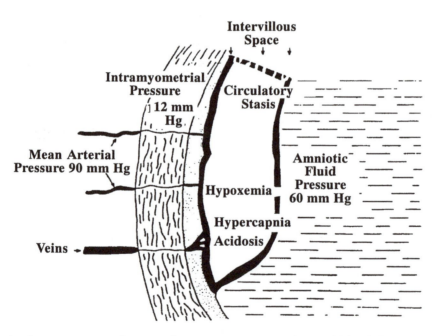

At the acme, or peak of a contraction of greater than 50 mmHg, uteroplacental blood flow ceases temporarily. This causes the fetus to be dependent upon placental reserve. There may be a brief alteration of contraction effectiveness.

FIGURE 2-1

Uteroplacental Blood Flow and the Influence of Intramyometrial Pressure
(Adapted from Freeman, Garite, & Nageotte, 1991; Poseiro, 1969)

fetal transfer (see Figure 2-2). Oxygen (O_2), carbon dioxide (CO_2), nutrients, and waste pass through spiral arteries directly into the intervillous space. Arterial pressures on one side of the intervillous space (the intramyometrial pressure), is balanced by the amniotic fluid pressure in the placenta (Greiss, 1967).

Fetal and maternal exchange happens by a variety of methods. These most commonly include diffusion, facilitated diffusion, active transport, bulk flow, and breaks in the integrity of the circulation (see Table 2-3). During the course of the pregnancy, especially during labor and delivery, these exchange mechanisms can be altered, affecting transfer of critical nutrients and gases to the fetus and causing the fetus to be adversely affected. Dehydration, maternal position, infection, and trauma are examples of these stressors. Changes in the maternal fetal exchange are reflected in the fetal heart rate.

Placental Influences

The placental structure and ability to function both affect the availability of oxygen for fetal use, and in turn affect the FHR. Key placental influences include the placental structure, the placental function, and placental blood flow.

Placental Structure

◆ Functional placental surface area is the amount of placental-fetal interface surface available for the exchange of nutrients (e.g., oxygen, amino acids, proteins, and glucose), elimination of fetal waste, and production of hormones and steroids (see Figure 2-3).

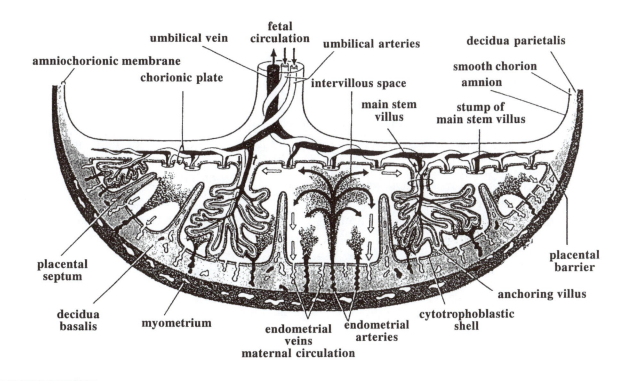

FIGURE 2-2

As Maternal Blood Enters the Intervillous Space, It Flows Upward from Uterine Spiral Arterioles and Spreads Laterally at Random

Note: From *The Developing Human*, by K. L. Moore, Copyright © 1993 by Elsevier Science. Reprinted with permission.

TABLE 2-3	
Maternal-Fetal Exchange Mechanisms	
Diffusion	Substances pass from gradients of high to low concentration (O_2, CO_2, Na, Cl)
Facilitated Diffusion	Energy may be present; fast exchange (Glucose, carbohydrates)
Active Transport	Energy is needed; transfer against gradient (Amino acids, calcium, iron)
Bulk Flow	Osmotic and/or hydrostatic gradient passes substances (H_2O, electrolytes)
Circulation Breaks	Integrity of intervillous space is disrupted. Mixing of maternal and fetal substances. (fetal Rh positive cells)

Adapted from Afriat, 1989; Meschia, 1999.

◆ Functional placental surface area depends on adequate maternal nutrients and maternal-uterine blood flow.

Placental Function

◆ Adequate placental function provides for the transport of oxygen to the fetus at levels above fetal basal needs (e.g., placental reserve) (Meschia, 1999).

◆ Compromised placental growth and development results in decreased placental function, and may, depending on the degree and timing of compromise, result in fetal growth restriction and, possibly, inadequate oxygenation (see Figure 2-4).

◆ Decreased placental function impairs the fetal ability to withstand the normal stresses of labor and birth (e.g., intrinsic fetal homeostatic mechanisms may be unable to compensate for normal degrees of hypoxemia seen with uterine activity).

◆ Depending upon the degree of loss of placental function, additional hypoxemic stresses usually tolerated by the healthy fetus may result in rapid decompensation.

◆ Compromised placental function also may be associated with a reduction of amniotic fluid volume, thus limiting protection of the fetus and umbilical cord (Clark, 1990; Phelan, 1989).

Placental Integrity Zones

Placental integrity affects the provision of fetal nutrients (e.g., oxygen, proteins, nutrients) to the fetus to allow for growth and development.

Placental blood flow and blood oxygen content affect oxygen delivery to the fetus.

◆ Approximately 70%–90% of uterine blood flow reaches the placenta. This percentage directly reflects the amount of oxygen available for maternal-fetal exchange (Harvey, 1999; Meschia, 1999; Parer, 1983).

◆ Substances cross the placenta by several mechanisms; oxygen is believed to cross the placenta predominantly by simple passive diffusion at a rate directly proportional to the placental area and to the differences in concentration and pressures of oxygen on either side.

◆ Fetal gas exchange occurs in the placental villi contained within the cotyledons (normally 15–20 in number) and depends on the

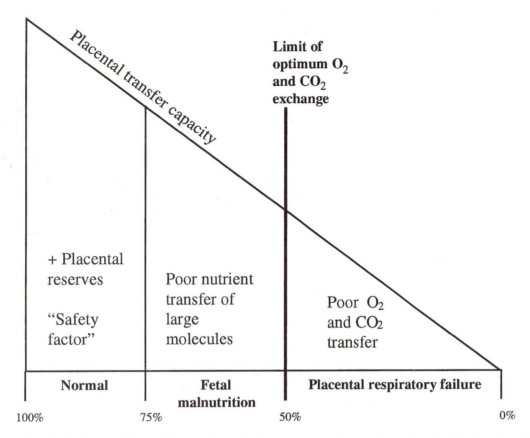

Placental integrity affects the provision of fetal nutrients (e.g., oxygen, proteins, nutrients) to the fetus to allow for growth and development.

FIGURE 2-3

Placental Transfer Capacity
(Adapted from Parer, 1983)

---

structural integrity of the placenta and the related placental blood flow. Placental structural integrity may be compromised by damage to the cotyledons (infarcts) as seen in maternal conditions such as inadequate nutrition, diabetes, smoking, or preeclampsia.

◆ Placental aging, partial abruption, and structural abnormalities, such as circumvallate placenta, also may compromise placental integrity, blood flow, and oxygen delivery.

These conditions may be observed and evaluated by ultrasound scan.

◆ Uteroplacental vessels have a marked capacity for constriction in response to either maternal sympathetic nervous system activation or vasoconstrictor drugs. The constricted vessels may result in reduced placental blood flow and reduced fetal gas exchange even in the presence of normal maternal hemoglobin and arterial oxygen saturation (Zuspan, O'Shaughnessy, & Iams, 1981).

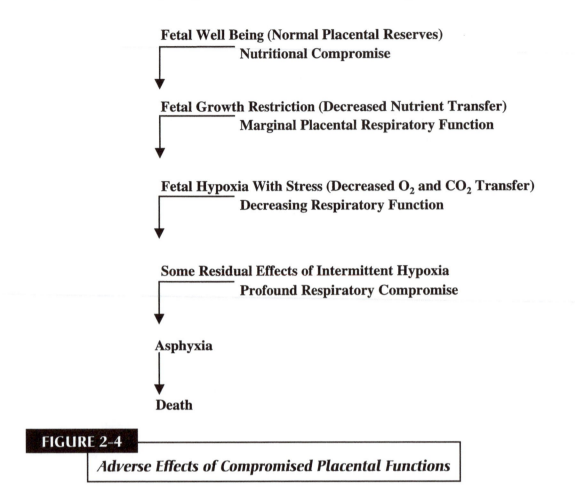

Fetal Well Being (Normal Placental Reserves)
Nutritional Compromise

Fetal Growth Restriction (Decreased Nutrient Transfer)
Marginal Placental Respiratory Function

Fetal Hypoxia With Stress (Decreased O_2 and CO_2 Transfer)
Decreasing Respiratory Function

Some Residual Effects of Intermittent Hypoxia
Profound Respiratory Compromise

Asphyxia

Death

FIGURE 2-4

Adverse Effects of Compromised Placental Functions

☞ UMBILICAL CORD INFLUENCES

The umbilical cord is the vascular connection between the placenta and fetus. The cord's contribution to fetal oxygenation and the subsequent FHR responses may be considered either as extrinsic or intrinsic factors. The umbilical cord vasculature is comprised of two arteries and one vein and has not been shown to have direct innervation (Beisher, Mackay, & Colditz, 1997). The vein is the thinner walled vessel and carries oxygenated blood from the maternal side of the placenta to the fetus. The vein is the first vessel to be compressed if the umbilical cord is compressed, resulting in a decrease of oxygenated blood to the fetus. The arteries are thicker walled vessels and carry deoxygenated blood from the fetus to the maternal side of the placenta. They are compressed after the vein resulting in an inability to transfer carbon dioxide to the maternal system. A gelatinous substance, Wharton's Jelly (see Figure 2-5), surrounds these structures as a means of protecting the vessels.

Alterations in blood flow may be attributed to structural, mechanical, or direct fetal myocardial influence (Zuspan, O'Shaughnessy, & Iams, 1981). Examples of structural alterations include true knots (see Figure 2-6), strictures, hematomas, or decreased number of vessels in the cord that may cause an acute or chronic impairment in blood flow. Sometimes, blood flow is impeded by mechanical conditions such as compression caused by maternal position, fetal body parts or loops of cord coiled around portions of the fetal body. Mechanical compression is found intermittently in many labor experiences.

FHR responses to umbilical cord compression have been shown to vary significantly, depending

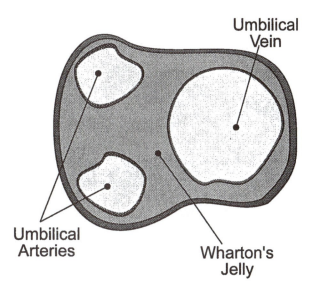

FIGURE 2-5

Vessels Surrounded by Wharton's Jelly, Providing Protection to Umbilical Vessels

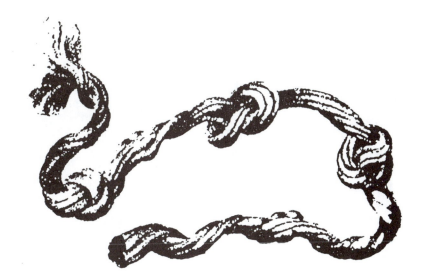

FIGURE 2-6

True Knots in the Umbilical Cord
(Maygrier, 1834)

upon the degree of occlusion and the resulting degree of reduction in blood flow (Itskovitz, La Gamma, & Rudolph, 1983). In a previously well-oxygenated fetus, partial cord occlusion that results in the occlusion of only the low-pressure umbilical vein may produce a decrease in fetal cardiac output and blood pressure, sympathetic stimulation, and result in an increase in the FHR (James et al., 1976). A transient hypoxemia in the fetus may occur, unless the occlusion is prolonged or chronic. Transient hypoxemia is often corrected with measures to relieve cord compression, such as change of position and hydration.

Complete prolonged cord compression results in an abrupt increase in fetal blood pressure that may stimulate fetal baroreceptors and produce an abrupt decrease in FHR; continuation of the complete cord occlusion is likely to result in hypoxemia, chemoreceptor response, and prolongation of decreased FHR. If unrelieved, complete cord compression, as seen with a prolapsed cord, may result in progressive hypoxia and acidosis (James et al., 1976).

☞ SUMMARY

It is important to understand the extrinsic influences in the fetal environment that affect the availability of oxygen and oxygen transportation to the fetus. Chapter 3 will further discuss fetal intrinsic factors that also affect fetal oxygenation. Understanding the normal physiology of pregnancy, uterine blood flow, placental blood flow, and umbilical blood flow can improve the nurse's ability to identify even the most subtle changes that affect the ability of the fetus to tolerate labor and effect a positive outcome.

☞ REFERENCES

Afriat, C. (1989). *Electronic fetal monitoring.* Rockville, MD: Aspen Publications.

Beischer, N. A., Mackay, E. V., & Colditz, P. B. (1997). Fetal and placental development. In N. A. Beischer, E. V. Mackay, & P. B. Colditz, (Eds.), *Obstetrics and the newborn* (3rd ed., pp. 38–52). London: W.B. Saunders

Bond, L. (1999). Physiology of pregnancy. In S. Mattson, & J. E. Smith, (Eds.), *Core curriculum for maternal-newborn nursing* (2nd ed, pp. 85–100). Philadelphia: W.B. Saunders.

Bonnar, J., McNichol, G. P. & Douglas, A. S. (1969). Fibrinolytic enzyme system and pregnancy. *British Medical Journal, 3,* 387–389.

Caldeyro-Barcia, R., & Poseiro, J. J. (1960). Physiology of the uterine contraction. *Clinical Obstetrics and Gynecology, 3,* 386–408.

Clark, S. (1990). How a modified NST improves fetal surveillance. *Contemporary OB/GYN, 35*(5), 45–48.

Clark, S. L., Cotton, D. B., Lee, W., Bishop, C., Hill, T., Southwick, J., Pivarnik, J., Spillman, T., DeVore, G. R., & Phelan, J. (1989). Central hemodynamic assessment of normal term pregnancy. *American Journal of Obstetrics and Gynecology, 161*(6, Pt. 1), 1439–1442.

Freeman, R. K., & Garite, T. J., & Nageotte, M. P. (1991). *Fetal heart rate monitoring* (2nd ed.). Baltimore: Williams and Wilkins.

Greiss, F. C. (1967). A clinical concept of uterine blood flow during pregnancy. *Obstetrics and Gynecology, 30*(4), 595–604.

Green, K. (1999). Prenatal Assessment. In C. N. Carcio (Ed.), *Advanced health assessment of women.* Philadelphia: Lippincott.

Harvey, M. G. (1999). Physiologic changes during pregnancy. In L. K. Mandeville. & N. H. Troiano (Eds.), *High-risk & critical care intrapartum nursing* (2nd ed., pp. 2–31). Philadelphia: Lippincott.

Hunter, S., & Robson, S. C. (1992). Adaptation of the maternal heart in pregnancy. *British Heart Journal, 68*(6), 540–543.

Itskovitz, J., La Gamma, E. F., & Rudolph, A. M. (1983). Heart rate and blood pressure responses to umbilical cord compression in fetal lambs with special reference to the mechanism of variable deceleration. *American Journal of Obstetrics and Gynecology, 147*(4), 451–457.

James, L. S., Yeh, M. N., Morishima, H. O., Daniel, S. S., Cartiis, S. N., Niemann, W. H., & Indyk, L. (1976). Umbilical vein occlusion and transient acceleration of the fetal heart. *American Journal of Obstetrics and Gynecology, 126*(2), 276–283.

King, T., & Parer, J. (2000). The physiology of fetal heart rate patterns and perinatal asphyxia. *Journal of Perinatal and Neonatal Nursing, 14*(3), 19–39.

Kirkinen, P., Jouppila, P., Koivula, A., Vuori, J., & Puukka, M. (1983). The effect of caffeine on placental and fetal blood flow in human pregnancy. *American Journal of Obstetrics and Gynecology, 147*(8), 939–942.

Martin, C. B., & Gingerich, B. (1976). Uteroplacental physiology. *Journal of Obstetric, Gynecologic, and Neonatal Nursing, 5*(suppl. 5), 16s–25s.

Maygrier, J. P. (1834). *Midwifery illustrated.* New York: Harper & Brothers. Facsimile Edition 1969, by Medical Heritage Press, Inc., Skokie, IL.

Mesa, A., Jessurun, C. Hernandez, A., Adam, K., Brown, D., Vaughn, W. K., & Wilansky, S. (1999). Left ventricular diastolic function in normal human pregnancy. *Circulation, 99*(4), 511–517.

Meschia, G. (1999). Placental respiratory gas exchange and fetal oxygenation. In R. K. Creasy & R. Resnick (Eds.), *Maternal-fetal medicine* (4th ed., pp. 260–269). Philadelphia: W.B. Saunders.

Moore, K. L. (1993). *The developing human* (2nd ed.). Philadelphia: W.B. Saunders.

Parer, J. T. (1983). Uteroplacental physiology and exchange. In *Handbook of fetal heart rate monitoring* (p. 15). Phildelphia: W.B. Saunders.

Phelan, J. (1989). The postdate pregnancy: An overview. *Clinical Obstetrics and Gynecology, 32*(2), 221–227.

Poseiro, J. J. (1969). Effect of uterine conractions on maternal blood flow through the placenta. *Perinatal factors affecting human development* (Pub. #185, pp. 161–171). Washington D.C.: Pan American Health Organization.

Resnick, R. (1999). Anatomic alterations in the reproductive tract. In R. K. Creasy & R. Resnick (Eds.), *Maternal-fetal medicine* (4th ed., pp. 90–94). Philadelphia: W.B. Saunders.

Scott, L. D. (1999). Gastrointestinal disease in pregnancy. In R. K. Creasy & R. Resnick (Eds.), *Maternal-fetal medicine* (4th ed., pp 1038–1053). Philadelphia: W.B. Saunders.

Torgersen, K. (2001). Maternal and fetal health. In S. M. Nettina, (Ed.), *Lippincott's manual for nursing practice* (7th ed., pp. 1098–1123). Philadelphia: Lippincott.

Zuspan, F. P., O'Shaughnessy, R., & Iams, J. D. (1981). The role of the adrenal gland and sympathetic nervous system in pregnancy. *Journal of Reproductive Medicine, 26*(9), 483–491.

CHAPTER 3

Intrinsic Influences on the Fetal Heart Rate

Nancy Feinstein
Jana L. Atterbury

When assessing the fetal heart rate (FHR) and uterine activity using intermittent auscultation or electronic fetal monitoring (EFM), it is critical to consider the potential underlying physiology for the FHR characteristics obtained. Accurate fetal heart monitoring assessment is based on understanding the physiology and pathophysiology of fetal heart responses to the intrauterine environment. These responses may be indirect indicators of fetal oxygenation. Although the study of maternal and fetal physiology remains an evolving science, research using animal models, coupled with the ongoing clinical evaluation of associations observed between FHR tracings and fetal outcomes has led to progressive improvement in understanding the process of fetal homeostasis. A focus on physiology is important, especially when the practitioner decides how to intervene when the FHR characteristics or patterns are nonreassuring. Physiology guides the interventions and the need for further evaluation of fetal oxygenation.

Physiologic controls of the FHR can be divided loosely into three types of FHR influences: those that are intrinsic to the fetus, those that are extrinsic, and those that represent the homeostatic interaction between the fetus and its environment.

Chapter 2 discusses extrinsic influences, including the fetal environment, maternal cardiovascular and uterine anatomy and physiology, and placental and umbilical cord structure and function. Intrinsic influences and homeostatic responses to the stressors in the fetal environment will be the primary focus of this chapter.

☞ PHYSIOLOGY UNDERLYING INTRINSIC INFLUENCES ON THE FHR

Maternal-Fetal Exchange

Oxygen (O_2), carbon dioxide (CO_2), and other substrates are transferred from the fetal to the maternal side through the placenta, which requires adequate functioning of the uterine vasculature, the intervillous space, and the placental and umbilical vessels (see Chapter 2). Oxygenated blood from the high-pressure maternal side is propelled into the low-resistance intervillous space by the spiral arteries; it then bathes the cotyledons until transferred by passive diffusion across the fetal capillary walls (Morriss, Boyd, & Manhendren, 1994). Blood flow into the intervillous space is regulated by (a) maternal blood pressure, (b) intrauterine pressure and the pattern of uterine activity (e.g., contractions and tone), and (c) flow to and from the intervillous space; the blood flow is decreased during contractions.

In addition, several interrelated factors are important in gas and nutrient exchange; each must function adequately, or transfer may be reduced or stopped, including maternal concentration of a substance, concentration gradients, maternal blood flow, placental area available for exchange, mechanism for transfer, placental metabolism, carrier proteins required or available, and fetal blood flow contractions (Ramsey & Davis, 1963). The primary factor mediating transfer of O_2 and CO_2 through the intervillous space is uteroplacental blood flow, but reduced exchange has been associated with other conditions. Causes of decreased uterine blood flow include decreased uterine perfusion, increased uterine pressure, reduced number or size of uteroplacental vessels, and changes in vascular resistance.

Most substances are readily transferred from maternal-placental-fetal circulations, and few substances will not cross the placental barrier over time (Hill & Longo, 1980). Oxygen, CO_2, water and most electrolytes are transferred transplacentally by passive diffusion, and different concentrations of substances on the maternal and fetal sides facilitate that transfer. Glucose, the major nutrient for fetal growth, is transferred by facilitated diffusion, whereas most amino acids require active transport and large molecular weight proteins (i.e., globulins) are transferred by pinocytosis and endocytosis. Hormones (such as insulin) and steroid hormones are transferred by diffusion but at much slower rates than gas exchange (Morriss et al., 1994).

The fetus is completely dependent on placental transfer of O_2 and nutrients; therefore, even minor reductions in placental perfusion can decrease O_2 and nutrient availability. However, several intrinsic fetal adaptations enhance metabolism during hypoxemic or other stress. For example, fetal cardiac output is increased over the adult, and fetal circulation shunts oxygenated blood to organs required for survival to maintain aerobic metabolism during hypoxemic stress (Rudolph &

Heymann, 1968). Fetal blood has increased O_2-binding affinity. Fetal hemoglobin is present in greater amounts than in the adult, whereas fetal blood has less affinity for CO_2 than maternal blood, which facilitates CO_2 exchange (de Verdier & Garby, 1969). The remainder of this chapter focuses on these and additional fetal intrinsic factors that influence FHR characteristics and patterns: fetal circulation, fetal hematologic adaptations, autonomic nervous system (ANS) influences, central nervous system (CNS) influences, baroreceptors, chemoreceptors, hormonal influences, fetal behavioral states, fetal reserve, and fetal homeostatic mechanisms.

Fetal Circulation

Fetal circulation transports blood from and to the placenta, which allows for the exchange of O_2, other respiratory gases, and nutrients and for the removal of fetal waste products. Fetal circulation differs from adult circulation in several important ways. The fetus is equipped with unique circulatory structures to meet oxygenation needs. These unique fetal structures include vessels that carry fetal blood away from and toward the placenta (the ductus venosus, two hypogastric arteries) and shunts that divert oxygenated blood from the right to the left side of the fetal heart, bypassing the lungs (the foramen ovale and the ductus arteriosus). The ductus venosus (DV) connects the umbilical vein (UV) to the inferior vena cava; the hypogastric arteries connect the internal iliac arteries and become known as the umbilical arteries where they enter the umbilical cord (Stables, 1999). The fetal shunts (foramen ovale, ductus arteriosus) allow for most of the fetal blood to bypass the liver and lungs. Also, the differential streaming of blood related to the unique characteristics of the fetal heart promotes less mixing of oxygenated and deoxygenated blood and preferential flow of more highly oxygenated blood to the brain and vital organs (Stables, 1999; Uckan & Townsend, 1999).

The fetal UV carries oxygenated blood from the fetal side of the placenta to the liver (see Figure 3-1). About half of the blood travels through the liver—through the hepatic veins—and then

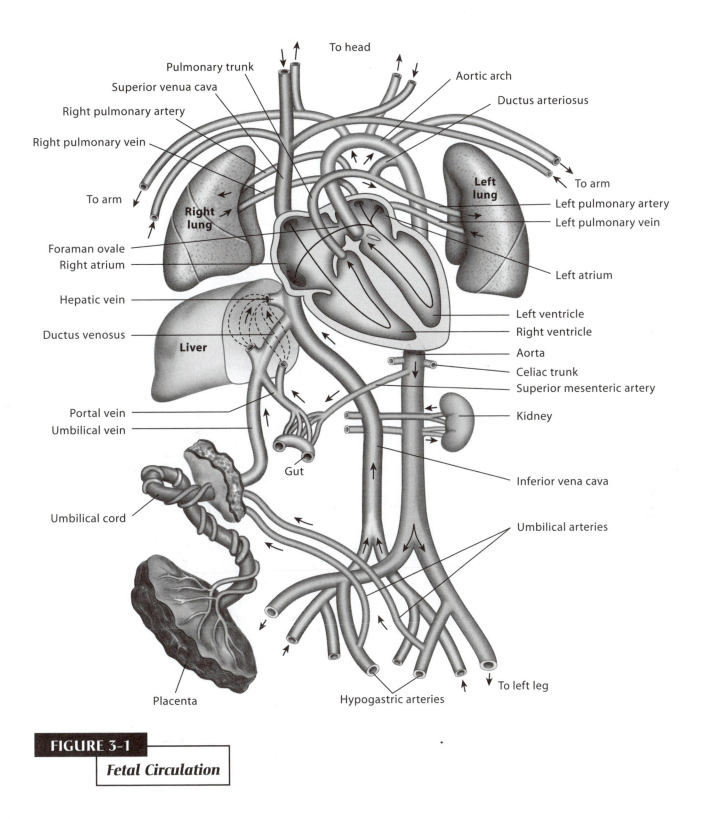

To head

Pulmonary trunk

Superior venua cava

Right pulmonary artery

Right pulmonary vein

Aortic arch

Ductus arteriosus

Left lung

To arm

Left pulmonary artery

Left pulmonary vein

To arm

Right lung

Foraman ovale

Right atrium

Left atrium

Hepatic vein

Ductus venosus

Liver

Left ventricle

Right ventricle

Aorta

Celiac trunk

Superior mesenteric artery

Portal vein

Umbilical vein

Kidney

Gut

Inferior vena cava

Umbilical cord

Umbilical arteries

Placenta

Hypogastric arteries

To left leg

FIGURE 3-1

Fetal Circulation

to the inferior vena cava (Stables, 1999). The O_2-rich blood from the UV mixes with the less oxygenated blood returning from the fetal gut through the portal vein in the liver. The rest of the highly oxygenated blood from the UV travels directly to the inferior vena cava through the DV (Stables, 1999). The DV, a vein that exists only in the fetus, diverts blood flow directly to the hepatic vein, bypassing the liver sinusoids (MacKenna & Callender, 1998). This more highly oxygenated blood then empties into the inferior vena cava, mixing with a small amount of deoxygenated blood returning from the lower fetal limbs.

The DV carries this mixture of blood to the inferior vena cava, which delivers the blood to the right side of the heart. The blood flow is then directed toward the left side of the heart through the foramen ovale and the ductus arteriosus, with the majority of blood flow by-passing the lungs. Specifically, as the blood enters the right atrium, the blood flow is separated into two streams.

The majority of the blood flows directly through the foramen ovale into the left atrium (right-to-left shunt), left ventricle, and aorta to deliver oxygenated blood to the head, trunk, and limbs (Stables, 1999). The second stream of blood enters the right atrium, where a small amount provides O_2 to the lung tissue. Most of the remaining second stream of blood (that does not go through the foramen ovale or to the lungs) flows into the aorta through the right ventricle and through the second right-to-left shunt, the ductus arteriosus. The right ventricle has less oxygenated blood (but higher O_2 levels than the normal neonate or adult right ventricle) that is directed through the ductus arteriosus and the aorta to the lower body. The left ventricle directs its more highly oxygenated blood through the aortic arch to the head (Stables, 1999).

From the aorta, blood flow is directed to fetal body tissues, with maximum flow of more highly oxygenated blood directed toward the brain, and with oxygenated blood flow directed toward body tissues. Deoxygenated blood from the head returns to the right atrium through the superior vena cava. Because this stream of deoxygenated blood crosses the stream from the inferior vena cava into the right heart, there is some mixing of blood. However, because of the shape of the atrium, the two streams remain mostly separate. Deoxygenated blood ultimately flows back to the placenta via the two umbilical arteries (MacKenna & Callender, 1998; Stables, 1999).

After the newborn's separation from the placenta, neonatal cardiovascular and respiratory system changes occur that ultimately result in these fetal structures (UV, DV, ductus arteriosus, foramen ovale, and hypogastric arteries) closing and becoming obsolete ligaments (Stables, 1999). For example, after birth the neonate uses his or her lungs to take in O_2. Therefore, for blood from the pulmonary artery to go to the lungs to pick up O_2, the ductus arteriosus needs to be closed. Normally, the ductus gradually narrows and closes in the first few hours to days after birth.

Hematologic Adaptations: Oxygen Carrying Capacity

Fetal blood levels of O_2 are much lower than maternal levels. However, as previously stated, fetal cardiac output is greater than in the adult (Rudolph & Heymann, 1968), which results in the delivery of more blood and O_2 per unit of body weight than in the adult (Jones et al., 1977; Uckan & Townsend, 1999).

Another fetal adaptation that promotes transport of large amounts of O_2 for use by the fetus includes the increased fetal hemoglobin levels. Fetal hemoglobin also has a higher affinity for O_2 than adult hemoglobin, thus it has an increased ability to combine with and to carry O_2. The oxyhemoglobin dissociation curve for the fetus demonstrates a shift to the left (see Figure 3-2).

The left shift means that at lower levels of O_2 pressures (PO_2), the fetus has a higher ability to saturate the hemoglobin with O_2 than the mother does. The maternal shift to the right for the mother during pregnancy means that she releases O_2 more quickly from the hemoglobin, which results in increased O_2 available to the fetus. Thus, O_2 is able to bind with hemoglobin at lower levels of O_2 saturation (PO_2).

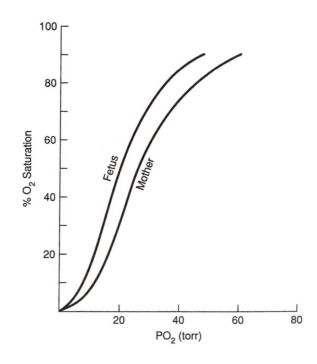

Autonomic Nervous System

The ANS has two branches, sympathetic and parasympathetic, which exert opposing influences on the FHR. Sympathetic stimulation increases the FHR, whereas parasympathetic stimulation decreases the FHR. The sympathetic and parasympathetic branches exert their influences in response to information on fetal oxygenation and blood pressure from the chemoreceptors and baroreceptors. Chemoreceptors are sensitive to changes in blood O_2, CO_2 and pH levels and are located in the aortic arch, carotid bodies, and medulla oblongata. Baroreceptors are sensitive to changes in blood pressure and are located in the aortic arch and carotid sinuses (see Figure 3-3; Table 3-1).

Parasympathetic Nervous System

The parasympathetic branch exerts its control of the FHR through the vagus nerve that originates in the medulla oblongata. The right and left branches of the vagus nerve innervate the sinoatrial (SA) and atrioventricular (AV) nodes within the fetal heart. Stimulation of the vagal nerve (e.g., by an increase in blood pressure) results in a decreased firing rate of the SA node and, thus, a decrease in the FHR. Parasympathetic stimulation also is thought to influence the presence of variability in the FHR (which can be assessed only with EFM). When vagal stimulation is blocked (e.g., with atropine), the FHR increases and loses its variability. As stated previously, parasympathetic tone increases with increasing gestational

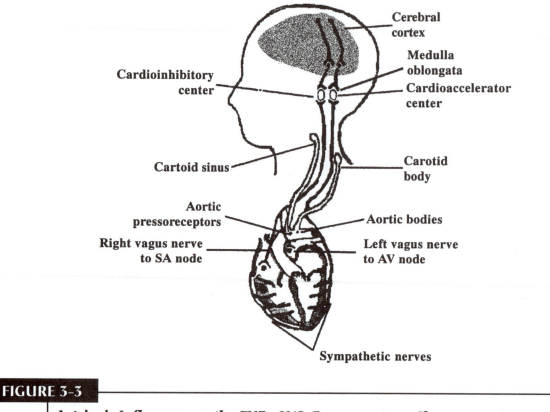

Cerebral
cortex

Medulla
oblongata

Cardioaccelerator
center

Cardioinhibitory
center

Carotid
body

Cartoid sinus

Aortic
pressoreceptors

Aortic bodies

Right vagus nerve
to SA node

Left vagus nerve
to AV node

Sympathetic nerves

FIGURE 3-3

Intrinsic Influences on the FHR: ANS, Baroreceptors, Chemoreceptors, and CNS

age, which results in a lower resting FHR baseline (Parer, 1997). The FHR decreases from an average of approximately 160 beats per minute (bpm) at 11 to 20 weeks gestation, to the 140s at 21 to 30 weeks, and to the 130s between 31 to 35 weeks gestation (Ibarra-Polo, Guiloff, & Gomez-Rogers, 1972). It is important to keep in mind that these are average rates. A rate of 110 bpm or even 100 bpm with other normal fetal heart characteristics may be a normal baseline rate associated with advanced fetal maturation (Feinstein, Sprague, & Trepanier, 2000).

Sympathetic Nervous System

The sympathetic branch of the ANS innervates the fetal heart via nerve fibers that are widely distributed in the fetal myocardium. Stimulation of the sympathetic nerve fibers produces an increase in the strength of the myocardial contraction of the heart and an increase in the FHR and cardiac output. In addition, sympathetic stimulation is thought to have some influence on FHR variability. When sympathetic stimulation is blocked, there is a decrease in the FHR and a small decrease in the variability (Feinstein et al., 2000; Parer, 1976).

Central Nervous System

The CNS also influences the FHR. The medulla oblongata controls the ANS through its action as an integrative center for central and peripheral nerve influences. The cardioaccelerator (sympathetic) nerves and cardiodecelerator (parasympathetic) nerves are controlled in this integrative center. When fetal heart characteristics are normal (e.g., normal baseline rate, increases or accelerations from the baseline), this normality indicates that the fetus has an intact and well-oxygenated brainstem, autonomic system, and fetal heart. In addition, there is evidence that the cerebral cortex exerts some control over FHR changes associated

TABLE 3-1

Intrinsic Influences on the Fetal Heart

AUTONOMIC NERVOUS SYSTEM INFLUENCES

Parasympathetic Nervous System Influences

Structure	Function
• Vagus nerve, originating in the medulla oblongata, innervates the sinoatrial (SA) and the atrioventricular (AV) nodes in the heart	• Stimulation slows SA node rate of firing, producing a decrease in the FHR. • Action occurs through release of norepinephrine. • Tone increases as gestation advances and produces a downward effect on baseline rate. • Parasympathetic nervous system influences are responsible for producing long-term variability (LTV) and short-term variability (STV) of the FHR, with the greatest influence on STV. • Effect on the FHR may be exaggerated during hypoxemia. • Blocking (e.g., with atropine) produces increased FHR and loss of variability.

Sympathetic Nervous System Influences

Structure	Function
• Nerves distributed widely in fetal myocardium	• Stimulation produces an increase in strength of myocardial contraction and an increase in the FHR. • Action occurs through release of norepinephrine. • The sympathetic nervous system influences are responsible for long-term baseline variability in conjunction with the parasympathetic system. • Blocking the sympathetic system, as with maternal medication, produces a decrease in the baseline FHR. • Effect on the FHR may be stimulated during hypoxemia.

Chemoreceptor Influences

Structure	Function
• Located peripherally (aortic bodies and carotid bodies) and centrally (medulla oblongata)	• Chemoreceptors respond to changes in O_2 and CO_2 tensions and in pH levels of blood or cerebrospinal fluid. • Stimulation caused by mild increases in CO_2 or mild decreases in O_2 produces an increase in fetal blood pressure and the FHR; more severe changes produces bradycardia.

(table continues)

TABLE 3-1 (cont.)

Intrinsic Influences on the Fetal Heart

AUTONOMIC NERVOUS SYSTEM INFLUENCES

Baroreceptor Influences

Structure	Function
• Stretch receptors located within vessel walls of the aortic arch and carotid sinus • Cardiac responses transmitted via vagus nerve and sympathetic nerves	• Baroreceptors respond rapidly to changes in fetal blood pressure. • An increase in fetal blood pressure produces a decrease in the FHR, which decreases fetal cardiac output and blood pressure. • A decrease in fetal blood pressure results in sympathetic stimulation to increase the FHR.

Central Nervous System Influences

Structure	Function
• Cerebral cortex • Medulla oblongata	• CNS is responsible for variations in the FHR and variability in response to fetal sleep state and body movements • CNS is the integrative center for central and peripheral neural influences that produces variability and net increase or decrease in baseline FHR.

Hormonal Influences

Hormone	Function
• Catecholamines	• Catecholamines facilitate hemodynamic changes in response to hypoxemia and adaptational changes in a neonate at birth (Lagercrantz & Slotkin, 1986; Parer, 1976, 1989).
• Epinephrine	• Epinephrine is secreted by adrenal medulla (in significantly smaller amounts than norepinephrine). • Epinephrine increases the FHR and blood flow to skeletal muscle.
• Norepinephrine (Lagercrantz & Slotkin, 1986; Parer, 1999)	• Norepinephrine is the predominant hormone secreted by adrenal medulla and is secreted by sympathetic nerves. • Norepinephrine is associated with initial increase in the FHR.

(table continues)

TABLE 3-1 (cont.)

Intrinsic Influences on the Fetal Heart

AUTONOMIC NERVOUS SYSTEM INFLUENCES	
Hormonal Influences *(cont.)*	
Hormone	*Function*
• Norepinephrine (cont.)	• Norepinephrine increases blood flow to vital organs (brain, heart, adrenals) and away from nonvital organs (e.g., gastrointestinal tract and periphery). • The hemodynamic changes elevate blood pressure and may cause a parasympathetic response that is reflected by a decreased FHR. Norepinephrine cannot overcome this parasympathetic response. • This hormone is secreted in greater amounts than that found in a resting adult.
• Vasopressin (also known as arginine vasopressin hormone [AVH]) (Bissonnette, 1991; Heymann, 1989; Lagercrantz & Slotkin, 1986; Parer, 1989)	• Vasopressin is secreted by the pituitary. Release increases during hypoxemia and hemorrhage (little influence in unstressed fetus). • Vasopressin helps regulate blood pressure. • Vasopressin produces a rise in blood pressure by increasing peripheral vascular resistance and decreasing FHR. • Vasopressin decreases blood flow to nonvital organs (e.g., gastrointestinal tract and periphery).
Renin-Angiotensin System	
• Renin	• Renin is secreted by the kidneys. Release increases in response to hemorrhage (hypovolemia).
• Angiotensin II (Bissonnette, 1991; Heymann, 1999; Lagercrantz & Slotkin, 1986)	• Angiotensin II is secreted by kidneys. Release increases in response to hemorrhage and hypoxemia. • Angiotensin II exerts tonic vasoconstricting effect on peripheral vascular bed, resulting in maintenance of systemic arterial blood pressure and umbilical-placental blood flow. • Increased release produces marked increase in blood pressure with an initial decrease in the FHR followed by an increase to higher than the previous FHR. Increased release produces increased cardiac output and blood flow to heart. • Angiotensin II decreases renal blood flow.

with increased fetal activity and sleep (Murray, 1997; Parer, 1976). As the gestational age increases, the fetal behavioral wake and sleep states (quiet sleep [QS], active sleep [AS], quiet awake, and active awake) become more distinct, and the number of accelerations in the FHR increase as gestational age increases (Feinstein, Sprague, & Trepanier, 2000; Parer, 1997).

Baroreceptors

Fetal baroreceptors respond to changes in the fetal blood pressure. Stretch receptors are located within the vessel walls of the aortic arch and carotid sinus. When fetal arterial blood pressure increases, the aortic and carotid baroreceptors respond, which results in vagal stimulation, reflex bradycardia, depression of myocardial contractility and output, and peripheral vasodilation (Rudolph, 1998). With a decrease in fetal blood pressure, there may be sympathetic stimulation to increase the FHR. In studies with fetal lambs, the baroreflex response has been shown to increase with gestational age and to be fully operative in regulating fetal arterial pressure in the term fetus (Rudolph, 1998).

Chemoreceptors

Fetal chemoreceptors respond to biochemical changes, particularly O_2 tension, CO_2 tension, and acid-base balance. Peripheral chemoreceptors are located in the aortic bodies and carotid bodies. Central chemoreceptors are located in the medulla oblongata. When there are decreased levels of O_2, CO_2, or pH levels in the blood or cerebral spinal fluid, the fetal chemoreceptors respond. Fetal lamb studies have shown that stimulation of the peripheral aortic chemoreceptors results in parasympathetic stimulation and bradycardia, with a concurrent fall in arterial blood pressure. In contrast, stimulation of the carotid chemoreceptors may produce varied responses: tachycardia with an increase in blood pressure, occasional bradycardia with hypotension, and respiratory responses or attempts of respiratory efforts (Rudolph, 1998).

Hormonal Influences

Hormones also have been shown to influence heart rate. The release of hormones by the adrenal glands, sympathetic nerves, hypothalamus, pituitary gland, and other fetal organs is believed to play an important role in fetal hemodynamic compensatory responses to stressors. The fetus responds to decreases in O_2 delivery or to decreased uteroplacental blood flow by releasing hormones that result in maximizing blood flow to vital organs, primarily the fetal brain, heart, and adrenal glands. Some of the key hormones that influence the FHR include epinephrine, norepinephrine, vasopressin, and hormones in the renin-angiotensin system. Additional hormonal influences exist and are being studied as well (Rudolph, 1998).

When the fetus is stressed by lower PO_2 or a decreased pH, there is a chemoreceptor response followed by a catecholamine response (the release of epinephrine and norepinephrine). Epinephrine is secreted from the adrenal medulla and is associated with an increase in the FHR. Norepinephrine, also secreted by the adrenal medulla and by the sympathetic nerve endings, stimulates an increase in the FHR as well. This compensatory response shunts blood away from the less vital organs and toward the brain, heart and adrenal glands (Copper & Goldenberg, 1990; Lagercrantz & Slotkin, 1986) (Figure 3-4). These hemodynamic changes increase the fetal blood pressure, which also may result in a parasympathetic response that decreases the blood pressure and thus results in a lower FHR.

Animal studies have demonstrated that vasopressin is formed in the hypothalamus and released from the pituitary gland in response to hypoxemia and hypovolemia (Kullama et al., 1992; Murray, 1997). This antidiuretic hormone is thought to regulate blood pressure by acting on the kidneys to increase intravascular volume and to increase peripheral resistance (vasoconstriction) (Kullama et al., 1992; Murray, 1997). The net result is an increase in blood pressure and stabilization of the hemodynamic system.

Renin and angiotensin, components of the renin-angiotensin system, are secreted by the kid-

Oxygen Deprivation

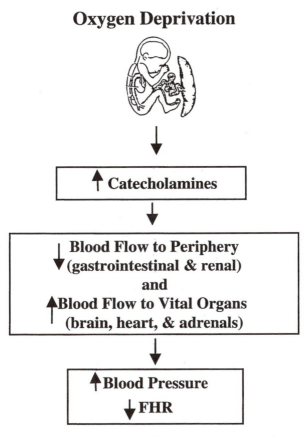

Increased catecholamine levels cause the peripheral blood flow to decrease while the blood flow to vital organs increases. These flow changes along with the increased catecholamine secretions increase the blood pressure and slow the heart rate.

FIGURE 3-4

Intrinsic Fetal Response to O₂ Deprivation: Redistribution of Blood Flow
(Lagercrantz & Slotkin, 1986.)

---

neys. Renin stimulates the production of angio-tensin, which is a vasopressor. These hormones produce vasoconstriction in response to hypo-volemia through retention of sodium and fluid to minimize blood pressure changes in the fetus (Bis-sonnette, 1991; Heymann, 1999).

Studies also suggest that the placenta and umbilical cord secrete hormones (e.g., prostacy-clins and thromboxanes). These hormones cause vasodilation and vasoconstriction of the placental and umbilical cord vessels. When hypoxemia oc-curs, there is an increase in the hormones that increase vasodilation (Rothstein & Longo, 1998). Additional effects of hormones are being explored.

The baroreceptors and chemoreceptors (sen-sors), the sympathetic and parasympathetic nerves (effectors), and the hormonal responses all inter-act and influence blood flow to promote oxygena-tion and to protect vital organs. Adequate fetal hemoglobin levels also affect the ability of the fetus to carry oxygenated blood.

Fetal Behavioral States

Fetal behavioral states also may influence the FHR. One of the earliest activities of the fetal CNS is organization of physiologic responses and gross movement into distinct behavioral states. A substantial body of evidence supports the existence of a relationship between fetal state organization and neurologic development (Groome & Watson, 1992). Although a wide spectrum of behavior can be evaluated in the newborn, the fetus can be observed only with ultrasound and noninvasive heart rate recording, which thus limits the scope of fetal physiologic assessment (Groome, Swiber, Atterbury, Bentz, & Holland, 1997). Research concerning fetal behavior followed newborn studies that demonstrated an association between abnormal state organization and subsequent neurologic dysfunction (Tynan, 1986). In an expansion on the definitions of newborn behavior states by physiologic variables, fetal behavior states were described by fetal physiologic criteria similar to those of the infant (Nijhuis, Prechtl, Martin, & Bots, 1982). Behavioral state organization is thought to mirror neurologic development of the fetus, and analysis of fetal behavior may provide information about fetal CNS development, function, and maturity.

Coordination of state variables begins gradually during the third trimester (Groome, Benanti, Bentz, & Singh, 1996), and although individual parameters have been described in fetuses as early as 32 weeks, no state can be identified reliably before 36 weeks (Visser, Poelmann-Weesjes, Cohen, & Bekedam, 1987). After that, the amount of time spent in a specific state progressively increases until 40 weeks, so that by 40 weeks nearly 90% of fetal behavior can be classified as a specific state (Groome, Swiber, et al., 1997). The states of QS or AS are the primary behaviors observed, with nearly twice as much time spent in AS as in QS. After 36 weeks, the periods when a fetal state cannot be identified is less than 10% (Groome, Bentz, & Singh, 1995). In addition, there is consistency between the fetal and neonatal periods; fetuses who moved at a certain rate, moved at a similar rate as newborns (Groome et al., 1999; Pillai & James, 1990), and the proportion of time spent in QS and AS was nearly equal for both ages (Groome, Mooney, Holland, Smith, & Atterbury, 1997).

As the fetus matures neurologically, progressively more time is spent in QS than AS, and the presence of QS heralds the development of higher-order CNS structures (Berg & Berg, 1987). Poor state regulation may serve as a marker for CNS dysfunction or fetal immaturity because inconsistent behavior states have been reported in neurologically impaired newborns or normal infants experiencing stress (Groome & Watson, 1992). In humans, structural changes in the CNS can significantly affect behavior state control, and abnormal regulation has been reported in fetuses with hydrocephalus (Arduini, Rizzo, Caforio, & Mancuso, 1987), exposure to ethanol or cocaine (Hume, O'Donnell, Stranger, Killian, & Gingras, 1989; Mulder, Kamstra, O'Brien, Visser, & Prechtl, 1986), growth restriction (van Vliet, Martin, Nijhuis, & Prechtl, 1985), and diabetic mothers (Mulder, Visser, Bekedam, & Prechtl, 1987). Specifically, fetuses of insulin-dependent diabetic mothers are in a potentially hostile environment and are, therefore, at risk for neurologic dysfunction. Even those infants of diabetic mothers who appear structurally normal and who had adequate glucose control during pregnancy are less likely to have synchronized sleep-wake cycles at 36 weeks. At 38 and 40 weeks, those infants are significantly less likely to enter recognizable behavior states than normal fetuses (Mulder et al., 1987). Impaired fetal growth can be attributed to decreased uteroplacental blood flow. Although the fetus shunts oxygenated blood to the organs needed to survive, there are possibly periods when hypoxia (lack of O_2 in the fetal tissue) occurs in the CNS. As a result, growth-restricted fetuses have significantly less behavior state control than normal fetuses, and fewer than 40% have identifiable states at 40 weeks (Rizzo, Arduini, Pennesstrí, Romanini, & Mancuso, 1987; van Vliet et al., 1985).

FHR Control

The FHR arises from a variety of neural and hormonal influences that undergo several changes during development. The FHR is audible with Doppler at 8 weeks gestation, and cardiac motion has been recorded by high-resolution sonography at 37 days postconception age. Before 20 weeks, the FHR is relatively stable, and the percentage of low variation (fluctuation) is three times greater than high variation. Both high and low FHR variation are recorded in nearly equal proportions until 27–34 weeks, when the proportion of high variation increases while the percentage of low variation remains constant. The increase in high variation FHR coincides with the onset of parasympathetic system influence (Dawes, Houghton, Redman, & Visser, 1982; Guinn, Kimberlin, Wigton, Socol, & Frederiksen, 1998).

The sinoatrial node of the fetal heart, like that of the adult, is the primary pacemaker for regulating the FHR. The average instrinsic FHR at term is 110 to 160 bpm (Parer, 1997). Studies demonstrate that as the fetus matures, the average FHR baseline decreases (Ibarra-Polo et al. 1972; Murray, 1997). This decrease is believed to be the result of increasing maturation and influence of the parasympathetic nervous system over the course of gestation.

Regulation of cardiac output in the fetus is thought to be related in part to the heart rate and the stroke volume. The volume of cardiac output determines the force of the heart contractions (the Frank-Starling mechanism); a rise in volume increases heart muscle contractility and increases the force of the contraction, with the stroke volume also increasing. Studies of fetal and adult sheep have shown that the fetal myocardium demonstrates less contractility (Rudolph, 1998). In turn, it is thought that cardiac output may be more dependent on the FHR because the immature contractile ability of the fetal heart is less than that of an adult and does not effectively alter the stroke volume when additional cardiac output may be needed.

Fetal Reserves

It is interesting to note the adaptive capabilities of the maternal-fetal unit. In the healthy maternal-fetal unit, the placenta provides the fetus with O_2 and nutrition delivery beyond the basal needs of the fetus. Placental reserve is a term commonly used to describe the reserve of O_2 available to the fetus. This O_2 reserve allows the fetus to withstand the temporary changes in blood flow and

oxygenation that are common during labor (Parer, 1997). Specifically, the term refers to the degree of hypoxemia that the fetus can tolerate before tissue hypoxia and subsequent acidosis will occur.

Fetal reserve is affected by two components: placental transfer capacity (the capacity of the placenta to transfer O_2) and fetal adaptive homeostatic compensatory mechanisms. Fetal compensatory mechanisms affect the ability of the fetus to maintain homeostasis when it is physiologically stressed.

Approximately twice as much O_2 and nutrients are provided to the fetus as would be required normally in the healthy maternal-fetal unit (Figure 3-5). Normally, O_2 perfusion of fetal organs is greater than normally required by the fetus. The amount of O_2 available to the fetus is decreased in situations of intrinsic uteroplacental insufficiency (e.g., in intrauterine growth restriction). When O_2 is decreased, preferential blood flow to vital organs can compensate for diminishing fetal reserves, but only as long as there is sufficient O_2 to allow the ANS and other compensatory mechanisms to function normally.

Studies of fetal lambs demonstrate that the fetus compensates and responds to maternal hypoxemia and to decreased uterine blood flow by shunting more blood through the ductus venosus (increasing blood flow to the fetal heart and decreasing flow to the body) (Rudolph, 1998). In another example of adaptation, the fetus maintains a normoxic status in high altitude or lower PO_2 environments by placental changes, increases in fetal and maternal hemoglobin, and increases in maternal hyperventilation (Rothstein & Longo, 1998). As previously discussed, the sensors (baroreceptors and chemoreceptors), effectors (sympathetic and parasympathetic nerves), and hormonal responses interact to increase or decrease blood flow and to promote optimal perfusion to vital organs (Feinstein et al., 2000).

The normal, healthy fetus is well equipped to withstand uterine contractions and the repeated transient hypoxemia that results from labor. However, when the placental reserves of O_2 are decreased or depleted, the fetus may not be able to adapt to or tolerate even brief episodes of decreased blood flow and O_2 delivery associated with

Placental Integrity Zones

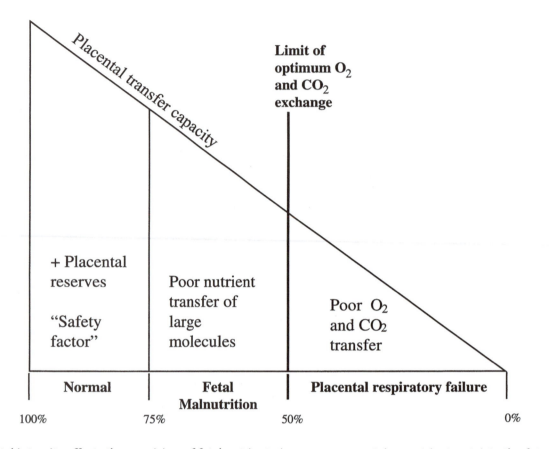

Placental integrity affects the provision of fetal nutrients (e.g., oxygen, proteins, nutrients, etc.) to the fetus to allow for growth and development.

FIGURE 3-5

Placental Transfer Capacity
(Adapted from *Handbook of Fetal Heart Rate Monitoring*, J. Parer, p. 30, © 1983 with permission from Elsevier Sciences.)

---

contractions (spontaneous or induced) or umbilical compression. When the placenta does not function adequately, even normal changes in uterine flow that occur during labor can deplete fetal reserves. This situation can be just as compromising to the fetus as acute, sudden, physiologic insults that also deplete fetal resources. Normally, fetal blood flow is not altered significantly when there is a sudden, short duration interruption of blood flow related to umbilical cord compression (Rudolph, 1998). However, when there is also

reduced uterine and placental blood flow, the fetal blood distribution to the peripheral circulation is decreased with umbilical cord compression. With more severely decreased uterine and placental blood flow, causing a more than 50% decrease in O_2 delivery, the proportion of blood flow to the less vital organs and peripheral circulation is reduced to a greater degree (Rudolph, 1998). Examples of the multiple conditions that may affect placental reserves include, but are not limited to, maternal vascular diseases or hypertensive disorders of pregnancy (Rothstein & Longo, 1998). In one example, Doppler flow studies have shown that hypertensive disorders are associated with decreased placental blood flow, as well as with increased resistance to blood flow in the vessels.

🖙 FETAL HOMEOSTATIC MECHANISMS

Fetal adaptation to the normal or abnormal stresses of labor and birth occurs through homeostatic mechanisms. These mechanisms provide for reflex responses to nonhypoxemic and hypoxemic stress. The normal healthy fetus is well equipped to withstand the repeated, transient hypoxemia that results from uterine contractions. However, prolonged or repeated hypoxemia, or a lack of fetal reserves before labor, may deplete fetal resources and result in decompensation.

Interpretation of FHR data requires the ability to differentiate among three types of FHR changes:

those that result from nonhypoxemic reflex responses, those that result from compensatory responses to hypoxemia, and those that result from impending decompensation. The responses of the fetal heart result from the interplay of intrinsic and extrinsic forces. The fetal physiologic status frequently changes as the fetus responds to the changing environment and the availability of intrinsic resources for homeostasis. This Dynamic Physiologic Response model is illustrated in Figure 3-6. As these patterns are defined and discussed in Chapter 6 and 7, the dynamic nature of changes will become evident.

Fetal heart patterns can reflect—

◆ A nonhypoxic response (such as an acceleration),

◆ A compensatory response (such as variable decelerations), or

◆ An impending decompensation (such as late decelerations).

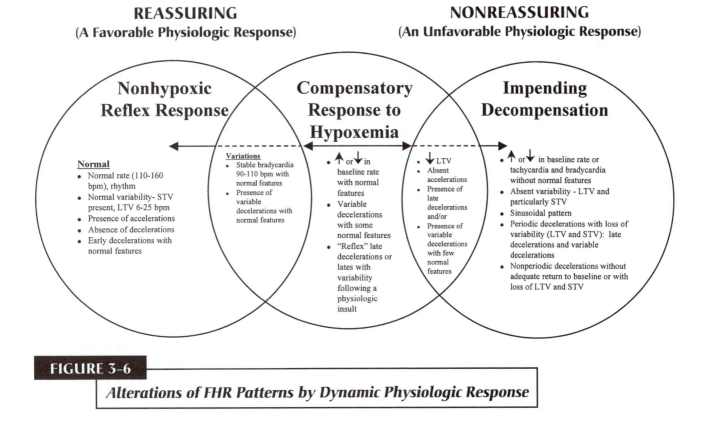

REASSURING
(A Favorable Physiologic Response)

NONREASSURING
(An Unfavorable Physiologic Response)

Nonhypoxic Reflex Response

Compensatory Response to Hypoxemia

Impending Decompensation

Normal
- Normal rate (110-160 bpm), rhythm
- Normal variability- STV present, LTV 6-25 bpm
- Presence of accelerations
- Absence of decelerations
- Early decelerations with normal features

Variations
- Stable bradycardia 90-110 bpm with normal features
- Presence of variable decelerations with normal features

- ↑ or ↓ in baseline rate with normal features
- Variable decelerations with some normal features
- "Reflex" late decelerations or lates with variability following a physiologic insult

- ↓ LTV
- Absent accelerations
- Presence of late decelerations and/or Presence of variable decelerations with few normal features

- ↑ or ↓ in baseline rate or tachycardia and bradycardia without normal features
- Absent variability - LTV and particularly STV
- Sinusoidal pattern
- Periodic decelerations with loss of variability (LTV and STV): late decelerations and variable decelerations
- Nonperiodic decelerations without adequate return to baseline or with loss of LTV and STV

FIGURE 3-6

Alterations of FHR Patterns by Dynamic Physiologic Response

The nursing assessment that begins with the collection of the maternal-fetal history assists the nurse in evaluating the fetal heart information and deciding whether he or she is reassured or not reassured by the FHR pattern. Some patterns are clearly reassuring or nonreassuring. Others are dynamic and changing. When the reserves are depleted, the result can be fetal compromise. It is important, then, to interpret fetal heart data accurately and to differentiate among the various FHR and pattern changes (see Chapters 6 and 7).

Nonhypoxic Responses

Several conditions or events have been shown to result in nonhypoxemic reflex responses of the FHR. The respective FHR changes may be the result of direct vagal stimulation, catecholamine release or baroreceptor response to temporary blood pressure changes in the fetus. Examples of circumstances in which those nonhypoxemic reflex changes in the FHR may occur include the following:

◆ Fetal movement of sufficient intensity and duration may be associated with a temporary increase in the FHR secondary to sympathetic nerve stimulation.

◆ Brief, acute occlusion of the umbilical cord may be associated with a brief increase or decrease in the FHR secondary to fetal blood pressure changes alone (prolonged cord occlusion may lead to hypoxemia and chemoreceptor stimulation).

◆ Head compression occurring at certain periods of labor may be associated with a temporary decrease in the FHR in direct correlation with the intensity and duration of a uterine contraction via vagal stimulation.

Compensatory Responses to Hypoxemia

The primary objective of a compensatory response to hypoxemia is maintenance of circulation to the fetal brain (brain sparing) and the heart to ensure the integrity of cardiac function. Acute hypoxemia in the previously normoxic fetus may produce sympathetic stimulation and acceleration in the FHR (e.g., with acute venous compression in the umbilical cord). Acute hypoxemia also may produce vagal stimulation, with an abrupt decrease in the FHR and decreased O_2 delivery. Baroreceptors, chemoreceptors, and hormonal responses may be involved.

Chronic hypoxemia causes prolonged use of physiologic mechanisms and biochemical resources that may result in an inability to compensate when acute hypoxemic events occur. FHR patterns preceding death in the chronically hypoxemic fetus cannot be defined specifically, but all have demonstrated a loss of short-term variability (STV). However, a fetus also may demonstrate the loss of STV without being hypoxemic (e.g., certain dysrhythmias) (See Chapter 13).

Changes in Fetal Circulation

Anatomic shunts, as previously described, enable the oxygenated blood from the placenta to reach the fetal systemic circulation. Those shunts also support preferential blood flow and streaming patterns, which limit the mixing of oxygenated and deoxygenated blood and provide a compensatory response mechanism for decreased umbilical blood flow and hypoxemia (Meschia, 1989). Animal studies demonstrate that circulatory patterns change in response to significant decreases in blood flow by selectively redistributing that blood flow (Meschia, 1999). Blood flow is increased to the brain, heart and adrenal glands (decreased vascular resistance), whereas vasoconstriction in peripheral vessels results in decreased blood flow to less vital organs. Those circulatory responses are interrelated with autonomic nervous system, chemoreceptor and baroreceptor, and hormonal responses (see Table 3-1 and Figure 3-7).

Studies with fetal lambs have demonstrated that the fetus can adapt and meet metabolic needs with up to 50% less O_2 than is normally available (Rudolph, 1998). As hypoxemia continues, cardiac output is redistributed to the heart, brain, and adrenal glands. With decreased cerebral vascular resistance and increased peripheral vasoconstriction, less blood flows to the periphery. Fetal hemoglobin affinity and the left shift in the

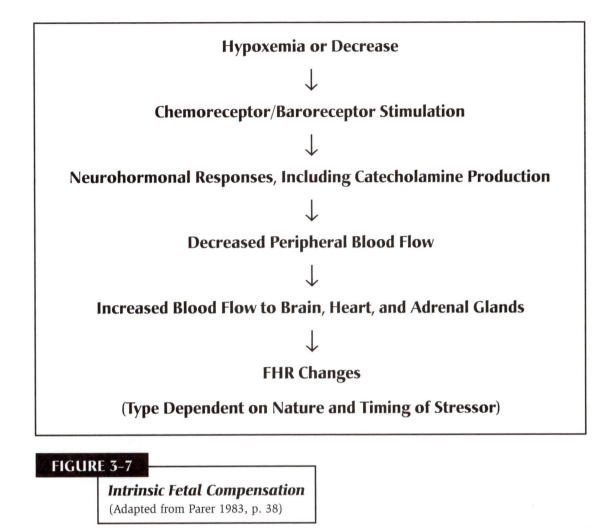

Hypoxemia or Decrease

↓

Chemoreceptor/Baroreceptor Stimulation

↓

Neurohormonal Responses, Including Catecholamine Production

↓

Decreased Peripheral Blood Flow

↓

Increased Blood Flow to Brain, Heart, and Adrenal Glands

↓

FHR Changes

(Type Dependent on Nature and Timing of Stressor)

FIGURE 3-7

Intrinsic Fetal Compensation
(Adapted from Parer 1983, p. 38)

dissociation curve continue to favor oxygenation of the fetus.

Neurohormonal Response

The fetus responds to hypoxemia with neurohormonal responses. As previously described, chemoreceptors detect low PO_2 and pH in the fetal blood. Baroreceptors detect changes in blood pressure. The stimulation of these receptors results in the appropriate sympathetic and parasympathetic response to compensate for changes associated with hypoxemia (see Table 3-1).

Hormones are also secreted. Arginine vasopressin is released in response to changes in fetal blood volume or pressures (Parer, 1999). Catecholamine levels rise with secretion of adrenocortico-tropic hormone and cortisol. Increased catecholamine levels cause the peripheral blood flow to decrease while the blood flow to vital organs increases. These flow changes and increased catecholamine secretion increase the blood pressure and slow the heart rate (see Table 3-1 and Figure 3-7). The actual FHR changes will depend on the insult.

Aerobic versus Anaerobic Metabolism

Normally, the fetus can withstand brief periods of hypoxemia, which allows the fetus to continue with aerobic metabolism. If hypoxemia progresses and fetal O_2 reserves are diminished, the fetus enters a stage of anaerobic metabolism. If lactic acid accumulates because of anaerobic metabolism, there can be progressive decrease in pH, increase in base deficit, and eventually metabolic acidosis (see Chapter 8 for further discussion of fetal oxygenation and acidemia). The fetus can still increase the compensatory shift of blood flow to vital organs (brain, heart and adrenal glands) by extracting more O_2 from the hemoglobin (Gu, Jones, & Parer, 1985; Uckan & Townsend, 1999; Wilkening & Meschia, 1983).

Impending Decompensation

If hypoxia is severe or prolonged, the fetus may no longer be able to extract further O_2 to meet metabolic needs (see Figure 3-8). The priority of providing vital organs with O_2 may not be adequately maintained, and the fetus may no longer compensate.

☞ SUMMARY

In summary, the fetus depends on adequate oxygenation of the mother, adequate blood flow to the placenta, adequate uteroplacental circulation, adequate umbilical circulation, and, finally, its innate ability to initiate compensatory mechanisms to regulate the FHR when challenged by labor and other stressors.

From this brief discussion of intrinsic and extrinsic factors that influence fetal oxygenation, it is apparent that multiple factors can place the fetus at risk for compromise during the labor process. An understanding of fetal circulation, hematologic adaptations, autonomic and CNS influences, baroreceptor and chemoreceptor influences, fetal behavioral states, fetal reserves, and

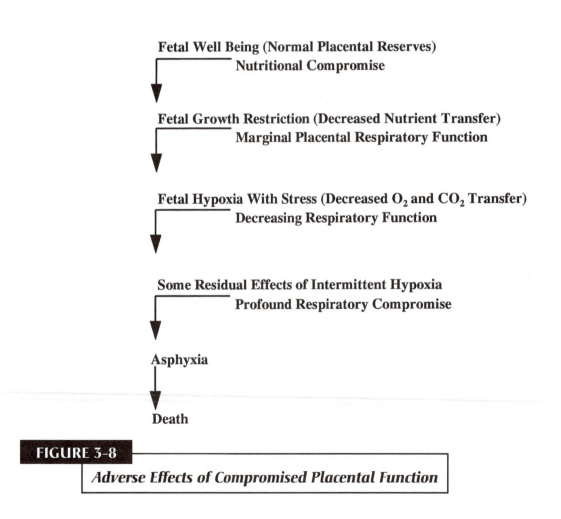

Fetal Well Being (Normal Placental Reserves)
    Nutritional Compromise

Fetal Growth Restriction (Decreased Nutrient Transfer)
    Marginal Placental Respiratory Function

Fetal Hypoxia With Stress (Decreased O_2 and CO_2 Transfer)
    Decreasing Respiratory Function

Some Residual Effects of Intermittent Hypoxia
    Profound Respiratory Compromise

Asphyxia

Death

FIGURE 3-8

Adverse Effects of Compromised Placental Function

homeostatic mechanisms provides a physiologic foundation for understanding fetal heart responses. A careful assessment of the maternal and fetal history provides the health care provider with insight into possible physiologic explanations for FHR characteristics and patterns. Identification of potential physiologic factors that may affect maternal-fetal oxygenation and subsequently affect FHR characteristics also informs care providers' selection of appropriate interventions to address non-reassuring fetal heart characteristics.

🔖 REFERENCES

Arduini, D., Rizzo, G., Caforio, L., & Mancuso, S. (1987). Development of behavioral states in hydrocephalic fetuses. *Fetal Therapy, 2*(3), 135–143.

Berg, W. K., & Berg, K. M. (1987). Psychophysiological development in infancy: State, startle, and attention. In J. D. Osofsky (Ed.), *Handbook of infant development* (2nd ed., pp. 238–317). New York: John Wiley & Sons.

Bissonnette, J. (1991). Placental and fetal physiology. In S. Gabbe, J. Niebyl, & J. Simpson (Eds.), *Obstetrics: Normal and problem pregnancies* (2nd ed., p. 3). New York: Churchill.

Copper, R. L., & Goldenberg, R. L. (1990). Catecholamine secretion in fetal adaptation to stress. *Journal of Obstetric, Gynecologic, and Neonatal Nursing, 19,* 223–226.

Dawes, G. S., Houghton, C. R. S., Redman, C. W. G., & Visser, G. H. A. (1982). Pattern of normal fetal heart rate. *British Journal of Obstetrics and Gynaecology, 89*(4), 276–284.

de Verdier, C. H., & Garby, L. (1969). Low binding of 2,3-diphosphoglycerate to hemoglobin F: A contribution to the knowledge of the binding site and an explanation for the high oxygen affinity of foetal blood. *Scandinavian Journal of Clinical and Laboratory Investigation, 23*(2), 149–151.

Feinstein, N. F., Sprague, A., & Trepanier, M. J. (2000). Fetal heart rate auscultation. Washington, DC: Association of Women's Health, Obstetric and Neonatal Nurses.

Groome, L. J., Benanti, J. M., Bentz, L. S., & Singh, K. P. (1996). Morphology of active sleep—quiet sleep transitions in normal human term fetuses. *Journal of Perinatal Medicine, 24*(2), 171–176.

Groome, L. J., Bentz, L. S., & Singh, K. P. (1995). Behavioral state organization in normal human term fetuses: The relationship between periods of undefined state and other characteristics of state control. *Sleep, 18*(2), 77–81.

Groome, L. J., Mooney, D. M., Holland, S. B., Smith, Y. D., & Atterbury, J. L. (1997). Heart rate response

in individual human fetuses to stimulation with a low-intensity speech sound. *Journal of Maternal-Fetal Investigation, 7,* 105–110.

Groome, L. J., Swiber, M. J., Atterbury, J. L., Bentz, L. S., & Holland, S. B. (1997). Similarities and differences in behavioral state organization during sleep periods in the perinatal infant before and after birth. *Child Development, 68*(1), 1–11.

Groome, L. J., Swiber, M. J., Holland, S. B., Bentz, L. S., Atterbury, J. L., & Trimm, R. F., III. (1999). Spontaneous motor activity in the perinatal infant before and after birth: Stability in individual differences. *Developmental Psychobiology, 35*(1), 15–24.

Groome, L. J., & Watson, J. E. (1992). Assessment of in utero neurobehavioral development. I. Fetal behavioral states. *Journal of Maternal-Fetal Investigation, 2,* 183–194.

Gu, W., Jones, C. T., & Parer, J. T. (1985). Metabolic and cardiovascular effects on fetal sheep of sustained reduction of uterine blood flow. *Journal of Physiology, 368,* 109–129.

Guinn, D. A., Kimberlin, D. F., Wigton, T. R., Socol, M. L., & Frederiksen, M. C. (1998). Fetal heart rate characteristics at 25 to 28 weeks' gestation. *American Journal of Perinatology, 15*(8), 507–510.

Heymann, M. (1999). Fetal cardiovascular physiology. In R. K. Creasy & R. Resnik (Eds.), *Maternal fetal medicine: Principles and practice* (4th ed., p. 249–259). Philadelphia: W. B. Saunders.

Hill, E. P., & Longo, L. D. (1980). Dynamics of maternal-fetal nutrient transfer. *Federation Proceedings, 39*(2), 239–244.

Hume, R. F., O'Donnell, K. J., Stranger, C. L., Killian, A. P., & Gingras, J. L. (1989). In utero cocaine exposure: Observations of fetal behavioral state may predict neonatal outcome. *American Journal of Obstetrics and Gynecology, 161*(3), 685–690.

Ibarra-Polo, A. A., Guiloff, E., & Gomez-Rogers, C. (1972). Fetal heart rate throughout pregnancy. *American Journal of Obstetrics and Gynecology, 113*(6), 814–818.

Jones, M., Sheldon, R. E., Peeters, L. L., Meschia, G., Battaglia, F. C., & Makowski, E. L. (1977). Fetal cerebral oxygen consumption at different levels of oxygenation. *Journal of Applied Physiology, 43*(6), 1080–1084.

Kullama, L. K., Ross, M. G., Lam, R., Leake, R. D., Ervin, M. G., & Fisher, D. A. (1992). Ovine maternal and fetal renal vasopressin receptor response to maternal dehydration. *American Journal of Obstetrics and Gynecology, 167*(6), 1717–1722.

Lagercrantz, H., & Slotkin, T. A. (1986). The "stress" of being born. *Scientific American, 254*(4), 100–107.

MacKenna, B. R., & Callender, R. (1998). *Illustrated physiology* (6th ed.). Edinburgh, Scotland: Churchill Livingstone.

Meschia, G. (1999). Placental respiratory gas exchange and fetal oxygenation. In R. K. Creasy & R. Resnik

(Eds.), *Maternal fetal medicine: Principles and practice* (4th ed., pp. 260–269). Philadelphia: W. B. Saunders.

Morriss, F. H., Jr., Boyd, R. D. H., & Manhendren, D. (1994). Placental transport. In E. Knobil & J. Neill, (Eds.), *The physiology of reproduction* (Volume II) (pp. 813–861). New York: Raven.

Mulder, E. J., Kamstra, A., O'Brien, M. J., Visser, G. H., & Prechtl, H. F. (1986). Abnormal fetal behavioural state regulation in a case of high maternal alcohol intake during pregnancy. *Early Human Development, 4*(3–4), 321–326.

Mulder, E. J., Visser, G. H., Bekedam, D. J., & Prechtl, H. F. (1987). Emergence of behavioural states in fetuses of type-1-diabetic women. *Early Human Development, 15*(4), 231–251.

Murray, M. (1997). *Antepartal and intrapartal fetal monitoring.* Albuquerque, NM: Learning Resources International, Inc.

Nijhuis, J. G., Prechtl, H. F., Martin, C. B., Jr., & Bots, R. S. (1982). Are there behavioural states in the human fetus? *Early Human Development, 6*(2), 177–195.

Parer, J. T. (1976). Physiological regulation of the fetal heart rate. *Journal of Obstetric, Gynecologic, and Neonatal Nursing, 5*(Suppl 5), 26s–29s.

Parer, J. T. (1983) *Handbook of fetal heart rate monitoring.* New York: Elsevier Sciences.

Parer, J. T. (1997). *Handbook of fetal heart rate monitoring* (2nd ed.). Philadelphia: W. B. Saunders.

Parer, J. T. (1999). Fetal heart rate. In R. K. Creasy & R. Resnik (Eds.), *Maternal fetal medicine* (4th ed., pp. 270–300). Philadelphia: W. B. Saunders.

Pillai, M., & James, D. (1990). Are the behavioral states of the newborn comparable to those of the fetus? *Early Human Development, 22*(1), 39–49.

Ramsey, E. M., & Davis, R. W. (1963). A composite drawing of the placenta to show its structure and circulation. *Anatomical Record, 145,* 366.

Rothstein, R. W., & Longo, L. D. (1998). Respiration in the fetal-placental unit. In R. M. Cowett (Ed.), *Principles of perinatal-neonatal metabolism* (2nd ed., pp. 451–485). New York: Springer.

Rizzo, G., Arduini, D., Pennesstrí, F., Romanini, C., & Mancuso, S. (1987). Fetal behaviour in growth retardation: Its relationship to fetal blood flow. *Prenatal Diagnosis, 7*(4), 229–238.

Rudolph, A. M. (1998). Circulation in the fetal-placental unit. In R. M. Cowett (Ed.), *Principles of perinatal-neonatal metabolism* (2nd ed., pp. 487–510). New York: Springer.

Rudolph, A. M., & Heymann, M. A. (1968). The fetal circulation. *Annual Review of Medicine, 19,* 195–206.

Stables, D. (1999). *Physiology in childbearing with anatomy and related biosciences.* Edinburgh, United Kingdom: Bailliere Tindall.

Uckan, E., & Townsend, N. (1999). Fetal adaptation. In L. Mandeville & N. Troiano, (Eds.), *AWHONN's high-risk & critical care intrapartum nursing* (2nd ed., pp. 32–50). Philadelphia: Lippincott.

van Vliet, M. A., Martin, C. B., Jr., Nijhuis, J. G., & Prechtl, H. F. (1985). Behavioural states in growth-retarded human fetuses. *Early Human Development, 12*(2), 183–197.

Visser, G. H., Poelmann-Weesjes, G., Cohen, T. M., & Bekedam, D. J. (1987). Fetal behavior at 30 to 32 weeks gestation. *Pediatric Research, 22*(6), 655–658.

Wilkening, R. B., & Meschia, G. (1983). Fetal oxygen uptake, oxygenation, and acid-base balance as a function of uterine blood flow. *American Journal of Physiology, 244*(6), 749–755.

SECTION THREE

Maternal-Fetal Assessment: Development of the Nursing Database

CHAPTER 4

Maternal-Fetal Assessment

Kathleen Mahoney
Keiko L. Torgersen
Nancy Feinstein

☛ INTRODUCTION TO MATERNAL-FETAL ASSESSMENT

Maternal-fetal assessment begins during the prenatal period and continues throughout the intrapartum period (see Figure 4-1). The maternal-fetal database should be current and should reflect the status of the dyad on a continuum. Each institution should address regulatory agency requirements for patient assessment in its policies and protocols, provide a means of communicating the requirements to its staff members, and plan for the implementation of those requirements. Also, each institution should consider developing policies relevant to pregnant patients with non-obstetric problems. Staff members should agree as to which conditions are best treated in the labor and delivery unit and which conditions need to be treated elsewhere in the institution (i.e., the emergency room or acute care clinic) or in the community. The priority of the evaluation and the site of care should be determined by the needs of the patient and by the institution's ability to care for such needs (American Academy of Pediatrics [AAP] & American College of Obstetricians and Gynecologists [ACOG], 2002).

Data collection methods include review of the prenatal record, interviews during admission, and initial and ongoing assessments of the maternal-fetal dyad. A review of the maternal medical, surgical, obstetric, gynecologic, and family histories should be included in the data collection. That information should then provide the means to identify maternal-fetal risk factors for maternal or neonatal morbidity or mortality. See Box 4-1 for a summary of maternal-fetal assessment components.

☛ PRENATAL RECORDS

The prenatal record provides an important source of information that directs the assessment of the maternal-fetal dyad. Basic initial laboratory results, trended vital signs, weight records, and documentation of significant events often are included in the prenatal record. In many institutions, those records are available in labor and delivery units after 34 weeks gestation. The record should be reviewed and updated during the course of the woman's pregnancy and with each admission to provide the most current information.

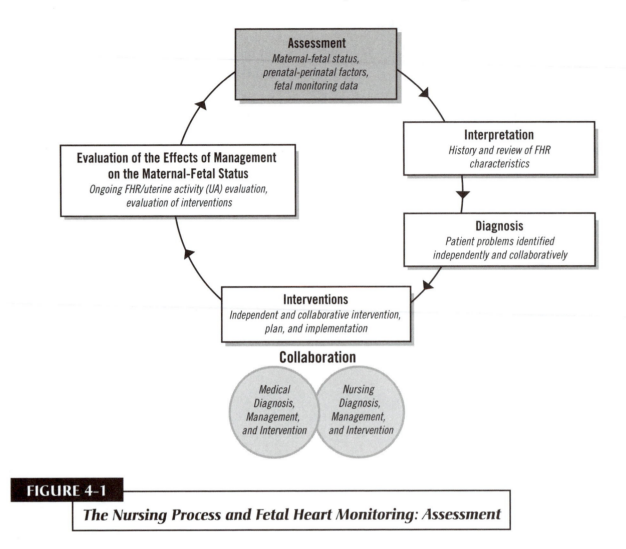

FIGURE 4-1

The Nursing Process and Fetal Heart Monitoring: Assessment

☞ INTERVIEWS

Pregnancy is a dynamic state, and both social and physical changes may occur from day to day. Building on the information already available in the prenatal record often contributes to a smooth transition through the continuum of care. Interviewing patients or using interactive bedside computers to access records will provide additional, more current information that may not be available in the prenatal record. Interviews should be conducted at each admission to any health care facility. Privacy should be maintained during the interview process.

The patient is a primary source of information, and she should be asked if she would like to include her significant other in the interview.

Optimally, patients should be interviewed without significant others present, which should increase the ease of answering potentially sensitive questions on topics such as domestic violence or undisclosed sexual history or pregnancies. However, if the patient is unable to provide information because of an altered level of consciousness, a significant other may be able to provide critical and reliable information. Whenever possible, the interview should be conducted in the language that the patient is most comfortable speaking and understanding. Institutions should have protocols that accommodate the language interpretation needs of patients and their families.

Basic patients' rights should be respected. Attention to those rights ultimately can improve the quality of data collection, decrease the mother's

BOX 4-1

Outline of Maternal-Fetal Assessment

I. **Prenatal record review**

II. **Patient and family interviews**

III. **Maternal–fetal historical data**
- A. Demographic factors
- B. Socioeconomic factors
- C. Medical and surgical history
- D. Obstetric history
  - 1. Past
  - 2. Current
  - 3. Gestational age assessment
  - 4. Fetal activity
  - 5. Leopold's maneuvers
    - a. Fetal lie
    - b. Fetal attitude
    - c. Fetal presentation
    - d. Fetal presenting part
- E. Psychosocial assessment
  - 1. Cultural diversity
  - 2. Resources and support systems
  - 3. Domestic violence screening
  - 4. Substance abuse screening
  - 5. Health coping mechanisms

IV. **Physical examination**
- A. Clinical assessment of maternal vital signs
  - 1. Temperature
  - 2. Pulse
  - 3. Blood pressure
  - 4. Respirations
  - 5. Pain
- B. Maternal height, weight, weight gain
- C. Nutritional status
- D. Uterine activity
  - 1. Contraction assessment
  - 2. Fetal response to contractions
- E. Membrane status
- F. Vaginal examination
  - 1. Vaginal bleeding or discharge
    - a. Color
    - b. Amount
    - c. Precipitating factors
    - d. Timing

(Box continues)

BOX 4-1 (cont.)

Outline of Maternal-Fetal Assessment

    2. Cervical examination
        a. Dilation
        b. Effacement
        c. Station
        d. Presenting part
G. Biochemical assessment (may vary depending on institutional policy and patient condition)
    1. Labs
        a. Complete blood count
        b. Blood group, Rh, and antibody screening
        c. Glucose screening
        d. Toxicology screen, if indicated
        e. Urine analysis
        f. Dipstick urine for protein and glucose
    2. Infectious disease evaluation
        a. Chlamydia
        b. Cytomegalovirus
        c. Group Beta Streptococcus
        d. Hepatitis A, B, and C
        e. Herpes
        f. HIV
        g. Rubella
        h. Syphilis
        i. Toxoplasmosis
        j. Trichomonas
        k. Tuberculosis

V. Fetal assessment
A. Gestational age determination
    1. Last menstrual period
    2. Fetal movement assessment
    3. Dating sonogram
B. Fetal activity
    1. Fetal movement by maternal report
    2. Fetal movement felt through palpation
C. Antenatal assessment
    1. Nonstress test
    2. Contraction stress test
    3. Biophysical profile (BPP) or modified BPP
    4. Ultrasound reports
        a. Amniotic fluid index and volume determination
        b. Placental location
D. Method of monitoring
    1. Auscultation

(Box continues)

BOX 4-1 (cont.)

Outline of Maternal-Fetal Assessment

  a. Rate
  b. Rhythm
  c. Increases or decreases in fetal heart rate (FHR)
  d. Interventions
  e. Response to interventions
 2. External
  a. Ultrasound
   (1) Baseline FHR
   (2) Variability
   (3) Accelerations or decelerations
   (4) Interventions
   (5) Response to interventions
  b. Tocodynamometer
   (1) Frequency
   (2) Duration
   (3) Intensity (per palpation)
   (4) Resting tone (per palpation)
   (5) Interventions
   (6) Response to interventions

 3. Internal
  a. Fetal spiral electrode
   (1) Baseline FHR
   (2) Variability
   (3) Accelerations or decelerations
   (4) Interventions
   (5) Response to interventions
  b. Intrauterine pressure catheter
   (Fluid-filled or Sensor-tipped)
   (1) Frequency
   (2) Duration
   (3) Intensity
   (4) Resting tone
   (5) Interventions
   (6) Response to interventions

Note: Adapted from Association of Women's Health, Obstetric and Neonatal Nurses [AWHONN] (1999). *Basic, High-Risk and Critical Care Intrapartum Nursing: Clinical Competencies and Education Guide* (3rd ed.). Washington, D.C.: Author

---

and her family's anxiety, and allow the mother to concentrate on the work of childbearing. For example, patients with disabilities should be provided the resources needed to participate fully in the births of their infants. If the mother is hearing impaired, she may require a sign language interpreter. If the patient is blind, she may require instructions in Braille as well as special provisions for the safety of both the mother and baby. The cultural and spiritual needs of the patient and her family should be identified and respected to facilitate the family's full participation in the birth.

🖳 HISTORICAL DATA

Maternal-fetal historical data are gathered from demographic and socioeconomic information; medical, surgical, obstetric, and gynecologic histories; psychosocial assessments; and physical examinations of both mother and fetus.

Demographic Factors

Data that may directly affect the outcome of the pregnancy include race, age, number of pregnancies, place of residence, and workplace. For example, pregnancy occurring before 19 years of age or after 35 years of age places mother and fetus at increased risk for age-related complications such as preeclampsia, poor nutrition, intrauterine growth restriction, gestational diabetes, placental disorders, chromosomal disorders, and conception problems (Deitch, 2000).

Where an individual lives and works directly affects quality of life and the availability and accessibility of needed services. For example, undocumented families from other countries may not seek prenatal care for fear of deportation. Environmental conditions may increase the risk of environmental toxin exposure and may increase the potential for fetal problems.

Socioeconomic Factors

Collection of socioeconomic historical data for the database is important. In this context, maternal data collection begins the process of planning for the discharge of the mother and her infant and helps guide their subsequent integration into the family. It is essential not only to identify risk factors that were present throughout the pregnancy, but also to know the extent to which those risks were alleviated or eliminated or the extent to which they may influence the outcome of the pregnancy. Socioeconomic factors include but may not be limited to, (a) exposure to domestic violence; (b) number of sexual partners; (c) lack of adequate housing or no housing; (d) lack of financial resources to provide food, clothing, and other infant needs; (e) lack of access to appropriate health care and social services; and (f) voiced fears or anxieties regarding pregnancy, delivery, and neonatal care (Smith & Mattson, 2000). Additionally, past or present exposure to risk-laden behaviors may surface, such as smoking or tobacco use, alcohol or drug use, or history of multiple unprotected sexual encounters. Other issues may also arise, such as the planning and spacing of pregnancies, including the issue of emotional acceptance of the current pregnancy.

The nurse should assess the potential effect of the risk on the current pregnancy, how much and to what degree the family is able to receive needed services, and how those services may help address or solve ongoing problems. Collection of such data will help the care provider form a care plan for the patient and family, as well as to assess the need for additional services. All of that information provides the opportunity for health teaching and for potentially improved maternal and neonatal outcomes.

Medical and Surgical History

Although the prenatal record should contain the patient's medical and surgical history, admission to labor and delivery provides another opportunity for the nurse to complete or update that information. The onset of labor often results in the communication of information that may not have been obtained during the prenatal period. Chronic medical conditions should be assessed and recorded because they may have an effect not only on the pregnancy, labor, and birth outcomes, but also on the postpartum recovery. Using a systems approach provides an organized and efficient method of collecting the data. No standard for gathering information has been set; however, to help ensure that no important information is missed, each nurse should ideally establish a routine method for her or his own personal use. For example, a head-to-toe assessment of the mother may be followed by followed by a complete head-to-toe assessment of the fetus. Individual patient circumstances and conditions may influence how and when patient data is collected.

Women with life-threatening congenital diseases or significant chronic illnesses usually have targeted assessment needs. Therefore, aspects of their disease state and related surgeries, hospitalizations and medications should be assessed to facilitate identification of additional risk factors. For example, heart transplant recipients and cystic fibrosis patients require not only a complete history including disease state, but also information such as disease specific medications taken during pregnancy and the various specialists who have consulted with the primary obstetrician (Sauer & Krening, 1997).

In addition to asking about prescribed medicines, women should also be questioned about the use of non-prescription and complimentary alternative medications. Use of complementary alternative medicines (CAM), including herbal therapies, has increased significantly in the past 5 years (ACOG, 2000; Kuhn, 1999). Mothers should be asked about herbs, natural vitamins, teas, tonics, tinctures, or any other substances that were used during the pregnancy. Many herbal preparations have been found to alter platelet function, thereby altering clotting factors that may contribute to postpartum hemorrhage (Fetrow & Avila, 2001). Thus, it is generally recommended that if a mother is taking herbal preparations containing gingko, ginger root, or garlic, she should stop a minimum of 2 weeks before her expected delivery date (American Society of Anesthesiologists, 1999; Thatcher, 2001).

Obstetric History
Current and Past

Past pregnancy experiences and outcomes may significantly influence the progress and outcome of a current pregnancy. History of prior pregnancy-specific states such as preeclampsia, gestational (Type II) diabetes, preterm labor, placental abnormalities, and difficult or operative deliveries can provide valuable insight about potential concerns relating to the current pregnancy. Table 4-1 provides a summary of selected medical, obstetric and psychosocial conditions or risk factors with associated implications for fetal and neonatal well-being.

When she enters labor and delivery, the mother should be asked about her estimated due date and her reason for presenting to the unit. She should also be questioned regarding allergies; medications taken during pregnancy (time, dosage, frequency); and illnesses during the pregnancy. The mother should be questioned regarding the total number of times she has been pregnant (gravida), the number of live births she has had, the length of gestation before her prior children were born, and the number of voluntary terminations or miscarriages she has had. The nurse should also question the mother about the type of births she has had (i.e.,

vaginal, cesarean, forceps, or vacuum extraction) and any known complications she or the fetus or newborn experienced. If the mother has had cesarean births, the history should include the number of cesarean births and whether vaginal birth after cesarean was attempted, with outcomes.

Following questions regarding the mother's obstetric history, the physical examination should provide additional information.

Gestational Age Assessment

The initial assessment of the estimated date of confinement (EDC) is done at the first prenatal visit. Use of Nägele's rule (the date of the last normal menstrual period, minus 3 months, plus 7 days) provides an initial estimate of EDC.

When trended over time, fundal height measurements provide a noninvasive and relatively reliable way of determining the gestational age. At 20 weeks gestation, the fundus should be at about the level of the umbilicus (when measured from the top of the symphysis pubis to the top of the fundus). From 22 weeks gestation until term, the fundal height in centimeters is approximately equal to the gestational age in weeks. Multiple gestation, malnutrition, and obesity reduce the reliability of this method (McKinney et al., 2000).

An early ultrasound that measures the crown to rump length between 7 and 10 weeks offers a more exact calculation of the EDC. Determining the exact date of conception with an embryo transfer date can provide an even more accurate due date for those undergoing assisted reproductive technology. Overall, only 5% of women deliver on the EDC (McKinney et al., 2000). Assessment of the gestational age at the time of admission helps direct the care and urgency of interventions.

Fetal Activity

A history taken from the mother at the time she is admitted regarding fetal movement will provide valuable information to the database. Non-perception of movement coupled with a history of any condition that may affect placental well-being should prompt further assessment of fetal status. The mother should be questioned regarding the

TABLE 4-1

Selected Maternal Conditions or Risk Factors with Associated Fetal and Neonatal Implications*

MATERNAL CONDITIONS OR RISK FACTORS	POTENTIAL FETAL/NEONATAL RISKS	POTENTIAL FHR ALTERATIONS

Cardiac
Underlying cardiac disease
  Anemia
  History of cardiac insufficiency
Hypertensive disorders
  Chronic hypertension
  Preeclampsia
  Kidney disease
  HELLP syndrome
	SGA/IUGR
	Hydrops
	Hypoxemia
	Decreased amniotic fluid
	Preterm labor/birth
	Placental abruption
		Tachycardia
		Bradycardia
		Decreased variability
		Lack of accelerations
		Late decelerations
		Variable decelerations
		Sinusoidal patterns

Respiratory Smoking Asthma Infections	SGA/IUGR Hypoxemia Presence of meconium Preterm labor/birth	Tachycardia Bradycardia Decreased variability Late decelerations
Neurological Stroke Underlying neurological disease	Placental abruption Hypoxemia	Bradycardia Decreased variability Late decelerations
Renal Infection Development of calculi Fluid/electrolyte imbalance Anemia Dialysis complications	SGA/IUGR Decreased amniotic fluid Decreased/reverse umbilical blood flow Preterm labor/birth	Tachycardia Decreased variability Variable decelerations Late decelerations Prolonged decelerations
Gastrointestinal Nutritional compromise Constipation/hemorrhoids Gall bladder disease Electrolyte imbalance	SGA/IUGR Altered electrolytes may adversely affect fetus if prolonged	Bradycardia Decreased variability
Hematologic Anemia Deep vein thrombosis Antiphospholipid antibody syndrome Thrombocytopenia	SGA/IUGR Preterm labor/birth Hypoxemia	Bradycardia Late decelerations Decreased variability

(Box continues)

TABLE 4-1 (cont.)		
*Selected Maternal Conditions or Risk Factors with Associated Fetal and Neonatal Implications**		
MATERNAL CONDITIONS OR RISK FACTORS	**POTENTIAL FETAL/NEONATAL RISKS**	**POTENTIAL FHR ALTERATIONS**

Psychosocial/Mental Health
Lack of prenatal care
Effects of prescribed/
  nonprecribed medications
Malnutrition
Substance abuse
  Alcohol
  Illicit drugs
Increased stress
Domestic violence
	SGA/IUGR
	Congenital anomalies
	Poor tolerance of labor
	Placental abnormalities
	Preterm labor/birth
	Neonatal infection
	Decreased amniotic fluid
	Preterm labor/birth
	Hypoxemia
		Tachycardia
		Marked or saltatory variability
		Decreased variability
		Variable decelerations
		Late decelerations

* This is not an all inclusive summary nor does it imply cause and effect. This summary is presented to illustrate some of the potential fetal or neonatal implications of selected maternal conditions or risk factors

Adapted from: Gabbe, S. G., Neibyl, J. R. & Simpson, J. L. (2001). *Obstetrics: Normal and problem pregnancies* (3rd ed.). New York: Churchill-Livingston.
Mandeville, L. & Troiano, N. (1999). *High Risk and Critical Care Intrapartum Nursing* (2nd ed.). Philadelphia, PA: Lippincott.
Simpson, K. R. & Creehan, P. A. (2001). *Perinatal Nursing* (2nd ed.). Philadelphia, PA: Lippincott.

last time of fetal movement and the type of fetal movement. See Chapter 12 for a more detailed discussion of fetal movement counting.

Leopold's Maneuvers

Leopold's maneuvers is an assessment technique used to determine the presentation and position of the fetus. Besides providing valuable assessment information, the initial "touching" of the patient and her fetus may provide the basis for the nurse-patient relationship. For a complete description and discussion of Leopold's maneuvers, refer to Chapter 5.

Psychosocial Assessment

When completing the psychosocial assessment, the nurse should focus on collecting data con-cerning cultural mores that may influence how care is provided in labor and during the postpartum period. For example, Asian American women tend to be very stoic in labor, and it may be challenging for the nurse to accurately assess pain and how the mother is tolerating labor (Enang, Wojnar & Harper, 2002; Williams, 2002). Another example is women of Islamic faith, who traditionally, may not be permitted to be touched by men other than their husbands (Baljon, 1996; Mattson, 2000). Such cultural differences could make the labor and delivery process difficult to manage if female primary obstetric care providers are not available. Cultural diversity issues should ideally be addressed before the patient enters labor and delivery to permit accommodation of patient and family preferences.

Screening for domestic violence and substance abuse are also important components of both the psychosocial and physical assessment that can influence perinatal outcomes. A number of useful tools are available in the medical and nursing arena, and each institution should have policies that address assessment of domestic violence and substance abuse. Completing screenings during the interview can also assist the nurse in observing how the mother and her family cope in stressful situations (e.g., labor and delivery).

The labor and birth process can result in increased anxiety and feelings of loss of control for the mother. The nurse should be attentive to signs of positive and negative adaptive behavior and the presence and quality of family or significant other support.

☛ PHYSICAL EXAMINATION

The physical examination should include a complete physical assessment of the mother and the fetus and should focus on four essential forces of labor:

◆ Power (assessment of uterine contractions)

◆ Passage (vaginal and pelvic examination)

◆ Passenger (fetal assessment)

◆ Psyche (assessment of maternal emotional status)

The physical examination thus includes assessment of maternal vital signs, uterine activity and fetal well-being; assessment of fetal presentation and station, membrane status, date and time that the primary obstetric care provider was notified; estimated fetal weight, and presence or absence of vaginal bleeding and laboratory evaluation. Maternal-fetal condition may influence the prioritization of elements of the physical assessment.

The primary obstetric care provider should be notified if the physical examination reveals risk factors such as (a) vaginal bleeding, (b) acute abdominal pain, (c) temperature equal to or greater than 100.4°F (38°C), (d) preterm labor, (e) premature rupture of membranes, (f) hypertension (blood pressure equal to or greater than 140/90), or (g) nonreassuring fetal heart rate.

Clinical Assessment of Maternal Vital Signs

Assessment of maternal vital signs is a primary component of the physical examination and ongoing assessment. These include temperature, blood pressure, pulse, respiration, and pain assessment. Pain assessment should include information about acute and chronic sources of pain, as well as patient and family expectations regarding pain relief or control during labor.

Evaluation of the effectiveness of pain management strategies should be done at regular intervals during labor and birth. Assessing pain on a continuum may also yield information about unusual manifestations of pain such as epigastric pain or unremitting uterine contractions that may indicate potential maternal-fetal compromise.

Pain relief measures can be accomplished and evaluated in a variety of ways, as addressed in Box 4-2.

Vital signs outside of the normal range for pregnancy and unrelieved or unusual pain should be reported to the primary obstetric care provider.

Maternal Height, Weight, and Weight Gain

Maternal height and weight, weight of previous infants (if applicable), and current pregnancy weight gain can provide the nurse with additional information in formulating potential risks for the laboring woman. If the estimated fetal weight of the current pregnancy falls into the large for gestational age category, the risk of cephalopelvic disproportion may be increased. If the mother is obese (greater than 20% or more in excess of ideal body weight), her labor can be affected by preeclampsia, diabetes, wound complications, thromboembolism, urinary tract infections, prolonged labor, macrosomic infants, and postpartum hemorrhage (Balcazar & Mattson, 2000). Pregnancy is not the time to lose weight. Low carbohydrate or low calorie diets are ketogenic and can cause glucose deprivation to the fetal brain (Balcazar & Mattson, 2000) and ketonuria, which has been correlated with preterm labor (Worthington-Roberts, 1997).

BOX 4-2

Pain Management Methods

I. **Nonpharmacologic methods**
  A. Labor support
  B. Cognitive techniques
    1. Relaxation
    2. Breathing
    3. Imagery
    4. Music
  C. Movement and positioning
  D. Hydrotherapy
  E. Superficial heat and cold
  F. Touch
    1. Counterpressure
    2. Effleurage
    3. Massage
    4. Acupressure

II. **Analgesia and anesthesia**
  A. Parenteral medications
    1. Classification
    2. Indications and contraindications
    3. Effects of medication on mother, fetus, and labor
    4. Nursing intervention for side effects, adverse reactions, or both
  B. Regional analgesia and anesthesia
    1. Types
      a. Local infiltration
      b. Paracervical block
      c. Pudendal block
      d. Epidural block
      e. Intrathecal block
    2. Indications and contraindications
    3. Effect of medication and method on mother, fetus, and labor
    4. Nursing care and maternal-fetal monitoring
    5. Nursing intervention for side effects, adverse reactions, or both
  C. General anesthesia
    1. Medications used
    2. Indications and contraindications
    3. Effect of general anesthesia on mother, fetus, and labor
    4. Nursing care and maternal-fetal monitoring
    5. Nursing intervention for side effects, adverse reactions, or both

Note: Adapted from: Association of Women's Health, Obstetric and Neonatal Nurses [AWHONN] (1999). *Basic, High-Risk and Critical Care Intrapartum Nursing: Clinical Competencies and Education Guide* (3rd ed.). Washington, D.C.: Author.

Nutritional Status

If the nutritional status of the mother is compromised there is an increased risk that the baby will be small for gestational age or suffer intrauterine growth restriction (Balcazar & Mattson, 2000; Torgersen, 2001). Additionally, mothers should be assessed for eating disorders that may also affect their energy level during labor.

Uterine Activity

Subjective and objective data are used to assess uterine contraction status. The mother should be asked about the onset, timing (frequency and duration), and intensity of her contractions. The nurse should also assess contraction frequency, duration, intensity, and resting tone by directly palpating the uterus before, during, and after contractions. Contraction frequency is measured from the beginning of one contraction to the beginning of the next contraction and is described in minutes. Duration is the length of the contraction and is described in seconds. Intensity refers to the strength of the contraction and is described as mild, moderate, or strong by palpation. Resting tone is described as soft or firm by palpation (Simpson & Creehan, 2001).

Membrane Status

Membrane status is assessed by history, objective assessment, or a combination of both. The mother may report rupture of membranes as a gush of fluid or a small leak. If that is the case, the time of rupture or onset of leaking should be determined, along with assessment of the color of fluid, presence of blood, and odor.

In that instance, a sterile speculum examination may be performed, and fluid from the vaginal vault may be tested with nitrazine (pH) paper and ferning. After insertion of the sterile speculum, the fluid is swabbed and placed on nitrazine (pH) paper. The nitrazine (pH) paper will turn blue or blue-green if the membranes have ruptured. However, the reliability of that test can be compromised by the presence of blood, urine, semen, vaginal infection, or incorrect application. Thus, a "ferning" test may also be performed to validate the nitrazine paper test. The vaginal fluid obtained from the speculum examination is applied to a slide, dried, and evaluated under a microscope. When the membranes are ruptured, a distinctive fern-like pattern known as "ferning" is observed (Mandeville & Troiano, 1999).

Once the membranes have ruptured, the risk for infection and chorioamnionitis increases. Therefore, vaginal examinations should be performed as indicated by maternal or fetal status versus regularly timed intervals (ACOG & AAP, 2002). Attention to perineal hygiene is important and may help to decrease the risk of infection (ACOG & AAP, 2002). Signs of chorioamnionitis may include maternal fever equal to or greater than 100.4°F (38°C), fetal tachycardia (greater than 160 beats per minute), increased maternal white blood cell count, uterine tenderness, and foul-smelling vaginal discharge (Mandeville & Troiano, 1999; Simpson & Creehan, 2001).

Vaginal Examination

Vaginal Bleeding or Discharge

The nurse's assessment should include evaluation of vaginal bleeding or discharge and identification of related potential risk factors in the patient's history. If the patient states that she has vaginal bleeding, vaginal examinations should not be performed until further evaluation is undertaken to rule out significant bleeding problems such as placenta previa. In addition, the nurse should question the patient regarding the onset of bleeding; amount, color, and type of blood (i.e., presence or absence of clots); pain or absence of pain with the bleeding; and precipitating events, if any. For example, questions may include these: Was the bleeding precipitated by sexual intercourse, a fall, or blunt trauma? Are you now having or did you have uterine contractions with the bleeding?

The underlying cause of vaginal bleeding may be bloody show (blood-tinged mucous accompanied with mucous strands) which is a normal indicator of cervical dilation. However, vaginal bleeding may result from more serious disorders such as placenta previa, placental abruption, or ruptured uterus, which can alter uteroplacental perfusion and significantly compromise maternal and fetal well-being.

The color and character of vaginal blood is an important diagnostic indicator. Bright red, painless vaginal bleeding may be an indication of placenta previa or low-lying placenta. The dark red bleeding with clots, or board-like abdomen typical of placental abruption may indicate accumulated blood loss. However, overt placental abruptions and uterine ruptures can also occur without vaginal evidence of bleeding. In those instances, maternal vital signs and fetal heart rate assessments will provide critical information.

Signs of hemorrhage or hypovolemia include cool, clammy skin; pallor; increased capillary refill time (greater than 3 seconds); restlessness and apprehension; increased pulse rate; decreased blood pressure; narrowing pulse pressure (narrowed difference between systolic and diastolic blood pressure); decreased mean arterial blood pressure; and decreased urine output. Fetal status should be assessed for the presence of a tachycardic or bradycardic fetal heart rate (FHR) and for nonreassuring FHR patterns. If not already done, an ultrasound evaluation by a qualified provider may be performed to assess the placenta and its location.

As the pregnancy nears completion, vaginal discharge normally increases (Torgersen, 2001). However, vaginal discharge that is copious, malodorous or discolored indicates risk of infection and should be evaluated further. The woman should be questioned about the onset, color, amount, and odor of vaginal discharge, and about other unusual symptoms, such as vaginal itching, that might signify a monilial or other infection.

Cervical Examination

A vaginal examination is performed to assess cervical status. The examination includes assessment of the cervix for dilation, effacement, cervical position, and station of the presenting part. It is accomplished through performing a gloved digital examination or, in the case of ruptured membranes without labor, premature rupture of membranes (PROM), or preterm PROM (PPROM), by sterile speculum examination or both. At times, this examination may be preceded by an ultrasound evaluation to determine placental location.

The nurse should explain the vaginal examination procedure to the family and the patient. The patient should determine if the significant other will remain with her during the examination. The patient should be draped for minimal exposure and positioned to maximize fetal oxygenation, avoiding the supine position. It may not necessary to place the mother in the lithotomy position because the examination can also be accomplished in a variety of positions (including squatting). Increased maternal cooperation and decreased discomfort can be gained by having the mother take slow deep breaths through a wide-opened mouth.

Cervical dilation is reported in a range between 0 and 10 centimeters. Cervical dilation of 10 centimeters is commonly referred to as "complete" dilation. Effacement is reported as a percentage between 0% and 100%. One hundred percent effacement is also referred to as "complete" effacement. Cervical position is reported as posterior, midposition, or anterior. Fetal station is reported as a numerical number between −4 (floating) and +4 (on the perineum). The presenting part is the part of the fetus that is presenting and felt through the cervix (Torgersen, 2001).

Biochemical Assessment

Laboratory Values

Each institution should establish its own policy addressing required laboratory tests for pregnant patients admitted to labor and delivery or perinatal units. Typically, the following basic tests should be performed and evaluated:

◆ Complete blood count or hemoglobin & hematocrit with differential

◆ Blood group, Rh and antibody screen (if not already done)

◆ Urine analysis for protein and glucose

The maternal condition and the presence of risk factors such as preeclampsia, infection, or diabetes will determine the need for additional laboratory assessments. For example, a patient presenting with preeclampsia may have additional preeclampsia panel laboratory tests drawn, such as liver enzymes, coagulation profile and 24-hour urine (National Institutes of Health, 2000).

Infectious Disease Evaluation

When a patient presents with a history of sexually transmitted disease (STD) or other infection during her pregnancy, or if she presents with symptoms of an STD or infection, an evaluation should be completed to further evaluate or evaluate findings. Health care facilities should determine infectious disease policies appropriate for their perinatal patient population and consistent with federal, state and local regulatory agency requirements.

🖳 FETAL ASSESSMENT

The assessment of fetal status is a key component of perinatal care. Fetal assessment begins at the first prenatal visit with gestational age determination and continues during subsequent visits to include fetal activity assessment, antenatal testing (as indicated by maternal or fetal needs), and, finally, by assessment of the fetus during labor either by auscultation or by external or internal fetal monitoring.

Fetal Activity

Another method used to validate gestational age is fetal movement assessment. Between 16 and 20 weeks of gestation, the mother usually perceives fetal movement; however, multiparous women may feel movement sooner as a result of previous pregnancy experience. By 28 weeks of gestation, the healthy fetus usually exhibits a recognizable pattern of movements that increases over time. Mothers have been reported to perceive 70–80% of gross fetal movements (Druzin, Gabbe & Reed, 2002). In addition to the mother's account of fetal movement, the nurse should palpate the pregnant uterus to assess for fetal movement and should document her or his findings in the medical record. Chapter 12 includes detailed information about fetal movement assessment.

Antenatal Assessment

A variety of methods are available that enable ongoing assessment of fetal well-being during pregnancy. The methods include but are not limited to the nonstress test, contraction stress test using nipple stimulation or oxytocin infusion, the biophysical profile (BPP), and modified BPP. An in-depth discussion of antepartum assessment methods is presented in Chapter 12. In addition, ultrasound performed by a skilled and credentialed sonographer can provide critical information regarding amniotic fluid index (AFI) and amniotic fluid volume (AFV). Evidence of oligohydramnios (AFI less than 5 cm) may result in variable decelerations as a result of a lack of cushioning for the umbilical cord. On the one hand, the nurse can then be prepared to intervene with amnioinfusion. On the other hand, evidence of polyhydramnios (AFI greater than 25 cm) can forewarn the nurse to the potential for cord compromise if rupture of membranes occurs prior to engagement of the presenting part and possible variable or prolonged decelerations. Further information regarding the maternal and fetal causes of variable and prolonged decelerations can be found in Chapter 6.

Besides AFI/AFV determination, the ultrasound can provide essential information about placental location. That information becomes essential when the patient presents with undiagnosed vaginal bleeding or documented low-lying placenta accompanied by vaginal bleeding. With such information, the nurse can be alert to the potential for uteroplacental insufficiency secondary to blood loss, especially if the fetal heart rate tracing shows late decelerations and decreased variability. Further information regarding the maternal and fetal causes and manifestations of uteroplacental insufficiency can be found in Chapter 6.

Method of Fetal Monitoring

The method of fetal monitoring used to assess fetal status during labor (via auscultation, external, or internal EFM mode) should be identified and documented. Each method has benefits and limitations as discussed in detail in Chapter 5.

When using auscultation, the nurse can assess the fetal heart rate and rhythm and increases and decreases in the FHR. On the basis of those findings, interventions are planned, and responses to interventions can be assessed and documented.

For both external and internal modes of electronic monitoring, the baseline FHR, variability, accelerations, and decelerations can be assessed. When the internal mode of monitoring (i.e., fetal spiral electrode and intrauterine pressure catheter) is used, the information about uterine activity relayed by the fetal monitor should be validated through palpation by the nurse. Based on the information obtained with auscultation or the electronic fetal monitor, coupled with ongoing assessment of maternal physical and emotional status, interventions can be planned and responses to interventions can be assessed and documented. Chapter 7 includes a detailed discussion of interventions related to fetal assessment by auscultation and electronic fetal monitoring.

☞ SUMMARY

Maternal-fetal assessment begins at the first prenatal visit and continues through birth as a process on a continuum of care. Ongoing assessment of the physical and emotional condition of the mother and the physical condition of the fetus are key to ensuring appropriate care during the perinatal period. Gathering essential data assists the nursing and medical staff in formulating the patient and family care plan, anticipating potential problems, and intervening on behalf of mother and fetus in a timely manner. Maternal-fetal assessment data is derived from many sources including but not limited to the prenatal record and information gathered through test results or interviews. Accessing a variety of information sources may be needed to gain a clear understanding of the physical and psychosocial needs of the mother and her fetus.

Chapter 5 provides detailed information about fetal assessment techniques that are needed to further assess the maternal-fetal dyad and to establish the plan of care.

☞ REFERENCES

American Academy of Pediatrics & American College of Obstetricians and Gynecologists. (2002). *Guidelines for perinatal care* (5th ed.). Elk Grove, IL: Authors.

American College of Obstetricians and Gynecologists. (2000). *Complementary and alternative medicine.* Committee Opinion No. 227. Washington, DC: Author.

American Society of Anesthesiologists. (1999). *Anesthesiologists warn: If you're taking herbal products, tell your doctor before surgery* (online http://www.asahq.org/PatientEducation/herbal.htm).

Association of Women's Health, Obstetric and Neonatal Nurses (AWHONN). (1999). *Basic, High-Risk, and Critical Care Intrapartum Nursing: Clinical Competencies and Education Guide.* Washington, D.C.: Author.

Balcazar, H., & Mattson, S. (2000). Nutrition. In S. Mattson & J. E. Smith (Eds.), *Core curriculum for maternal newborn nursing* (2nd ed., pp. 161–182). Philadelphia: W.B. Saunders.

Baljon, J. (1996). Indo-Pakistani and Egyptian muftis on medical issues. *Muslim World* (Hartford) 86, 85–95.

Deitch, K. V. (2000). Age-related concerns. In S. Mattson & J. E. Smith (Eds.), *Core curriculum for maternal newborn nursing* (2nd ed., pp. 116–126). Philadelphia: W.B. Saunders.

Druzin, M. L, Gabbe, S. G., & Reed, K. L. (2002). Antepartum fetal evaluation. In S. G. Gabbe, J. R. Neibyl, & J. L. Simpson (Eds.), *Obstetrics: Normal and problem pregnancies* (4th ed.). New York: Churchill Livingstone.

Enang, J. E., Wojnar, D., & Harper, F. D. (2002). Childbearing among diverse populations: How one hospital is providing multicultural care. *AWHONN Lifelines, 6,* 153–158.

Fetrow, C. W., & Avila, J. R. (2001). *Complementary and alternative medicines* (2nd ed.). Springhouse, PA: Springhouse Corporation.

Kuhn, M. A. (1999). *Complementary therapies for health care providers.* Baltimore: Lippincott Williams & Wilkins.

Mandeville, L., & Troiano, N. (1999). *High risk and critical care intrapartum nursing* (2nd ed.). Philadelphia: Lippincott.

Mattson, S. (2000). Providing culturally competent care: Strategies and approaches for perinatal clients. *AWHONN Lifelines, 4,* 37–39.

McKinney, E., Ashweil, J., Murray, S., James, S., Gorrie, T., & Drokse, S. (2000). *Maternal child nursing.* Philadelphia: W.B. Saunders.

National Institutes of Health. (2000, July). *Working Group Report on High Blood Pressure in Pregnancy* (Publication No. 00-3029). Rockville, MD: Author

Sauer, P., & Krening, C. (1997). *High risk pregnancy: Chronic medical conditions.* White Plains, NY: March of Dimes Birth Defects Foundation.

Simpson, K. R., & Creehan, P. (2001). *Perinatal nursing* (2nd ed.). Philadelphia: Lippincott.

Smith, J. E., & Mattson, S. (2000). Domestic Violence. In S. Mattson & J. E. Smith (Eds.), *Core curriculum for maternal newborn nursing* (2nd ed., pp. 376–390). Philadelphia: W.B. Saunders.

Thatcher, T. (2001). The proverbial herb. *American Journal of Nursing, 101,* 36–43.

Torgersen, K. L. (2001). Maternal child nursing. In: *Lippincott's Manual for Nursing Practice* (7th ed.). Philadelphia: Lippincott.

Williams, D. B. (2002). Dealing with special needs populations. *Lippincott's Case Management, 7,* 137.

Worthington-Roberts, B. (1997). The role of maternal nutrition in the prevention of birth defects. *Journal of the American Dietitic Association.* 10 (Suppl. 2), pp. 184–185.

CHAPTER 5

Techniques for Fetal Heart Assessment

Faith Wight Moffatt
Nancy Feinstein

🖙 INTRODUCTION

The primary purpose of intrapartum fetal surveillance is to assess fetal well-being and the FHR response to labor to make appropriate physiologic-based clinical decisions. Many factors need to be taken into consideration when selecting the appropriate method of fetal monitoring (e.g., fetal/maternal status, preferences of the mother and the care provider, institutional and national guidelines). Regardless of the fetal heart monitoring (FHM) method selected for a given patient, the nurse is accountable for knowing how to interpret and respond to auditory as well as electronically obtained FHR data. FHR data are incomplete without uterine activity assessment. The nurse also needs to know how to recognize and respond to both palpated and electronically obtained uterine activity data. Developing skills in these methods enables the nurse to select and combine techniques to provide appropriate care for individual patients.

This chapter focuses on non-electronic and electronic techniques for assessing the fetal heart and uterine activity. As the history of the development of these techniques is outlined in Chapter 1, this section will address the current state of the science for auscultation, palpation, and electronic

fetal monitoring, beginning with the non-electronic methods of auscultation and palpation, progressing to the electronic detection of the FHR, ending with electronic detection of uterine activity. The techniques, capabilities, limitations, procedures, and troubleshooting strategies for each monitoring method are discussed.

🖙 AUSCULTATION

Auscultation of the fetal heart is the practice of using a device to listen to the fetal heart sounds and requires attention to the audible FHR characteristics. Intermittent auscultation (IA) refers to the auditory assessment of the FHR characteristics at selected intervals over time. A summary of the research describing IA outcomes is included with a description of this method.

Auscultation as Compared to EFM

Although IA has been used for many years, EFM has become the predominant method of intrapartum fetal surveillance since its inception in the 1960s. In 2000, EFM was the most prevalent obstetric procedure, associated with 84% of all live births in the United States (Martin, Hamilton, Ventura, Menaker, & Park, 2002). In a recent U.S. national survey of women, 93% reported having fetal monitoring during their labor (Maternity Center Association, 2002). Most of the women reported having external monitors and continuous monitoring, whereas 6% stated that a hand-held Doppler or stethoscope was used exclusively to monitor their fetus. In Canada, EFM was used by about 75% of laboring women (Davies et al., 1993; Levitt, Hanvey, Avard, Chance, & Kaczorowski, 1995). Another study of two tertiary and two secondary hospitals in one Canadian province reported EFM use in that region in 90% of labors in 1995 (Davies et al., 2002). After implementation of tailored hospital interventions to promote transfer of evidence into practice (including the use of IA), post-intervention EFM use rates in hospitals ranged between 51–85% in the intervention hospitals, and 58.5 to 83.5% in the control hospitals (Davies et al., 2002). However, one Canadian quality improvement project reported an EFM rate of 80.7% from 1995 to 1996, with a reduction in EFM use to 69.5% in 1997 (Grzybowski et al., 1998).

When EFM was introduced in the 1960s, the prevailing belief was that continuous EFM would prevent fetal deaths and cerebral palsy (Neilson, 1994a). Therefore, EFM became firmly established as the primary method of fetal assessment during labor. However, the effectiveness of EFM versus IA was not established prior to widespread use of the technology.

The randomized controlled trials (RCTs) comparing outcomes with IA and EFM were based primarily on a 1:1 nurse-to-patient ratio. The most common procedure for IA used in these studies was use of a fetoscope or Doppler device to assess the FHR every 15 minutes during the first stage of labor, regardless of the patient's risk status. Researchers generally counted the FHR for 30 to 60 seconds after a uterine contraction and between contractions for 30 to 60 seconds (Feinstein, Sprague, & Trepanier, 2000).

Results of meta-analyses of RCTs comparing fetal and maternal outcomes associated with EFM and IA have been reported throughout the literature (Grant, 1992; Neilson, 1994a, 1994b; Thacker

& Stroup, 1998; Thacker, Stroup, & Peterson, 1995, 1997; Vintzileos et al., 1995). Summaries of individual studies and findings exist in these and additional resources (Enkin et al., 2000; Feinstein, 2000; Feinstein, Sprague, & Trepanier, 2000).

Overall, IA has been reported as equivalent to EFM in terms of neonatal morbidity and mortality outcomes based on RCTs and meta-analyses to date (Grant, 1992; Neilson, 1994a, b, c; Thacker & Stroup, 1998). In one meta-analysis of RCTs that were conducted between 1966 and 1994, a protective effect of using routine EFM was found for 1-minute Apgar scores less than 4 (Thacker & Stroup, 1998). However, this effect was only found in non-United-States studies. Although one meta-analysis reported decreased neonatal seizures in the EFM group, longer-term negative neurologic effects associated with seizures were not apparent (Thacker et al., 1995). For women, more cesarean deliveries were performed when EFM was used versus IA (Thacker et al., 1995).

Therefore, professional organizations have stated that IA is an appropriate method for monitoring and is equivalent to EFM, particularly for the low risk patient (AAP & ACOG, 2002; ACOG, 1995; SOGC, 2002a). Based on the best available evidence, we cannot conclude what effect EFM has on outcomes such as intrapartum death and cerebral palsy, nor would we conclude that IA is inadequate or negligent in a normal labor (Enkin et al., 2000; Neilson, 1994c). ACOG has stated that "Well-controlled studies have shown that IA of the FHR is equivalent to continuous electronic monitoring in assessing fetal condition when performed at specific intervals with a 1:1 nurse-to-patient ratio" (1995, p. 2). In Canada, the SOGC has stated that IA is recommended as the preferred method of fetal surveillance in healthy pregnancies during the active phase of labor (SOGC, 2002a). When abnormal fetal heart characteristics are detected with IA and are unresponsive to interventions, increased surveillance with continuous EFM or fetal scalp sampling or delivery should be initiated (SOGC, 2002a). Regardless of the method of monitoring, women in active labor desire and should receive close support from appropriately trained professionals (Hodnett, 2002; Maternity Center Association [MCA] 2002; SOGC, 2002a).

Auscultation Devices and Techniques

Non-electronic devices for auscultation (e.g., fetoscope, Leffscope, or Pinard stethoscope) allow a health care provider to hear the fetal heart sounds associated with the opening and closing of ventricular valves. In practice, however, a hand-held Doppler device or the transducer of the fetal monitor is frequently used to assess fetal heart characteristics (ACOG, 1995; SOGC, 2002). The Doppler device detects fetal heart motion such as the moving heart walls or valves and converts the ultrasound information into a sound that represents the cardiac activity. Although the two methods obtain information differently, both are appropriate choices in most IA clinical situations. Based on the current findings of RCTs, both methods of auscultation are recommended by AWHONN (2000a), ACOG (1995), and SOGC (1995, 2002a). However, SOGC (1995) promotes the use of a Doppler for IA. Some smaller studies have found improved ability to assess the FHR with the Doppler device (Simpson, Siren, & Oppenheimer, 1995; Simpson et al., 1999). Some devices provide a digital, as well as an audio, representation of the FHR. More recently, Doppler devices have been developed that can be submerged under water for use in women choosing use of the labor tub (Feinstein et al., 2000).

Regardless of the device used in auscultation, skill in sound differentiation is required. The regular rhythm of the FHR must be distinguished from the somewhat similar sounds produced by the maternal vessels (uterine bruit or uterine souffle), sounds that are synchronous with the maternal pulse. Either sound may present clinical problems if confused with the FHR, which may lead to erroneous conclusions regarding fetal status. An elevated maternal heart rate could be mistaken for a normal FHR and result in failure to assess the fetus at all. The passage of blood through the umbilical arteries also produces a double sound (funic souffle). The sound usually has a "swooshing" or "hissing" quality, similar to the heart sounds. Routine assessment of the maternal pulse simultaneously with FHR auscultation is the primary approach that is used to avoid confusion. Also, when the possibility of fetal arrhythmia exists, use of a non-electronic device will validate heart sounds and rhythms, as compared with the heart motion detected by ultrasound devices.

Capabilities

What Can Be Assessed?

Based on the available research, it is appropriate to assess the FHR baseline rate, rhythm, and increases or decreases from the baseline. Auscultation can be used to assess spontaneous accelerations (Miller, Pearse, & Paul, 1984; O'Leary, Mendenhall, & Andrinopoulos 1980; Paine, Benedict, Strobino, Gregor, & Larson, 1992; Paine, Johnson, Turner, & Payton, 1986). Baseline variability and types of decelerations should not be assessed with auscultation (ACOG, 1995; AWHONN, 1997a; SOGC, 2002a).

The baseline rate is assessed between palpated uterine contractions and when the fetus is not moving, the same as with EFM. Tachycardia and bradycardia also can be assessed with IA. Because baseline rates are established in a minimum 10-minute span, it would be appropriate to auscultate more often when a tachycardic or bradycardic rate is heard, to establish a baseline. It is important to determine whether the fetus is experiencing a brief, isolated increase or decrease from the baseline or an actual change in the baseline rate (Feinstein et al., 2000).

Baseline rhythm is assessed for regularity and is described as either regular or irregular. When an irregular heart rate is audible, further assessment with a fetoscope-type device, or other methods (e.g., ultrasound, cardiography) may be warranted to rule out artifact or determine the type of dysrhythmia present. Most dysrhthmias are benign and often revert to a normal rhythm during or after birth. However, all dysrhythmias should be reported to the care provider.

Auscultation can be used to identify increases from the baseline FHR. Auscultation has been used to detect accelerations in nonstress testing in studies comparing auscultation and EFM (Paine, Benedict, et al., 1992; Paine, Johnson, et al., 1986; Paine, Zanardi, et al., 2001). Abrupt or gradual decreases from the baseline can be assessed

(SOGC, 2002a; Feinstein et al., 2000). However, deceleration patterns that can be visually assessed with EFM cannot be identified based on an auditory decreases in the fetal heart rate.

Auscultation is a useful method to assess the FHR prior to initiation of EFM or to validate EFM findings (Murray, 1997; Parer, 1997; Simpson & Creehan, 2001). Maternal and fetal heart rates can be differentiated by palpating the maternal pulse during abdominal auscultation. For example, when there has been a fetal demise, a spiral electrode can transmit the maternal signal despite the absence of the fetal heart signal. Or when the Doppler EFM is audible at a supraventricular tachycardic rate, the tracing records at one-half the audible rate. In both of these cases, auscultation, along with checking the maternal pulse, can be used to rule out artifact and clarify the source of the signal. See Table 5-1 for a list of capabilities.

What Cannot Be Assessed?

Evidence does not support the ability of an individual to accurately and reliably assess FHR baseline variability or discriminate FHR deceleration patterns (Feinstein et al., 2000; Murray, 1997; Parer, 1997). Although health care providers have become accustomed to using labels to describe these fetal heart characteristics and may believe that counting for more frequent intervals will allow them to assess for variability or detect subtle deceleration patterns, there is no research to support this practice. While health care providers may be uncomfortable with the inability to assess these characteristics with IA, the RCTs provide evidence that outcomes for low-risk pregnancies are similar for IA and EFM fetal surveillance (ACOG, 1995; Feinstein et al., 2000; SOGC, 2000a). It is appropriate to use other methods of assessment of fetal well-being as adjuncts to IA, such as fetal stimulation and fetal capillary sampling. However, it is important to follow an established protocol of fetal surveillance (SOGC, 2002a).

Auscultation Benefits and Limitations

A list of benefits and limitations associated with IA are included in Table 5-1. Some items appear as both a benefit and as a limitation, depending on the perspectives of the care provider and patient.

Frequency of Assessment

Recommendations for the frequency of IA assessment during the latent phase of labor is a subject of debate, given the lack of a clear base of evidence to support specific recommendations (SOGC, 2002a). If a woman is being assessed for the possibility of early labor, the FHR may be assessed at least as often as the maternal vital signs. Also, if a woman experiences a change in condition during latent labor, then it is recommended by SOGC (2002a) that the fetal heart rate should be assessed and documented on a regular basis. Changes in condition include rupture of the membranes, the onset of bleeding, or other clinically important events (SOGC, 2002a).

National professional organizations have provided general guidelines for frequency of assessment during active and second stage of labor based on existing evidence (ACOG, 1995; AWHONN, 2000a; SOGC, 2002a). In the absence of risk factors for the intrapartum woman, it has been suggested that auscultation be done every 30 minutes during the active phase of the first stage of labor, and every 15 minutes during the second stage (ACOG, 1995; AWHONN, 2000a). In the presence of risk factors, auscultation should occur at 15-minute intervals during the active phase and at 5-minute intervals during the second stage (ACOG, 1995; AWHONN, 2000a). The SOGC has recommended that a reasonable protocol for auscultation assessment would be every 15 to 30 minutes in active labor for all patients and every 5 minutes during the active stage of second stage labor (SOGC, 2002a). SOGC also further states that although they recommend assessment at 5-minute intervals, that there are no studies to compare outcomes at 5, 10, or 15-minute intervals during the second stage of labor (2002a). The frequency of assessment may be increased when nonreassuring FHR characteristics are heard and before or after events such as rupture of membranes or administration of medication (SOGC, 2002a; AWHONN, 1997a) (see Table 5-2). SOGC further states that although there is insufficient evidence to indicate specific situations, if any, where EFM might result

TABLE 5-1

Fetal Heart Auscultation: Capabilities, Benefits and Limitations, and Troubleshooting/Corrective Actions

CAPABILITIES OF AUSCULTATION DEVICES	
Fetoscope can be used to	*Doppler can be used to*
• Detect FHR baseline • Detect FHR rhythm • Verify the presence of a dysrhythmia visualized on EFM tracing • Detect ↑ and ↓ from FHR baseline • Clarify halving or doubling on the EFM tracing • Differentiate fetal and maternal heart rates, eliminating errors related to fetal demise and EFM equipment errors	• Detect FHR baseline • Detect FHR rhythm • Detect ↑ and ↓ from FHR baseline

BENEFITS AND LIMITATIONS	
Benefits	*Limitations*
• Neonatal outcomes are comparable to those with EFM based on current RCTs. • Lower cesarean birth rates have been associated with auscultation than EFM in some RCTs. • The technique is noninvasive. • Widespread application is possible. • Patient's freedom of movement and ambulation is increased. • The technology allows for fetal heart assessment if the patient is immersed in water. • The equipment is less costly than EFM. • Auscultation is not automatically documented on paper (often a source of debate in legal situations). • A caregiver must be present by the bedside to allow for the 1:1 nurse-to-patient ratio that is recommended based on RCTs comparing auscultation and EFM; increased hands-on time with patient.	• Use of a fetoscope may limit the ability to hear the FHR, e.g., in cases of obesity or increased amniotic fluid volume, maternal or fetal movement. • Uterine tension disrupts assessment. • Certain FHR characteristics associated with EFM, e.g., variability and types of decelerations, cannot be detected. • Some patients may feel that auscultation is more intrusive. • Auscultation is not automatically documented on paper (as EFM is, which is perceived as an important piece of documentation by many practitioners), for collaborative decision making and record keeping. • There is a potential need to increase or realign staff to meet the 1:1 nurse-to-patient ratio that is recommended based on RCTs comparing auscultation and EFM. • Requires education, practice, and skill in auditory assessment.

TROUBLESHOOTING/CORRECTIVE ACTIONS	
Problem	*Action*
• When you cannot hear with the fetoscope or leffscope • Twins: Ensure that you are assessing each twin's fetal heart rate • When you hear the funic souffle of maternal placental vessels or the umbilical cord blood flow	• Check equipment functioning, patient and fetal position (Leopold's) and consider use of a Doppler device • Palpate maternal pulse, use 2 different devices simultaneously to assess FHRs • Reposition and re-evaluate; palpate maternal pulse simultaneously with fetal heart assessment

TABLE 5-2

Frequency of Auscultation: Recommended Assessment and Documentation

	LATENT PHASE	ACTIVE PHASE	SECOND STAGE
ACOG[a] Low risk High risk	— —	q 30 minutes q 15 minutes	q 15 minutes q 5 minutes
AWHONN[b] Low risk High risk	— —	q 30 minutes q 15 minutes	q 15 minutes q 5 minutes
SOGC[c]	Regularly after rupture of membranes or other clinically significant change	q 15 minutes	q 5 minutes once pushing is initiated

Assess FHR before	*Assess FHR after*
• Initiation of labor enhancing procedures (e.g., amniotomy) • Ambulation • Administration of medications • Administration or initiation of analgesia or anesthesia • Transfer or discharge of patient	• Admission of patient • Artificial or spontaneous rupture of membranes • Vaginal examination • Ambulation • Recognition of abnormal uterine activity patterns • Administration of medication

[a] American College of Obstetricians and Gynecologists, 1995
[b] Association of Women's Health, Obstetric, and Neonatal Nurses, 2000
[c] Society of Obstetricians and Gynaecologists of Canada, 2002a

in better outcomes than IA, they recommend use of continuous EFM for "a) for pregnancies where there is an increased risk of perinatal death, cerebral palsy, or neonatal encephalopthy (IIIC); b) when oxytocin is being used for augmentation of labour (I-A); c) when oxytocin is being used for induction of labour." (SOGC, 2002a, p. 6).

Auscultation Procedure

Each facility needs to develop a procedure for IA that is consistent with state, province, or national guidelines or regulations on when to listen to and document the fetal heart rate in relation to uterine activity. Based on the protocols used in the RCTs, ACOG (1995) and SOGC (2002a) have

recommended listening to the FHR immediately after uterine contractions for 30 and 60 seconds, respectively. An example of a suggested procedure for IA is included in Table 5-3. While listening and counting during uterine contractions may be difficult, was not used in the RCTs, and is not required, it may be helpful in clarifying unclear auscultated findings (Tucker, 2000). However, it is inappropriate to attempt to determine types of decelerations based on these assessments.

During auscultation to establish a baseline, the fetal heart rate should be listened to for a full 60 seconds. Goodwin (2000) suggested that the count for 60 seconds is more accurate than counting for less time. Theoretically, slight errors in counting for shorter times would be magnified by

	TABLE 5-3	

Auscultation Procedure

PROCEDURE	RATIONALE
1. Explain the procedure to the woman and her support person(s).	1. Allays fears and anxiety; offers opportunity for emotional and informational support.
2. Assist the woman to a semi-Fowler's or wedged lateral position.	2. Prevents supine hypotension syndrome and promotes comfort.
3. Palpate the maternal abdomen and perform Leopold's maneuvers.	3. Locates the fetal vertex, buttocks and back, and determines the best location for auscultation (fetal heart sounds are usually best heard through the fetal back).
4. Assess uterine contractions (frequency, duration, intensity) and uterine resting tone by palpation.	4. Determines the FHR response to uterine activity.
5. Apply conduction gel to underside of the Doppler, if used.	5. Provides an airtight seal and aids in the transmission of ultrasound waves.
6. Position the bell of fetoscope or Doppler on the area of maximum intensity of the fetal heart sounds (usually over the fetal back). Use firm pressure if using the fetoscope.	6. Obtains the strongest fetal heart rate signal.
7. Place a finger on woman's radial pulse.	7. Differentiates maternal from fetal heart rate.
8. Count the FHR after uterine contractions for at least 30–60 seconds (60 seconds per SOGC, 2002b).	8. Identifies the baseline FHR (in bpm), the rhythm (regular or irregular) and the presence or absence of accelerations or decelerations between contractions.
9. In clarifying accelerations and decelerations, recounts for multiple, consecutive brief periods of 6–10 seconds (multiplied by 10 and 6 respectively) may be particularly helpful.	9. Clarifies the presence and the nature of FHR changes, such as abrupt versus gradual changes, and amplitude.
10. Interpret FHR findings and document as per protocol.	10. Provides record of assessments.
11. Share findings with woman and support person(s), and answer questions as needed.	11. Provides informational support.
12. Promote maternal comfort and continued fetal oxygenation.	12. Provides physical support and promotes fetal well-being.

multiplying. It should be noted, however, that randomized controlled clinical trials of auscultation versus electronic fetal monitoring which have been undertaken since the 1970s have used either 30- or 60-second auscultation times.

When preparing to use IA, it is appropriate to perform Leopold's maneuvers to determine the best location for listening to the FHR. Palpation of uterine activity and the maternal pulse also assist the care provider in determining when to auscultate and in differentiating the FHR from the maternal heart rate, respectively.

Reassuring versus Nonreassuring Characteristics

Reassuring FHR characteristics are assumed to be associated with favorable fetal physiologic responses. FHR characteristics associated with a normoxic fetus include a normal baseline rate of 110–160 bpm, a regular rhythm, accelerations from the baseline rate, and absence of decreases from the baseline rate (ACOG, 1995; AWHONN; 1997a; SOGC, 2002a). Nonreassuring fetal heart characteristics include tachycardia of greater than 160 bpm for 10 minutes or longer, bradycardia of less than 110 bpm for 10 minutes or longer, irregular rhythm, or abrupt or gradual decreases in the FHR (ACOG, 1995; AWHONN, 1997a; SOGC, 2002a).

Clinical Management

Assessment of the FHR with IA is a part of the larger clinical picture and maternal/fetal assessment for a woman in labor. It is appropriate to consider the woman's clinical history and respond to assessed fetal heart characteristics in light of her individual history. For example, if the FHR baseline is normal, rhythmic, and accelerations are audible it is appropriate to continue to assess the FHR at the designated intervals while providing routine care and support for the laboring woman. When a change in the FHR baseline is auscultated, it is appropriate to reassess and confirm whether a change has occurred or is persistent. It is important to consider the potential physiologic reasons for the auscultated change (e.g., whether there is maternal fever in the case of tachycardia). When a decrease from the FHR baseline is audible, it is appropriate to reassess with the next contraction or two to confirm the finding. In addition, interventions to promote the physiologic goals of improving uterine blood flow, umbilical cord blood flow, and oxygenation, and reducing uterine activity are implemented as appropriate to the individual situation (Feinstein, Sprague, & Trepanier, 2000). Additional assessment of fetal oxygenation status for further reas-

surance of fetal well-being may include scalp stimulation or fetal blood sampling. When nonreassuring FHR characteristics are assessed, further assessment of oxygenation may be indicated and if persistent, EFM may be initiated (SOGC, 2002a) (see Figure 5-1).

Fetal heart characteristics and interventions are documented at the recommended assessment intervals (AAP & ACOG, 2002; ACOG, 1995; AWHONN, 2000; SOGC, 2002a). Flow sheets or equivalent formats are recommended at the intervals indicated by the facility's policies and procedures. The process of management and documentation is similar to that of EFM and should reflect assessment of the overall clinical picture, actions taken, and the evaluation of results of the interventions.

Barriers and Facilitators to IA Use

Barriers and facilitators to the implementation of IA for low-risk patients also should be considered. Barriers include the lack of consistent preparation for performing IA (Davies et al., 1993), lack of confidence, inadequate staffing, costs, and lack of support. In one study, 73% of randomly selected nurses received at least yearly inservice training related to EFM (Haggerty, 1999). However, it is not clear how many nurses received education on IA on a regular basis. In addition, Sandelowski (1993) questioned whether nurses lose important hands-on skills (such as IA) as they rely more heavily on technology, resulting in a "technological dependence." This can result in lack of confidence in implementing skills such as IA that require different auscultory and hands-on skills. Anecdotally, experienced nurses have verbally expressed discomfort with attempting the "new" skill of auscultation in an educational setting using audiotapes of recorded Doppler sounds that simulate the clinical situation. Although the simulated situation itself can create anxiety, nurses specifically stated that their lack of experience in using IA also produced anxiety.

Concern about inadequate levels of personnel to do IA and potential costs associated with a need for increased staffing are also stated barriers (Morrison et al., 1993). Lack of facility or clinical support for the use of IA can be a barrier to implementation. In Canada, the SOGC (2002) promotes

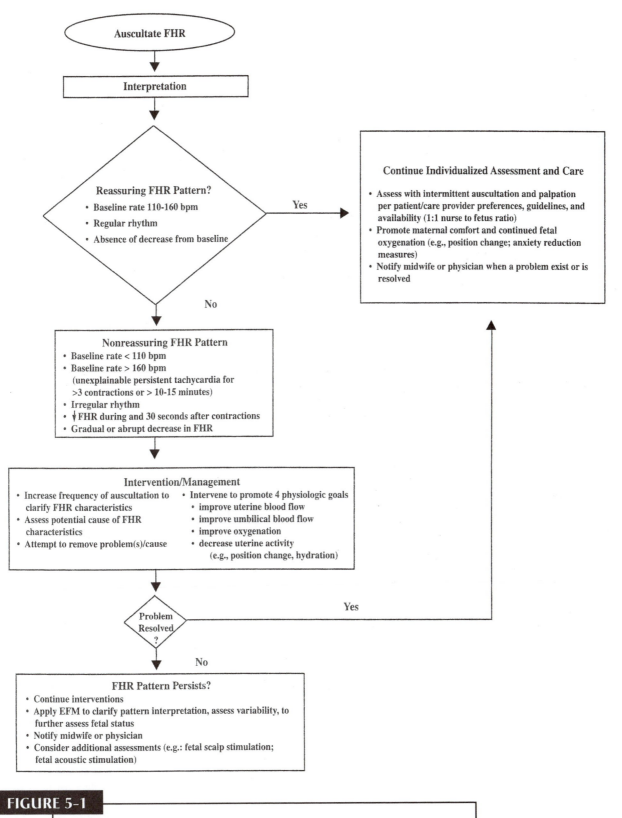

FIGURE 5-1

Auscultation Interpretation and Intervention Management

the use of IA as the primary fetal surveillance method for low-risk pregnancies. In conjunction with that view, the SOGC also recognizes the need for appropriate education to prepare clinicians and support the implementation of IA. Recently, a self-learning manual addressing fundamentals of IA and EFM was developed to address this need (Canadian Perinatal Regionalization Coalition, SOGC, & Perinatal Education Programs across Canada, 2002). Additional IA information and resources that can support development and evaluation of IA educational programs also exist throughout the literature (American Academy of Pediatrics & ACOG, 2002; AWHONN, 1997a; Feinstein, Sprague, & Trepanier, 2001; Simpson & Creehan, 1998). It is logical that administrative and clinical support for the use of IA in a particular setting is helpful (Davies et al., 2002). Research is needed to further explore appropriate staffing ratios and to demonstrate the cost effectiveness of IA. This information will be helpful to facilities investing in the use of IA during labor for low-risk pregnant women.

🖭 PALPATION

When the uterus contracts, its musculature becomes more firm and tense, which can be felt by the care provider when the fingertips are placed on the maternal uterine fundal area. This assessment can give information about the presence or absence of a contraction at a given point in time and about contraction duration and frequency, as well as a general indication of contraction strength or intensity. In addition, uterine palpation can provide information about uterine tenderness, fetal size, and fetal movement. Nursing assessment of contractions is essential for overall professional caregiving and provides important contextual data when considering fetal heart rate information during labor.

Palpation Technique

Palpation should be done throughout an entire contraction, from start of the contraction to the palpa-

tion of resting tone following that contraction. Palpation is used in conjunction with auscultation of the fetal heart. It also is used to confirm and supplement findings gathered from electronic uterine monitoring. The actual frequency of palpation may vary, depending on the status of labor, but should be at least as frequent as FHR assessments. The following are steps in palpation:

◆ Place fingertips on the maternal abdomen, over the area where changes in uterine firmness can be best felt (most commonly near the fundus). Fingertips are generally more sensitive than the palm of the hand

◆ Firmly, but gently attempt to indent the uterus with fingertips avoiding undue discomfort.

◆ Assess duration: from the beginning of increasing tone or tightening of uterus to the end of the tightening.

◆ Assess frequency: from beginning of one contraction to the beginning of the next contraction.

◆ Assess intensity: as mild, moderate, or strong. Although there is no standard measure for determining palpated contraction intensity (strength), the following comparison approach based on the degree to which the uterine muscle can be indented, is used by many antepartum and intrapartum nurses (see Tables 5-4 and 5-5).

Leopold's Maneuvers

Abdominal palpation using Leopold's maneuvers is a method of assessing fetal lie, presentation, and position, which may be confirmed by a vaginal examination. In review, fetal lie is the position of the long axis of the fetus and is described as being longitudinal, transverse, or oblique. Fetal presentation refers to the part of the fetus that is entering the pelvis, and is described as cephalic, breech, or shoulder. Fetal position describes the relationship of the presenting part to the pelvis and is described as anterior, posterior, or transverse.

Leopold's maneuvers include four maneuvers to assess the fetal part in the upper uterus, the

TABLE 5-4

Comparison Model for Palpation of Uterine Activity

PALPATION OF UTERUS	FEELS LIKE	CONTRACTION INTENSITY
• Easily indented	• Tip of nose	• Mild
• Can slightly indent	• Chin	• Moderate
• Cannot indent	• Forehead	• Strong

Note: Contraction intensity should be referred to using one of the above descriptive terms, rather than labeled as "good" or "satisfactory." (Adapted from Malinowski, Pedigo, & Phillips, 1989)

TABLE 5-5

Uterine Palpation

CAPABILITIES

- Detect relative uterine resting tone
- Detect relative frequency, duration, and relative strength of uterine contractions

BENEFITS AND LIMITATIONS

Benefits	*Limitations*
• Noninvasive; hands-on assessment and care of patient • Not limited by access to equipment; widely used • Provides information regarding relative frequency, duration, strength, and resting tone • Allows mother freedom of movement and ambulation • Use of touch may be reassuring to some women	• Palpation cannot be used to detect actual intrauterine pressures • Maternal size, large amount of adipose tissue, may limit ability to palpate contractions • Subjectivity may result in different interpretations of uterine activity characteristics • No permanent record

TROUBLESHOOTING/CORRECTIVE ACTIONS

Problem	*Action*
• If uterine contractions are not readily felt over the fundal area	• Attempt palpation over a variety of areas on the uterus to find best location

location of the fetal back, the presenting part, and the descent of the presenting part (see Figure 5-2). In relation to FHM, these four maneuvers provide a systematic approach to identifying the point of maximal sound intensity of the FHR. In general, the FHR is best heard over the curved part of the fetus that is closest to the anterior uterine wall. For example, if the fetus is in a vertex or breech presentation with an anterior position, the fetal heart is generally heard by placing the monitoring device over the fetal back. When there is a face or brow presentation, the fetal heart rate is often heard by placing the device over the fetal chest or small parts. Once the point for maximal sound intensity is identified, the auscultation device or the Doppler ultrasound transducer can be placed in the optimal position for fetal heart assessment. Placement of the device also depends on the degree of descent of the fetal presenting part. Additional information about performing Leopold's maneuvers is included in Chapter 10.

☞ ELECTRONIC FETAL HEART RATE MONITORING

Doppler Ultrasound

The Doppler ultrasound transducer is used to assess FHR characteristics and patterns. Multiple piezoelectric crystals within the ultrasound transducer generate sound waves that are transmitted toward the fetal heart and receive ultrasound waves reflected back from the fetal heart movements. The sound waves returning from moving structures are altered in frequency from those sound waves originally transmitted towards the moving structure. This frequency shift, called the Doppler Shift, is detected and amplified to produce the waveform, which is then interpreted by the computer in the fetal monitor. The monitor then produces an audible sound and tracing to reflect the detected FHR

In the evolution of the technology of Doppler FHR assessment, advances in the electronic processing of data have led to a discrimination between two generations of equipment (Boehm et al., 1986). To compensate for the complexity and

variation in waveforms, the first-generation monitors employed two mechanisms: use of a refractory window and maximum peak detection. To prevent the counting of both components of the fetal cardiac waveform as separate beats, a refractory window is used (Hutson & Petrie, 1986; Klapholz, 1978). This window of time is an inhibitory period in which the system does not attempt to count the incoming signal. This time period follows the moment of detection of the fetal cardiac waveform and is presumed to be the waveform's first component. The length of time, measured in milliseconds, of the refractory window is dynamic in that the time is set to vary according to the FHR. This variance, however, has limitations. Slow FHRs below 90 bpm may cause the second component of the waveform to occur after the refractory window period. This action will produce a double counting of a single waveform, leading to doubling on the FHR tracing. Rapid FHRs may cause a second waveform to occur within the refractory window period and produce halving of the FHR tracing because the second heart beat is not counted.

The complexity and variability of the first generation Doppler-generated waveforms made accurate counting of the same point in the fetal cardiac cycle difficult. The mechanism first-generation monitors used to compensate for this problem was maximum peak detection. When the movement of the fetal heart generates a waveform, the monitor detects its maximum peak and then counts the time interval between peaks. Problems with this technique are caused by Doppler signals from other anatomy, such as the umbilical cord, as well as variations in an early or late appearance of the peak in the waveform. These problems lead to false variability in the printed fetal heart tracing. Consequently, what is viewed on the tracing cannot be equated with the true status of the fetal heart's STV if a first generation monitor is used.

Second Generation Monitors and Autocorrelation

The major alteration in Doppler signal processing associated with second-generation fetal monitors is referred to as autocorrelation (Figure 5-3). This

Leopold's Maneuvers

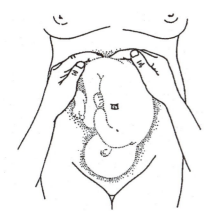

1st Maneuver
Assess part of fetus
in the upper uterus

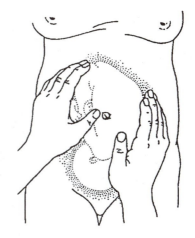

2nd Maneuver
Assess location
of the fetal back

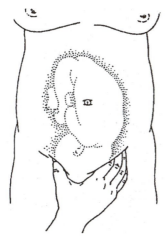

3rd Maneuver
Identify presenting part

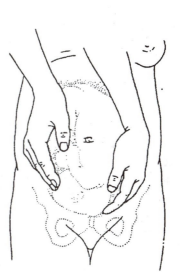

4th Maneuver
Determine the descent
of the presenting part

FIGURE 5-2

The Four Steps in Performing Leopold's Maneuvers
(Adapted from Oxorn, 1986; Simpson & Creehan, 1996)

Piezoelectric Effect

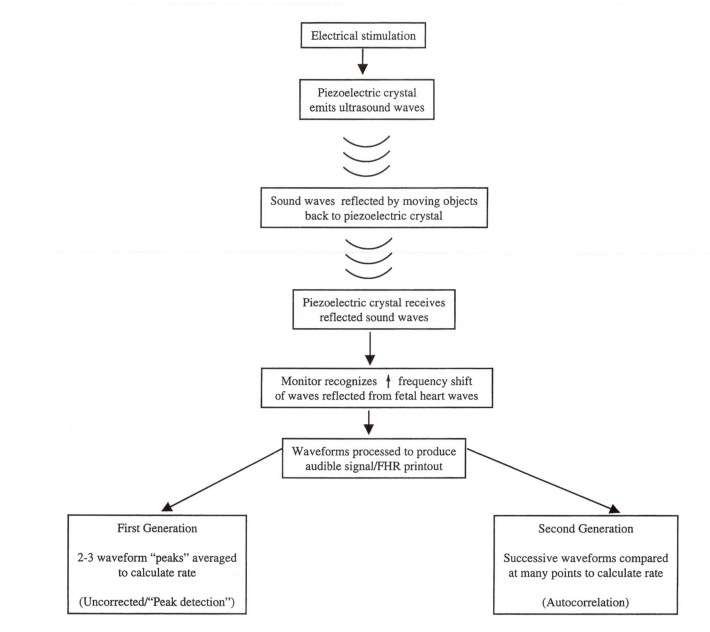

This is a linear view, but in fact, the piezoelectric crystal is emitting and receiving sound waves continually.

FIGURE 5-3

Linear Pictorial of Piezoelectric Effect
(Adapted from information in Hon, 1975; Klavan, Laver, & Boscola, 1977)

technique evolved from efforts to improve the quality of the processing of waveforms. The rapidly growing field of microprocessor technology has facilitated the development of this technique, which entails digitalizing and analyzing the reflection of ultrasound waveforms. Autocorrelation works by matching each incoming waveform with the previous one by repetitively analyzing small segments of the waveforms. In one model of this technique, during a 1.25-second time interval or envelope, 256 slices or digitalized points are taken (one every 5 milliseconds). The 256 points are then compared by means of a mathematical algorithm to the equivalent points obtained in the previous envelope. This process results in rejection of artifactual waveforms and a more accurate identification of the initiation of the fetal cardiac cycle than other techniques provide. Problems with amplitude variations of the waveforms are minimized, and the need for the traditional peak detection is eliminated (Hewlett-Packard, 1984). All of the monitors that use some form of autocorrelation have technical variations such as the length of time in which waveforms are retained in the memory system and how many waveforms are used for comparison. Further developments and improvements in this technology are ongoing.

The monitor may generate, detect, and print signals other than the FHR. The maternal heart rate may be picked up by the external ultrasound transducer, and this may be more likely if the fetus is active or if the mother is large (Schifrin, Harwell, Rubinstein, & Visser, 2001), or if a large maternal blood vessel is under the transducer (Freeman & Garite, 1981). Therefore, when placing the ultrasound transducer, the clinician should palpate the mother's pulse and compare it with the audible signal and printed rate to rule out inadvertent recording of the maternal pulse. Though it may be relatively easy to determine one from the other when they are both in normal ranges, an elevated maternal pulse rate may be more likely confused with a fetal heart rate, particularly during maternal pushing efforts in second stage labor. It is recommended that sudden changes in recorded heart rate be attended to, and that maternal pulse be assessed at times other than just whether a recorded heart rate appears to be bradycardic, to confirm whether the mother or the fetus is the signal source (Schifrin et al., 2001).

Artifact is a term used to describe irregular variation or absence of FHR on the fetal monitor record, resulting from mechanical limitations of the monitor or electrical interference problems, with "noise" being translated by the machine as a signal. A number of types of artifact are created by electronic fetal monitoring, including increased variability possible with external FHR monitoring, half-counting and double-counting of FHR, and recording of maternal heart rate. Half-counting of the fetal heart rate is most commonly seen with ultrasound use, when the fetal heart rate is rapid. Double-counting may also occur more commonly with external monitoring, with a slow fetal heart rate, but also may be seen with internal monitoring.

A summary of benefits, limitations, and troubleshooting actions to address common problems with ultrasound transducer use are included in Table 5-6.

Fetal Spiral Electrode

The fetal spiral electrode is viewed as the most accurate method of detecting fetal heart characteristics and patterns by directly deriving a signal from the fetal electrocardiogram. Direct FHR monitoring, when using the spiral electrode, uses electronic logic to detect and measure R- to R- wave intervals in consecutive QRS complexes to derive the FHR. The interval is recalculated with the detection of each new R-wave. This process allows for continuous detection of the FHR and provides a true representation of STV (see Figure 5-4). Major benefits for this method include the ability to detect short-term changes in the FHR (STV), detect dysrhythmias and obtain a continuous tracing of the FHR. Additional benefits and limitations are described in Table 5-7. When a spiral electrode is being used to assess FHR, a range of problems may require troubleshooting by the nurse to correct or improve the quality of monitor data being produced. Many common situations and suggestions for troubleshooting are included in Table 5-7. The electronic fetal monitor is, like any instrument, capable of equipment malfunc-

TABLE 5-6

Ultrasound (US) Transducer: Capabilities, Benefits and Limitations, Troubleshooting/Corrective Actions

CAPABILITIES

- Detect FHR baseline rate, long-term variability, accelerations, decelerations

BENEFITS AND LIMITATIONS

Benefits	*Limitations*
• Is noninvasive • Does not require rupture of membranes • Provides a permanent record	• Signal transmissions may be influenced by maternal obesity, occiput posterior, and anterior placenta, fetal movement (e.g., weak, absent, or false signal) • Restricts maternal movement • Maternal and fetal movement may interfere with continuous record • Artifact may artificially increase variability • Monitor may half- or double-count, especially in the presence of FHR tachycardia or bradycardia

TROUBLESHOOTING/CORRECTIVE ACTIONS

Problem	*Action*

■ Erratic recordings or gaps on the tracing paper
 • Potential causes
  —Inadequate conduction of ultrasound signal
  —Transducer may be displaced
  —Fetal or maternal movement
  —Dysrhythmia
  —Equipment malfunction
	• Evaluate potential causes
	• Assess whether a thin layer of ultrasonic gel is present under the transducer
	• Apply ultrasonic gel to the transducer as needed until a light seal is formed
	• Encourage maternal position changes to improve the signal
	• Determine whether the belt holding the transducer is snug around the abdomen; Tighten as needed to improve contact and signal detection
	• Reposition the transducer over the fetal back (determined by Leopold's maneuvers), as necessary
	• Check maternal pulse; auscultate as needed
	• Check the connection to the power source as well as the connections to the monitor
	• Check equipment according to manufacturer's directions
	• Apply fetal spiral electrode as appropriate

Interpretation of Short-Term Variability

- R-to-R intervals in consecutive QRS complexes to derive FHR
- Internal monitoring
- Fetal reserve
- Parasympathetic nervous system

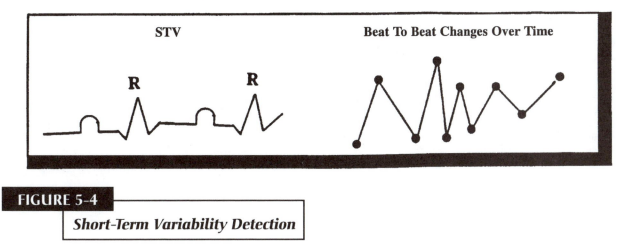

FIGURE 5-4

Short-Term Variability Detection

tion or error. It also is possible that the use of the instrument may be subject to incorrect procedure or human error. Although it is difficult to categorize or list all possible problems, some of them, with suggestions, are listed in Table 5-7.

The frequency for assessment of the FHR with either method of electronic monitoring (external or internal) is the same as for IA (AAP & ACOG, 2002; ACOG, 1995; SOGC, 2002a).

🖅 ELECTRONIC UTERINE ACTIVITY MONITORING

Tocodynamometer (Toco Transducer)

The contour of the uterus and abdomen changes somewhat with contractions. The tocodynamometer or toco transducer is the part of the electronic fetal monitor that externally detects abdominal pressure or contour changes resulting from uterine contractions. The pressure sensitive sensor, usually a button, should be placed on the abdomen over the uterine fundal region of the abdomen, with the particular location determined on the

basis of abdominal palpation, that is, where the contractions are best or more easily felt. The actual best location will vary from woman to woman, but may also change during a given labor. Computer technology then translates the degree of pressure detected by the sensor into an electrical signal and onto a numeric display on the monitor, as well as on the tracing paper. When the sensor is placed correctly, this mode of contraction assessment is useful in determining:

◆ Relative changes in abdominal pressure between uterine resting tone (tonus) and contractions

◆ Approximate duration (length) of contractions

◆ Approximate contraction frequency.

It is important to note that use of the external toco transducer does not allow for determination of the contraction strength (intensity), a fourth key element of contraction assessment. Therefore, palpation of the uterus during and between contractions, as well as input from the laboring woman is essential for the nurse to have a complete and adequate picture of contractions at a given point in time. Palpation is used in conjunction with elec-

TABLE 5-7

Fetal Spiral Electrode: Capabilities, Benefits and Limitations, Troubleshooting/Corrective Actions

CAPABILITIES

- Detect FHR baseline rate; variability, accelerations, decelerations
- Detect FHR dysrhythmias

BENEFITS AND LIMITATIONS

Benefits	*Limitations*
• Continuous detection of FHR • Accurately detects STV and LTV • Maternal position change does not alter ability to assess FHR or quality of tracing	• Invasive • Requires rupture of membranes, cervical dilatation, and accessible/appropriate fetal presenting part • Requires moist environment for detection of FHR • Potential small risk of infection and fetal hemorrhage or injury • May record maternal heart rate in presence of fetal demise • Fetal dysrhythmia may not be evident if logic or ECG button is engaged • Electronic interference and artifact may occur

TROUBLESHOOTING/CORRECTIVE ACTIONS

Problem	*Action*

■ Intermittent markings on the FHR tracing
  • Potential causes
    —Artifact
    —Failure to detect electrical activity
    —Fetal dysrhythmia
    —Monitor connections improperly attached
	• Evaluate potential causes
	• Confirm FHR with fetoscope
	• Check connections to the monitor, electrode cable
	• Check circuitry of the monitor
	• Turn off the logic or ECG deactivation switch
	• Check fetal spiral electrode placement on presenting part, if possible
	• Apply new fetal spiral electrode as indicated

■ Illegible FHR tracing
  • Potential causes
    —Artifact
    —Faulty electronic connection or monitor placement
	• Press the test button; check the numerical value
	• Check the connection to the power source and check all lead connections

■ Abnormal rate on the tracing
  • Potential causes
    —Doubling or halving of actual heart rate by monitor
	• Confirm/establish correct rate (e.g., auscultation with fetoscope)
	• Confirm maternal pulse simultaneously with FHR

TABLE 5-7 (cont.)

Fetal Spiral Electrode: Capabilities, Benefits and Limitations, Troubleshooting/Corrective Actions

TROUBLESHOOTING/CORRECTIVE ACTIONS (CONT.)	
Problem (cont.)	*Action (cont.)*

■ Abnormal rate on the tracing (cont.)
 • Potential causes (cont.)
  —Actual fetal tachycardia, bradycardia, or deceleration
  —Interference from maternal signal (e.g., fetal demise, fetal spiral electrode placement on maternal cervix)
  —Artifact
	• Refer to manufacturer's instruction manual for procedure for separating or distancing the maternal signal from the fetal ECG signal.
	 • Replace the fetal spiral electrode if necessary

■ FHR pattern compressed • Potential causes —Paper speed or scaling errors	• Verify paper speed (e.g., 3 cm per minute in the United States) • Confirm that paper being used has the appropriate calibrations for the monitor in use

■ INOP display
 • Potential causes
  —Signal cannot be received
  —Leads not connected to leg plate
  —Fetal spiral electrode may have a poor connection to the presenting part
  —Referencing electrode may not be operating
	• Check the lead connections to the monitor (gently remove the fetal spiral electrode wire) and check the EFM circuitry
	 • Vaginal secretions may be inadequate and an external reference electrode, if available, may need to be applied
	 • Palpate the maternal pulse and compare it with the audible signal and printed rate to rule out a recording of the maternal pulse

tronic uterine activity monitoring to validate uterine contraction intensity and confirm findings from electronic monitoring. Palpation also is used to assess uterine activity when the tocodynamometer is removed for ambulation (with auscultation) or during procedures such as epidural placement.

Caldeyro-Barcia and Poseiro (1960) described contractions as being abdominally palpable at a pressure of 10 mm Hg, which is a slightly lower pressure than the point at which the laboring woman feels the pain of contractions (15 mmHg). In most cases, toco transducers, in concert with palpation, provide satisfactory data to adequately assess uterine contraction patterns (LaCroix, 1968). Women may often be aware of the contrac-

tion before the toco transducer detects the contraction (Parer, 1997) (see Figure 5-5). On monitor tracings, the uterine activity portion of the tracing paper is marked off vertically in units of measure. Millimeters of mercury (mmHg) are the units of measure used in North America. Kilopascals are considered the standard measure for contraction strength in some other parts of the world. These measures have utility only when an intrauterine pressure catheter (IUPC) is used. Millimeters of mercury, as well as Montevideo units (MVUs) will be further addressed in the IUPC discussion in this chapter).

When the external toco transducer is in use, the numbers that represent uterine contraction

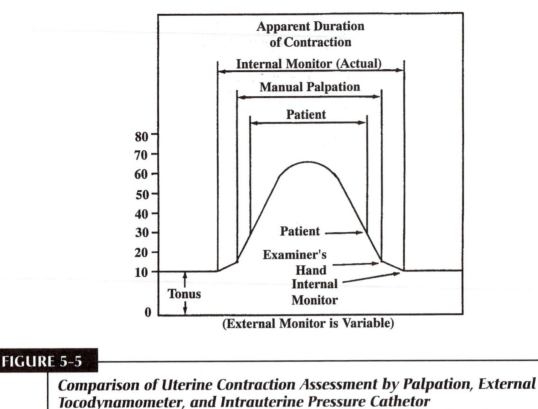

Apparent Duration of Contraction

Internal Monitor (Actual)

Manual Palpation

Patient

80
70
60
50
40
30
20
10
0

Patient

Examiner's Hand

Internal Monitor

Tonus

(External Monitor is Variable)

Comparison of Uterine Contraction Assessment by Palpation, External Tocodynamometer, and Intrauterine Pressure Cathetor
Note: From *Fetal Heart Rate Monitoring* (page 81), by R. K. Freeman, T. J. Garite, and Michael P. Nageotte, 1991, Baltimore: Williams & Wilkins, Copyright © 1991 by Williams and Wilkins, Reprinted with permission.

---

pressures on the uterine activity (UA) channel on the electronic fetal monitor are only arbitrary. The UA numbers should be set to 15 to 20 mmHg between contractions (Freeman & Garite, 1981), in order to facilitate the recorder's capturing of the relative contraction duration more fully. It is important that the toco transducer of the electronic fetal monitor be in use when the cardiotransducer is in use. This practice ensures that fetal heart rate patterns and responses can be considered in relation to the presence or absence, frequency, and duration of contractions. Also, it is important to ensure the time is being accurately documented on the tracing at regular intervals. Though most monitors currently print the time automatically, the nurse needs to ensure that the time is actually correctly shown.

Benefits and limitations as well as troubleshooting strategies to address common problems that may occur when using the tocodynamometer are summarized in Table 5-8 along with ways to improve the quality of the pressure signal information provided. Other problems are illustrated in Figure 5-6).

Intrauterine Pressure Catheters (IUPCs)

Intrauterine pressure catheters are inserted internally into the uterus via the vagina and cervix to objectively and quantitatively measure the pressures and characteristics of uterine contraction activity: resting tone and contraction, intensity, frequency, and duration. There are several types of IUPCs, which are divided into two categories: open-ended fluid-filled and solid sensor-tipped. Key concepts related to fluid-filled and solid sensor-tipped IUPCs are highlighted below.

The decision to use an IUPC is generally based on the clinical need for information beyond what

TABLE 5-8

Toco Transducer: Capabilities, Benefits and Limitations, Troubleshooting/Corrective Actions

CAPABILITIES
• Detect relative uterine resting tone • Detect relative frequency, duration of uterine contraction

BENEFITS AND LIMITATIONS	
Benefits	*Limitations*
• Noninvasive • Easily placed • Does not require ruptured amniotic membranes • Generates a tracing for future assessment and for a permanent medical record	• Subjective • Unable to detect uterine contraction intensity and resting tone • May be unable to accurately detect exact contraction frequency and duration, particulary if a woman is very large or is having preterm labor • Toco is location sensitive; placement can lead to false information • Sensitive to maternal or fetal motion that may be superimposed on the waveform • Transducer presence or position may be uncomfortable for the mother • Limits potential for maternal movement and ambulation during labor

TROUBLESHOOTING/CORRECTIVE ACTIONS	
Problem	*Action*
• Contractions not recording on the tracing	• Use manual palpation to validate presence of contractions • Confirm toco transducer is on abdomen & connected to monitor • Test calibration of the toco system by pushing firmly on the abdominal transducer button. The digital monitor display should show a particular numeric display (See operating manual for the monitor type you are using to confirm what the specific number should be) • Assure that placement of the tocodynamometer is firm, but not tight, on the maternal abdomen • Palpate the uterus for the area of strongest contraction and reposition the tocodynamometer over that point • When the uterus is relaxed, set the UA dial or button to 15–20 mmHg • Consider IUPC placement, as indicated

(table continues)

TABLE 5-8 (cont.)

Toco Transducer: Capabilities, Benefits and Limitations, Troubleshooting/Corrective Actions

TROUBLESHOOTING/CORRECTIVE ACTIONS (CONT.)	
Problem (cont.)	*Action (cont.)*
• Recording only portion of contractions	• Palpate the uterus for the area of strongest contraction intensity; reposition the tocodynamometer over that area • When the uterus is relaxed, set the uterine activity dial or button to 15–20 mmHg

• Other problems
  —Position
  —Pushing
  —Vomiting
	• Encourage position change as needed.
	• Palpate to verify uterine activity
	• If necessary, note uterine contractions on tracing using the event marker
	• Note clinical events (e.g., vomiting, pushing)

is available through maternal descriptors, abdominal palpation, and tocodynamometer data, or for amnioinfusion. Indications for intrauterine pressure monitoring include situations such as: (a) nonprogression of labor; (b) the presence of a uterine scar; (c) oxytocin induction or augmentation, if external methods of assessing uterine activity are inadequate; (d) circumstances in which amnioinfusion may be desirable, such as in the presence of thick meconium or variable deceleration patterns, and (e) to differentiate between early versus late decelerations, when external assessment of FHR changes in relation to contractions cannot otherwise be determined.

IUPC use is invasive and requires the consideration of potential risks and benefits of this mode of contraction assessment on a case-by-case basis (see Table 5-9). A sterile, flexible catheter inserted into the amniotic cavity of the uterus through a guide can be used after rupture of the membranes and cervical dilatation to monitor the intrauterine pressure directly. The proximal end of the catheter is attached to a pressure transducer.

The most common North American unit of IUPC measurement for contraction intensity is millimeters of mercury (mmHg). Uterine baseline resting tone and peak intrauterine pressure intensity can be described, using the actual mmHg measurement from the monitor tracing.

Alternate methods of describing uterine activity strength include determining the contraction amplitude by subtracting the difference in mmHg between the uterine tone before a contraction and the peak. Using this definition of amplitude, contraction strength tends to vary across a given labor, from 30 mmHg amplitude in early spontaneous labor, to 50 mmHg at the end of first stage, to 20 to 30 mmHg during second stage (Caldeyro-Barcia & Poseiro, 1959).

Another approach to quantify uterine contraction strength is to use Montevideo units (MVUs), a measurement defined in 1952 by Dr. Caldeyro-Barcia and colleagues from Montevideo, Uruguay. These units are calculated by measuring the peak intensity or amplitude (in mmHg) for each contraction occurring in a ten-minute window of time and adding the numbers together (Caldeyro-Barcia, Pose, & Alvarez, 1957). Contraction amplitude is the difference between the resting tone and the peak of the contraction (in mmHg). For example, if there are 3 contractions in 10 minutes, peaking 70, 80, and 75 mm Hg of intrauterine pressure,

Normal

1. Uterine contraction wave form.

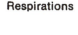

Respirations

2. Respiration may produce an undulating overlay.

Pushing

3. Valsalva maneuver with pushing effects during the second stage of labor may produce blunted spikes.

Vomiting seizures

4. Extreme maternal activity such as vomiting or a seizure may produce a series of sharp spikes.

Fetal activity

5. Fetal movement may produce sharp isolated spikes.

Sudden baseline shift

6. Sudden baseline shifts may be produced by maternal position change.

Obscured

7. Low baseline setting may obscure all but tip of contractions.

8. Certain placements of tocodynamometer may produce reversed waveform when uterus contracts away from the tocodynamometer

Inverted

FIGURE 5-6

Tocodynamometer Variations
(Adapted from information in Wagner and Cabaniss, unpublished.)

TABLE 5-9

Intrauterine Pressure Catheters: Capabilities, Benefits and Limitations, Troubleshooting/Corrective Actions

CAPABILITIES

Intrauterine pressure catheters can be used to

- Detect actual uterine resting tone
- Detect actual frequency, duration, and strength of uterine contractions
- Withdraw amniotic fluid for testing
- Perform amnioinfusion

BENEFITS AND LIMITATIONS

Benefits	*Limitations*
GENERAL • An objective method of assessing accurate uterine contraction frequency, duration, intensity, and resting tone • More accurate correlation of timing of FHR changes with uterine activity • Generates a tracing that is a permanent part of the medical record	GENERAL • Rupture of membranes and adequate cervical dilation are required • Procedure is invasive • Increased risk of uterine infection, uterine or placental perforation • Limits potential for maternal ambulation during labor • Use may be contraindicated with infections where rupture of membranes is discouraged to prevent maternal-fetal transmission (e.g., B-strep, herpes, HIV) • May be contraindicated in presence of vaginal bleeding • Increased risk of uterine perforation (rupture), placental abruption or perforation, infection, or umbilical cord prolapse (Usta, Mercer, & Sabai, 1999) • Differences in readings between fluid-filled and sensor-tipped catheters
FLUID-FILLED IUPC • Provides means for aspiration of amniotic fluid to assess for chorioamnionitis • Provides means for performing amnioinfusion	FLUID-FILLED IUPC • Catheter tip may become wedged against the uterine wall or fetal part and prevent the production of any pressure data or produce a distorted or truncated waveform • Catheter tip in relation to external pressure transducer position may affect pressures • Catheter may become obstructed with particulate matter such as meconium or blood • Pressure readings may be lower than sensor-tipped (or solid) transducers

TABLE 5-9 (cont.)

Intrauterine Pressure Catheters: Capabilities, Benefits and Limitations, Troubleshooting/Corrective Actions

BENEFITS AND LIMITATIONS (CONT.)

Benefits (cont.)	*Limitations (cont.)*
SOLID-STATE IUPC • Easily zeroed to atmospheric pressure: most can be re-zeroed • Most models allow for amnioinfusion and aspiration of amniotic fluid (see benefits of fluid-filled catheters) • Design avoids pressure artifacts that may be caused by a catheter that may contain air or become kinked	SOLID-STATE IUPC • Maternal position may change hydrostatic pressure within the uterus and may alter readings including resting tone • Pressure readings may be higher than with fluid-filled catheters

TROUBLESHOOTING/CORRECTIVE ACTIONS

Problem	*Actions*

■ No contractions recorded
  • Potential causes
    —Displacement of IUPC
    —Obstructed catheter
    —Incorrectly zeroed catheter
    —Uterine perforation
	• Evaluate potential causes
	• In verifying the position of the IUPC, ask patient to cough or perform Valsalva's maneuver; a spike should appear if the IUPC is positioned properly
	• Palpate to confirm presence of contractions
	• Check monitor for loose connections
	• Flush fluid-filled catheter
	• Verify calibration per detailed instructions in transducer manufacturer's operating manual (run monitor's self-test)
	• Zero/rezero the transducer according to manufacturer's operating manual and verify the position of the IUPC
	• In addition to troubleshooting for placement of IUPC, observe for signs of maternal shock, fetal compromise

■ Abnormal uterine contraction waveform appearance on tracing
  • Potential causes
    —The IUPC tip may be lodged against the uterine wall, placenta, or a fetal body part
    —Fluid-filled IUPC may be dry or incompletely filled with sterile water, thus permitting air to dampen the waveform
    —Catheter tip is above the diaphragm transducer level creating higher pressure readings; or if below, the reading may be artificially low
	• Evaluate potential causes
	• Palpate
	• Flush the IUPC, if applicable
	• Rotating the IUPC 180 degrees may change the relationship of the pressure-sensing device to the fetus and uterus
	• In addition to troubleshooting for placement of IUPC, observe for signs of maternal shock, fetal compromise

(table continues)

TABLE 5-9 (cont.)

Intrauterine Pressure Catheters: Capabilities, Benefits and Limitations, Troubleshooting/Corrective Actions

TROUBLESHOOTING/CORRECTIVE ACTIONS (CONT.)	
Problem (cont.)	*Actions*

■ Abnormal uterine contraction waveform appearance on tracing (cont.)
   • Potential causes (cont.)
     —Inadvertent insertion of the IUPC between the wall of the uterus and the membranes (Lind, 1999, case study)
     —Uterine perforation, placental abruption, or perforation	

■ Inverse tracing of uterine contractions
   • Potential causes
     —Uterine perforation
	• Evaluate potential causes
	• In addition to troubleshooting for placement of IUPC, observe for signs of maternal shock, fetal compromise

■ Uterine resting tone or baseline tonus is elevated or not tracing
   • Potential causes
     —Fluid-filled IUPC is sensitive to hydrostatic pressure and changes in hydrostatic pressure
     —Pressures may vary in different maternal positions
	• May need to rezero IUPC according to manufacturer's instructions
	• Record the uterine resting tone in all positions on insertion, especially when using those sensor-tipped IUPCs that cannot be rezeroed after insertion

---

and a baseline uterine tone of 10 mmHg, this would be calculated as $(70 - 10) + (80 - 10) + (75 - 10) = 60 + 70 + 65 = 195$ MVUs . It is important to note that these calculations are dependent on IUPC data. A contraction pattern totaling at least 200 MVUs per 10-minute period has been considered as adequate labor (Schifrin, 1974), and normal spontaneous labor activity is generally less than 280 MVUs (Caldeyro-Barcia, & Poseiro,1959), though MVUs can vary widely across spontaneous laboring women (Caldeyro-Barcia, et al, 1960). The American College of Obstetricians and Gynecologists (1995) has recommended that uterine contraction patterns should be at least 200 MVUs per 10 minutes for at least 2 hours without cervical change before arrest of first-stage labor can be diagnosed. Recent research findings by Rouse and colleagues (1999) suggest that at least 4 hours in active phase of labor may be more appropriate before such a diagnosis.

Fluid-Filled Intrauterine Pressure Catheter

The fluid-filled IUPC was the first type available for clinical use and is based on the assumption that fluid in the uterus and catheter forms a closed system. The catheter measures pressure within the uterine cavity caused by fluid being displaced, with increased pressure generated by a contraction and transmitted up the fluid column in the catheter. This displaced fluid exerts pressure against a diaphragm in the transducer, which generates changes in the electrical resistance of a series of wires. These electrical changes are converted to measures of pressure and displayed on the uterine activity channel of the chart record.

The accuracy of this system, therefore, depends on the fluid pool surrounding the catheter tip. Intrauterine pressures have been shown to vary by as much as 25% when measured at different areas of the uterus. Other factors also may influence the accuracy of measured pressures. Air in the closed system will cushion the pressure generated, producing dampened waveforms and inaccurate measurement of contractions. Leakage and obstruction of the catheter will distort the waveform (Hutson & Petrie, 1986; Klapholz, 1978). In particular, fluids containing heavy particulate matter, such as thick meconium, can lead to significant damping of waveforms in fluid-filled IUPCs (Devoe, Smith, & Stoker, 1993). Therefore, intermittent flushing of this type of IUPC catheter with normal saline (without preservatives) will likely be required.

See Table 5-9 for an overview of benefits, limitations, and troubleshooting issues regarding the use of the fluid-filled intrauterine pressure catheter.

Solid State Sensor-Tipped Intrauterine Pressure Catheters

The solid-state sensor tipped intrauterine pressure catheter was introduced in the 1980s as an alternative to the fluid-filled catheter systems (Strong & Paul, 1989). This technology uses a micro solid-state pressure transducer located at the catheter tip. Dual lumen versions that enable simultaneous amnioinfusion or sampling of amniotic fluid and rezeroing after insertion are also available.

The baseline reading of resting tone from a sensor-tipped IUPC can be affected by changes in maternal position and the hydrostatic pressures exerted on the catheter. The position of the IUPC tip in relation to the position of the patient may affect the amount of pressure exerted by the fluid above the catheter. Intrauterine hydrostatic pressure is altered by maternal position changes. Obtaining baseline pressure readings in the left, right, and supine with lateral tilt positions demonstrates

these alterations, and may prevent potential misinterpretations of resting tone pressures following subsequent position changes during labor. Knowing these baseline differences also may prevent erroneous conclusions regarding induction or augmentation management. See Figure 5-7.

MONITOR TRACING ISSUES

Although the focus of this section of the chapter is electronic fetal monitoring methods, it is important to address tracing and paper speed technology.

USA-scaled paper has markings from 30 to 240 bpm, with dividing lines at 10 bpm intervals. European-scaled paper has markings from 50 to 210 bpm, with dividing lines at 5 bpm intervals. These differences can affect interpretation of the FHR and variability.

Fetal monitor technology provides the capacity to set the tracing paper speed (as well as the visual tracing display) at a certain speed setting. In the United States, the recommended paper speed is 3 centimeters per minute (cm/min) (ACOG, 1995). Professional practice guidelines in other countries suggest other rates of paper speed. In Britain, for example, the recommended standard is 1 cm/min (Royal College of Obstetricians and Gynaecologists [RCOG], 2001), while other countries consider 2 cm/min as appropriate. The SOGC of Canada has not chosen to recommend a specific centimeter-per-minute speed (SOGC, 2002a). Despite these apparent differences, one recommendation is constant across professional practice organizations: They stress that standardization of paper speed within and across practice settings is essential for optimal interpretation by professional care providers (ACOG, 1995; RCOG, 2001; SOGC, 2002a). In this way, clinicians are more likely to recognize key FHR and uterine activity patterns (SOGC, 1995). Therefore, the switching of paper speeds during individual labors is not recommended. At any time fetal heart rate and uterine activity patterns appear compressed, it is important for the clinician to consider the possibility that a particular tracing is set at a slower per minute speed. The converse is also true.

It has been argued that a 1 or 2 centimeter speed is satisfactory in order to determine FHR pat-

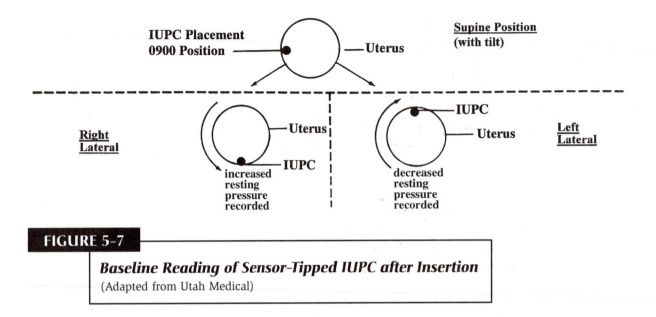

FIGURE 5-7

Baseline Reading of Sensor-Tipped IUPC after Insertion
(Adapted from Utah Medical)

terns, while at the same time limiting the volume of tracing paper required, and thus the storage space required. However, as computer archiving systems become more commonplace in intrapartum care units, this argument may carry less weight. One or 2 cm/min paper speed may provide an "overview" of the recording, but it is suggested that at such a paper speed, "'long-term' variability is artificially accentuated, 'short-term variability' is hardly recognizable and the time-relation between uterine contractions and decelerations is more difficult to assess" (Van Geijn, 1998, p. 1426). It is important to note, however, that scientific study of possible clinical influences of differences in paper speed has not been undertaken.

Despite the recommendations for a consistent paper speed, there are geographic differences regarding paper speed practices across North America. These differences may be related to historical tradition, the country or location in which particular nurses and physicians previously trained and practiced, and/or the argument that slower paper speeds save paper and maximize storage efficiency. This lack of consistency may make interpretation and communication more challenging; and such inconsistency may set the stage for misinterpretation of EFM data or miscommunication of that data. As communication issues often are key issues in cases of legal liability, development

of and adherence to national and institutional standards and guidelines for EFM paper speeds are essential. It is a nursing responsibility to be familiar with paper speed standards in your country, province/state, and clinical facility. The nurse should also know where the paper speed switch is located on the various monitors where (s)he works.

◻️ INTRAPARTUM FETAL SURVEILLANCE TECHNOLOGY AND THE NURSE'S ROLE

Maternal Responses to Monitoring

Studies of maternal responses to electronic fetal monitoring were undertaken early in its history, but sample sizes tended to be small and most were uncontrolled surveys, which limits generalizability of the findings. We do know that maternal movement in labor may be restricted with use of continuous EFM (Garcia, Corry, MacDonald, Elbourne, & Grant,1985; Hodnett, 1982), and restriction of movement may negatively influence a woman's sense of control in labor (Hodnett, 1982). Some women may consider continuous EFM in a negative light (Shields, 1978), whereas others may feel positive or reassured from the use of EFM (Molfese, Sunshine, & Bennett, 1982; Shields, 1978). In a more recent national survey in the United States, women reported having EFM (93%) along with other interventions including intravenous drips (85.6%), epidural analgesia (63%), artificially ruptured membranes (55%), and oxytocin to strengthen contractions (53%) (MCA, 2002). Most women also reported that they did not walk during labor related to being hooked up to instruments, having had pain medications, or because the care provider instructed them not to ambulate.

It is reassuring that most mothers described feeling positive about their birth experiences and satisfied with the care they received from their care providers. The majority felt that they generally understood what was happening (94%) and got the information that they needed (91%), while 89% stated they were as involved in decision making as they needed to be (MCA, 2002). However, it has been suggested that professional organizations, researchers, and health care agencies are challenged to determine whether the level of current evidence supports routine use of interventions and whether women are making informed choices (Maternity Wise, 2002; Sakala, Declercq, & Corry, 2002), and to continue research to address gaps in the evidence to support current practice.

Intrapartum Care Issues

Patient Education

Patient education regarding methods of fetal assessment is helpful to women in making fully informed mutual decisions with their nurses and other care providers.

The recent explosion in technological capabilities and the technological society within which we live and practice may influence patients' preferences for IA or EFM. More current studies regarding patient preferences or feelings about monitoring methods are warranted, although patients have reported that they prefer to have a supportive professional present during labor (Hodnett et al., 2002; Killien & Shy, 1989).

Labor Support Regardless of Monitoring Method

It has been stated that "to monitor is to observe closely and regularly or continuously" (McFadyen, 1993, p. 53). Both auscultation and palpation and electronic fetal monitoring require close observation and attention to the fetal data gathered as well as other ongoing maternal and fetal assessments. It is critical to keep in mind that the information obtained from electronic fetal monitoring technology is inadequate without close attention to both the data from the monitor and that gathered from other ongoing assessments and interaction with mother and fetus.

Clinicians and researchers have cautioned against nursing activities becoming more heavily focused on monitors and other machinery, rather than on the woman in labor (Hoerst & Fairman, 2000; McNiven, Hodnett, & O'Brien-Pallas, 1992; Sandelowski, 1998). EFM technology does not replace the need for care by experienced care providers and EFM should not be considered a replacement for skilled and supportive nursing care. Indeed, the Royal College of Obstetricians and Gynaecologists underlined that "Women should have the same level of care and support regardless of the mode of monitoring" (RCOG, 2001, p. 9; SOGC, 2002a). AWHONN also encourages professional nursing support of laboring women and encourages women to request that they receive support from a registered and/or advanced practice nurse (AWHONN, 2000b).

In a descriptive social history study of how nurses put EFM into use, Sandelowski described the complexity of the challenges facing nurses in implementing EFM and considering women's responses (2000). More recently, professional nurses have been described as providing supportive care simultaneously with surveillance of the mother and fetus (Miltner, 2002). However, this study found that emotional support was provided at higher rates than physical support (e.g., encouragement to ambulate) (Miltner, 2002) which seems to mirror women's reports of their labor experience. Women in a national survey in the U.S. stated that they had supportive care (99%) and rated supportive care provided by doulas and nurse midwives as the highest quality of support (MCA, 2002). The finding that women desire supportive care during labor is consistent in other research findings (Hodnett, 1997; Hodnett et al., 1997, 2002). In a meta-analysis of studies examining outcomes associated with labor support, versus usual care, there were short- and long-term benefits to the mother and neonate (less analgesia use, fewer operative deliveries, improved Apgar scores, increased breastfeeding, and less incidence of postpartum depression) (Hodnett, 1997). In a more recent RCT to examine the effect of nurses trained to provide supportive care in North America as compared to usual care, there were no significant differences found in cesarean delivery rates or other medical or psychosocial outcomes (Hodnett et al., 2002). The researchers stated that a plausible explanation for these findings is that the effects of birth environments with high medical intervention rates may have overpowered the effects of continuous support (Hodnett et al., 2002). However, comparisons of women's responses in the continuous support and usual care groups regarding their likes and dislikes and level of support desired in future labors favored the provision of continuous support. In summary, women desire supportive care and information regardless of the method of monitoring being used.

Institutional Policies

Individual facilities need to develop policies and procedures for IA, palpation, and electronic fetal monitoring that are consistent with their appropriate state, provincial, or national guidelines or regulations. Inclusion of key nursing personnel and development of collaborative teams are suggested for planning and implementing evidence-based practices (AWHONN, 1998a). Policies should address when it is appropriate to use IA and EFM, the frequency of assessment, and documentation of findings (AWHONN, 2000a). In addition, attention to the skill mix needed to perform IA and EFM is required. Additional position statements have described who should perform auscultation and the recommended frequency of auscultation (ACOG, 1995; AWHONN, 1998, 2000a; SOGC,

2002a). The initiation and ongoing assessment and interpretation of EFM and IA falls into the realm of registered nurses, advanced practice nurses, and physicians with professional expertise practice (AWHONN, 1998; 2000a).

Professional Education on Monitoring Methods

It is important for professionals to receive preparation for implementing fetal monitoring that includes the physiologic interpretation of data and its implications for care (AWHONN, 2000a; SOGC, 2002a). Facilitators to implementing evidence-based practice include education preparation, resources, and support (Davies et al., 2002). Whether new skills are being taught or existing skills reinforced, the level of the learner, novice to expert, needs to be considered (Benner, 1994). Educational programs that take into account adult learning principles and the levels of learners can assist care providers in increasing their IA skills.

Future Research

Additional research on methods of monitoring will continue to inform our use of monitoring methods, including identifying who needs to be monitored with EFM or IA and how frequent assessments should be (ACOG; 1995; AWHONN, 2000a; SOGC, 2002a, 2002b).

☞ SUMMARY

Fetal surveillance methods allow for gathering data to form an adequate assessment of fetal well-being and uterine activity. Clear assessment data are vital for accurate interpretation, nursing diagnosis, and subsequent interventions. Therefore, the methods used to assess the FHR and uterine activity may change, as labor progresses, depending upon the quality of information received for interpretation and what is needed for adequate assessment, interpretation, clinical interventions, and evaluation (see Figure 5-8). Understanding the methods, benefits, limitations, and troubleshooting measures of fetal surveillance are criti-

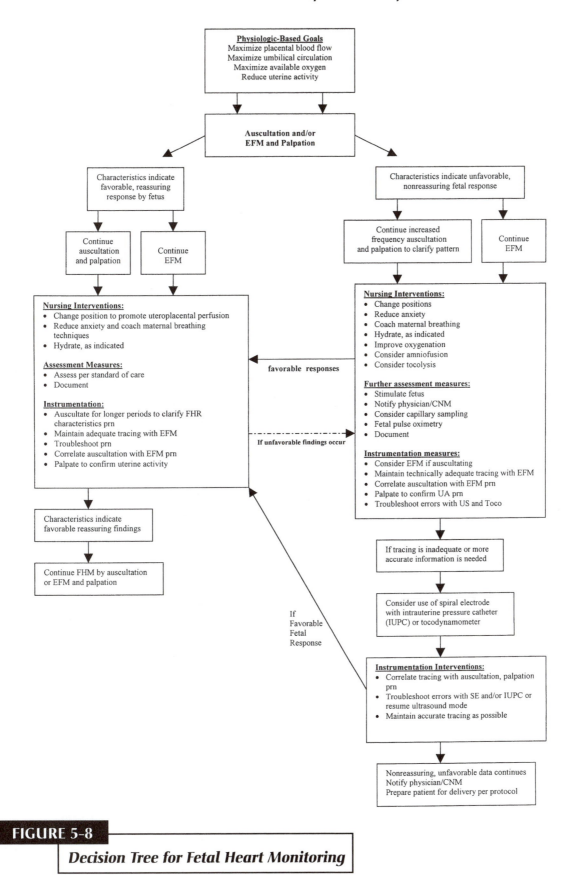

FIGURE 5-8

Decision Tree for Fetal Heart Monitoring

cal for informed decision making and skill in the use of these methods. Chapter 6 will continue with interpretation of the FHR characteristics.

☞ REFERENCES

American Academy of Pediatrics, & American College of Obstetricians & Gynecologists. (2002). *Guidelines for perinatal care* (5th ed.). Washington, D.C.: Authors.

American College of Obstetricians and Gynecologists. (1995). *Fetal heart rate patterns: Monitoring, interpretation, and management* (Technical Bulletin No. 207). Washington, D.C.: Author.

Association of Women's Health, Obstetric and Neonatal Nurses. (1997a). *Fetal heart monitoring principles and practices.* Washington, D.C.: Author.

Association of Women's Health, Obstetric and Neonatal Nurses. (1997b). *The role of unlicensed assistive personnel in the nursing care for women and newborns* (Clinical Position Statement). Washington, D.C.: Author.

Association of Women's Health, Obstetric and Neonatal Nurses. (2000a). *Fetal assessment* (Clinical Position Statement). Washington, D.C.: Author.

Association of Women's Health, Obstetric and Neonatal Nurses. (2000b). *Professional nursing support of laboring women* (Clinical Position Statement). Washington, D.C.: Author.

Benner, P. (1984). *From novice to expert. Excellence and power in clinical nursing practice.* Menlo Park: Addison-Wesley.

Boehm, F., Fields, L., Hutchison, J., Bowen, A. W., & Vaughn, W. K. (1986). The indirectly obtained fetal heart rate: Comparison of first and second generation electronic fetal monitors. *American Journal of Obstetrics and Gynecology, 155*(1), 10–14.

Caldeyro-Barcia, R., Pose, S., & Alvarez, H. (1957). Uterine contractility in polyhydramnios and the effects of withdrawal of the excess of amniotic fluid. *American Journal of Obstetrics and Gynecology, 73,* 1238.

Caldeyro-Barcia, R., & Poseiro, J. (1959). Oxytocin and contractility of the pregnant human uterus. *Annals of the New York Academy of Science, 72,* 813–830.

Caldeyro-Barcia, R., & Poseiro, J. (1960). Physiology of the uterine contraction. *Clinics in Obstetrics and Gynecology, 3,* 386.

Canadian Perinatal Regionalization Coalition, Society of Obstetricians & Gynaecologists of Canada, & Perinatal Educator Program. (2001). *Fundamentals of fetal health surveillance in labor: A self-learning manual.* Ottawa, Canada: Author.

Davies, B., Hodnett, E., Hannah, M., O'Brien-Pallas, L., Pringle, D., Wells, G., Perinatal Partnership Program of Eastern and Southeastern Ontario, & Society of Obstetricians and Gynaecologists of Canada. (2002). Fetal health surveillance: A community-wide approach versus a tailored intervention for the implementation of clinical practice guidelines. *Canadian Medical Association Journal, 167*(5), 469–474.

Davies, B. L., Niday, P. A., Nimrod, C. A., Drake, E. R., Sprague, A. E., & Trepanier, M. J. (1993). Electronic fetal monitoring: A Canadian survey. *Canadian Medical Association Journal, 148*(10), 1737–1742.

Devoe, L. D., Smith, R. P., & Stoker, R. (1993). Intrauterine pressure catheter performance in an in vitro uterine model: A stimulation of problems for intrapartum monitoring. *Obstetrics and Gynecology, 82*(2), 285–289.

Enkin, M., Keirse, M., Neilson, J., Crowther, C., Duley, L., Hodnett, E., & Hofmeyer, J. (2000). *A guide to effective care in pregnancy and childbirth* (3rd ed.). Oxford, UK: Oxford University Press.

Feinstein, N. F. (2000). Fetal heart rate auscultation: current and future practice. *Journal of Obstetric, Gynecologic, & Neonatal Nursing. 29*(3), 306–315.

Feinstein, N. F., Sprague, A., & Trepanier, M. J. (2000). *Fetal Heart Rate Auscultation.* Washington, D.C.: Association of Women's Health, Obstetric and Neonatal Nurses.

Freeman, R. K., & Garite, T. J. (1981). *Fetal heart rate monitoring.* Baltimore: Williams and Wilkens.

Freeman, R. K., Garite, T. J., & Nageotte, M. P. (1991). *Fetal heart rate monitoring.* Baltimore: Williams & Wilkins.

Garcia, J., Corry, M., MacDonald, D., Elbourne, D., & Grant, A. (1985). Mother's views of continuous electronic fetal monitoring and intermittent auscultation in a randomized controlled trial. *Birth, 12*(2), 79–86.

Goodwin, L. (2000). Intermittent auscultation of the fetal heart rate: A review of general principles. *Journal of Perinatal and Neonatal Nursing, 14*(3), 53–61.

Grant, A. M. (1992). EFM and scalp sampling versus intermittent auscultation in labor. In M. Enkin, M. Keirse, M. Renfrew, & J. Neilson (Eds.), Cochrane database of systematic reviews: Pregnancy and childbirth modules Review # 03297. Oxford: Update Software, Disk Issue 1.

Grzybowski, S., Harris, S., Buchinski, B., Pope, S., Swenerton, J., Peter, E., et al. (1998). *First Births Project manual: A continuous quality improvement project. Volume 1.* Vancouver, British Columbia: Women's Hospital and Health Centre.

Haggerty, L. A. (1999). Continuous electronic fetal monitoring: Contradictions between practice and research. *Journal of Obstetric, Gynecologic, and Neonatal Nursing, 28,* 409–416.

Hewlett Packard (1984). The technology within. Andover, MA: Author.

Hodnett, E. (1982). Patient control in labor: Effects of two types of fetal monitors. *Journal of Obstetric, Gynecologic, and Neonatal Nursing, 11,* 94–99.

Hodnett, E. (1994). Support from caregivers during childbirth. In M. Enkin, M., Keirse, M. Renfrew, & J. Neilson (Eds.), Cochrane Database of Systematic Reviews: Pregnancy and Childbirth Modules Review #03871. Oxford: Update Software, Disk Issue 1.

Hodnett, E. (1997). Support from caregivers during childbirth. (Cochrane review). In Cochrane Library, Issue 2. Oxford: Update Software, 1998.

Hodnett, E., Lowe, N., Hannah, M., Willan, A., Stevens, B., Ohlsson, A., Gafni, A., Muir, H., Myhr, T., & Stremler, R. (2002). Effectiveness of nurses as providers of birth labor in North America hospitals: A randomized controlled trial. *Journal of the American Medical Association, 288*(11), 1373–1381.

Hoerst, B. J., & Fairman, J. (2000). Social and professional influences of the technology of electronic fetal monitoring on obstetrical nursing. *Western Journal of Nursing Research, 22*(4), 475–491.

Hutson, J., & Petrie, R. (1986). Possible limitations of fetal monitoring. *Clinical Obstetrics and Gynecology, 29*(1), 104–113.

Killien, M. G., & Shy, K. (1989). A randomized clinical trial of electronic fetal monitoring in preterm labor: Mother's views. *Birth, 16*(1), 7–12.

Klapholz, H. (1978). Techniques of fetal heart monitoring. *Seminars in Perinatology, 2*(2), 1.

LaCroix, G. (1968). Monitoring labor by an external tocodynamometer. *American Journal of Obstetrics and Gynecology, 101,* 111.

Levitt, C., Hanvey, L., Avard, D., Chance, G., & Kaczorowski, J. (1995). *Survey of routine maternity care and practices on Canadian hospitals.* Ottawa: Health Canada and Canadian Institute of Child Health.

Lind, B. (1999). Complications caused by extramembranous placement of intrauterine pressure catheters. *American Journal of Obstetrics and Gynecology, 180*(4), 1034–1035.

Liston, R., Crane, J., Hughes, O., Kuling, S., MacKinnon, C., Milne, K., Richardson, B., & Trepanier, M. J. (2002). Fetal Health Surveillance Working Group. Fetal health surveillance in labour. *Journal of Obstetrics & Gynaecolog in Canada, 24*(4), 342–355.

Kaczorowski, J., Levitt, C., Harvey, L., Avard, D., & Chance, G. (1998). A national survey of use of obstetric procedures and technologies in Canadian hospitals: routine or based on existing evidence? *Birth, 25*(1), 11–18.

Malinowski, J., Pedigo, C., & Phillips, C. (1989). *Nursing care during the labor process* (3rd ed.). Philadelphia: F.A. Davis.

Martin, J. A., Hamilton, B. T., Ventura, S. J., Menacker, F., & Park, M. M. (2002). Birth: Final data for 2000. *National Vital Statistics Reports, 50*(5), 1–102.

Maternity Center Association. (2002). Listening to mothers: Report of the first national US survey of women's childbearing experiences. Retrieved 12/24/02.*http://www.maternitywise.org/listeningtomothers/*

McFadyen, I. (1993). Clinical applications of intrapartum monitoring. In J. Spencer & R. Ward (Eds.) *Intrapartum fetal surveillance* (pp. 53–63). London: RCOG Press.

McNiven, P., Hodnett, E., & O'Brien-Pallas, L. L. (1992). Supporting women in labor: A work sampling study of the activities of labor and delivery nurses. *Birth, 19*(1), 3–8.

Miller, F. C., Pearse, K. E., & Paul, R. H. (1984). Fetal heart pattern recognition by the method of auscultation. *Obstetrics & Gynecology, 64*(3), 332–336.

Miltner, R. S. (2002). More than support: Nursing interventions provided to women in labor. *Journal of Obstetric, Gynecologic, and Neonatal Nursing, 31,* 753–761.

Molfese, V., Sunshine, P., & Bennett, A. (1982). Reactions of women to intrapartum fetal monitoring. *Obstetrics and Gynecology, 59*(6), 705–709.

Morrison, J. C., Chez, B. F., Davis, I. D., Martin, R. W., Roberts, W. E., Martin, J. N., & Floyd, R. C. (1993). Intrapartum fetal heart rate assessment: Monitoring by auscultation or electronic means. American *Journal of Obstetrics and Gynecology, 168*(1 Pt 1), 63–66.

Murray, M. (1997). *Antepartal and intrapartal fetal monitoring.* Albuquerque, NM: Learning Resources International, Inc.

Neilson, J. (1994a). EFM versus intermittent auscultation in labour. In M. Enkin, M. Keirse, J. Renfrew, & J. Neilson (Eds.), Cochrane database of systematic reviews: pregnancy and childbirth modules Review #03884. Oxford: Update Software, Disk Issue 1.

Neilson, J. (1994b). EFM alone versus intermittent auscultation in labour. In EFM alone versus intermittent auscultation in labour. In M. Enkin, M. Keirse, J. Renfrew, & J. Neilson (Eds.), Cochrane Database of Systematic Reviews: Pregnancy and Childbirth Modules Review #003298. Oxford: Update Software, Disk Issue 1.

O'Leary, J. A., Mendenhall, H. W., & Andrinopoulos, G. C. (1980). Comparison of auditory versus electronic assessment of antenatal fetal welfare. *Obstetrics & Gynecology, 56*(2), 244–246.

Paine, L. L., Benedict, M. I., Strobino, D. M., Gegor, C. L., & Larson, E. L. (1992). A comparison of the auscultated acceleration test and the nonstress tests as predictors of perinatal outcomes. *Nursing Research, 41*(2), 87–91.

Paine, L. L., Johnson, T. R., Turner, M. H., & Payton, R. G. (1986). Auscultated fetal heart accelerations. Part II. An alternative to the nonstress test. *Journal of Nurse Midwifery, 31*(2), 73–77.

Paine, L. L., Zanardi, L. R., Johnson, T. R., Rorie, J. A., & Barger, M. K. (2001). A comparison of two time intervals for the auscultated acceleration test. *Journal of Midwifery and Women's Health, 46*(2), 98–102.

Parer, J. T. (1997). *Handbook of fetal heart rate monitoring* (2nd ed.). Philadelphia: W.B. Saunders.

Royal College of Obstetricians and Gynaecologists. (2001). The use of electronic fetal monitoring. *The use and interpretation of cardiotocography in intrapartum fetal surveillance.* (Evidence-based Clinical Guideline No. 8). London: Author.

Sakala, C., Declercq, E. R., & Corry, M. P. (2002). Listening to mothers: The first national U.S. survey of women's childbearing experiences. *Journal of Obstetric, Gynecologic, and Neonatal Nursing, 31*(6), 633–634.

Sandelowski, M. (1993). Toward a theory of technology dependence. *Nursing Outlook, 41*(1), 36–42.

Sandelowski, M. (1998). Looking to care or caring to look? Technology and the rise of spectacular nursing. *Holistic Nursing Practice, 12*(4), 1–11.

Sandelowski, M. (2000). Retrofitting technology to nursing: The case of electronic fetal monitoring, *Journal of Obstetric, Gynecologic, and Neonatal Nursing, 29*(3), 316–324.

Schifrin, B., Harwell, R., Rubinstein, T., & Visser, G. (2001). Maternal heart rate pattern: A confounding factor in intrapartum fetal surveillance. *Prenatal and Neonatal Medicine, 6,* 75–82.

Shields, D. (1978). Fetal and maternal monitoring: Maternal reactions to fetal monitoring. *American Journal of Nursing, 78*(12), 2110–2112.

Simpson, K. R., & Creehan, P. (2001). *Perinatal nursing* (2nd ed.). Philadelphia: Lippincott.

Simpson, N., Oppenheimer, L. W., Siren, A., Bland, E., McDonald, O., McDonald, D., & Dabrowski, A. (1999). Accuracy of strategies for monitoring fetal heart rate in labor. *American Journal of Perinatology, 16*(4), 167–173.

Simpson, N., Siren, A., & Oppenheimer, L. (1995). Seeing is believing: The way ahead in fetal auscultation. *Perinatal Newsletter, 12,* 1–4.

Snydal, S. (1988). Responses of laboring women to fetal heart rate monitoring. A critical review of the literature. *Journal of Nurse-Midwifery, 33*(5), 208–216.

Society of Obstetricians and Gynaecologists of Canada (SOGC). (1995). SOGC Policy Statement: Fetal health surveillance in labour. *Journal of Obstetrics and Gynaecology in Canada, 17*(9), 865–901.

Society of Obstetricians, and Gynaecologists of Canada. (2002a). Fetal health surveillance in labour (SOGC Clinical Practice Guidelines No. 112). *Journal of Obstetrics and Gynaecology in Canada, 112*(March), 1–13.

Society of Obstetricians, and Gynaecologists of Canada. (2002b). Fetal health surveillance in labour (SOGC Clinical Practice Guidelines No. 112). *Journal of Obstetrics and Gynaecology in Canada, 112*(April), 1–7.

Strong, T. H., & Paul, R. H. (1989). Intrapartum uterine activity evaluation of an intrauterine pressure catheter. *Obstetrics and Gynecology, 73*(3), 432–434.

Supplee, R. B., & Vezeau, T. M. (1996). Continuous electronic fetal monitoring: Does it belong in low-risk birth? *MCN American Journal of Maternal Child Nursing, 21*(6), 301–306.

Thacker, S. B., Stroup, D. F., & Peterson, H. B. (1995). Efficacy and safety of intrapartum electronic fetal monitoring: An update. *Obstetrics & Gynecology, 86*(4, Pt. 1), 613–620.

Thacker, S. B., Stroup, D. F., & Peterson, H. B. (1997). Continuous electronic fetal monitoring during labor. In J. Neilson, C. Crowther, E. Hodnett, G. Hofmeyr, & M. Keirse (Eds.), Pregnancy and Childbirth Module of the Cochrane Database of Systematic Reviews. Oxford: The Cochrane Collaboration, Issue 2, Update Software.

Thacker, S. B., & Stroup, D. F. (1998). Continuous electronic fetal heart rate monitoring during labor. (Cochrane Review). In: The Cochrane Library, Issue 3. Oxford Update Software.

Tucker, S. M. (2000). *Pocket guide to fetal monitoring and assessment* (4th ed.). St. Louis: Mosby.

Van Geijn, H. P. (1998). Cardiotocography. In A. Kurjak (Ed.), *Textbook of perinatal medicine* (vol. 2, pp. 1424–1428). New York: Parthenon.

Vintzileos, A. M., Nochimson, D. J., Guzman, E. R., Knuppel, R. A., Lake, M., & Schifrin, B. S. (1995). Intrapartum electronic fetal monitoring versus intermittent auscultation: A meta-analysis. *Obstetrics and Gynecology, 85*(1), 149–155.

SECTION FOUR

Fetal Monitoring: Nursing Diagnosis and Intervention

CHAPTER 6

Interpretation of Fetal Heart Rate Patterns

Rebecca L. Cypher
Donna Adelsperger
Keiko L. Torgersen

☞ INTRODUCTION

This chapter provides concepts for nursing process interpretation of fetal heart rate (FHR) characteristics (Figure 6-1). Interpretation includes the systematic analysis of maternal and fetal assessment data essential for collaborative diagnosis and intervention. The physiologic basis of FHR characteristics found on electronic fetal monitoring (EFM) tracings is emphasized.

Intrapartum monitoring of the fetus by either auscultation or continuous EFM can reduce the intrapartum fetal death rate from 1.76/1,000 births (approximately 18 per 10,000 births) to 0.5/1,000 births (5 deaths per 10,000 births) (ACOG, 1995b). By the early part of the last century, auscultation of the fetal heart was commonly used to evaluate fetal status during childbirth. During the past four decades, however, EFM has become the most common method used in North America to assess intrapartum fetal status (AWHONN, 1998a; Albers, 1994, Flamm, 1994). This widespread use of EFM remains controversial; several studies have shown that auscultation during labor and delivery in both low-risk and high-risk pregnancies provides the same outcome for the fetus (Thacker, Stroup, & Peterson, 1998). This chapter focuses on the use and interpretation of EFM data. For an in-depth discussion on auscultation methodology in intrapartum patients see Chapter 5.

The electronic fetal monitor is a piece of equipment that obtains, measures, and records the FHR and uterine activity on a continuing basis. The monitor provides assessment data for the fetus and mother in much the same way as any other automated devices such as a blood pressure cuff and pulse device, or even a hemodynamic monitor. Health care providers who use EFM need to know whether the data generated are valid. Also, the focus is not only on the data the monitor provides but also on the fetal and maternal physiologic status that the data imply. Knowledge of related fetal and maternal physiologic status is important to the interpretation of patterns.

Most professionals involved in interpreting FHR monitoring tracings agree that historically there has been a lack of consensus concerning agreed-upon and reproducible definitions or terminology in clinical trials and clinical practice (Beckmann, Van Mullem, Beckmann, & Broekhuizen, 1997; Lotgering, Wallenburg, & Schouten, 1982).

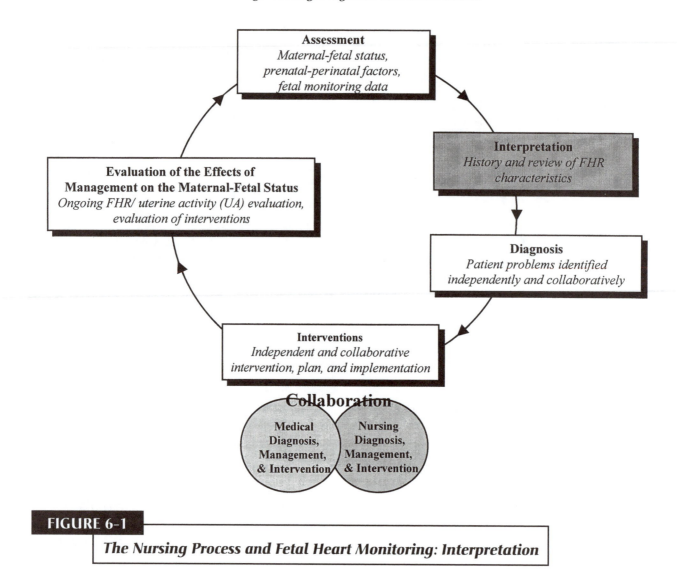

FIGURE 6-1

The Nursing Process and Fetal Heart Monitoring: Interpretation

In addition to the lack of standardized terminology, nonspecific words such as *fetal stress* and *distress* have been commonly used. Because these terms have no definitive meaning, their use to communicate the fetal status or the degree of concern may increase the risk of miscommunication (King & Simpson, 2001). In 1998, the American College of Obstetricians and Gynecologists (ACOG) issued a Committee Opinion on the inappropriate use of the traditional EFM terms fetal distress and birth asphyxia to promote the abandonment of such nonspecific terms (ACOG, 1998). The publication again addressed the obstacles due to the lack of agreed upon terminology and the mischaracterization of the fetal physiologic process when asphyxia is used in written or verbal communication. ACOG also recommended the use of the term *nonreassuring fetal status* rather than *fetal distress* (ACOG, 1998). The term nonreassuring fetal status is discussed in more detail later in this chapter.

In 1995–1996, the U.S. National Institutes of Health and Human Development (NICHD) brought together renowned experts in EFM to dicuss standardized EFM terminology for the purposes of fetal monitoring and assessment research and to recommend areas of future research. In 1997, the NICHD work group published new EFM terminology (or nomenclature) that was based on clinical, laboratory, manufacturing, and published research.

Because further research is needed before universal adoption of the NICHD nomenclature, the FHMPP workshop is presented using the same terminology presented in the second edition of this text. However, the NICHD nomenclature system is very similar to previous definitions and will be discussed in this text (Table 6-1).

Regardless of the practice setting or the terminology, the process of interpreting a FHR monitoring tracing includes (a) examining the tracing for trends of FHR and uterine activity parameters and (b) answering the question "At the present time, what is the likely status of this fetus?" In light of all the current literature, it is important to realize that FHR monitoring is one assessment for fetal well-being and is not a substitute for informed clinical judgment (ACOG, 1995b; SOGC, 2002).

When EFM was introduced more than 30 years ago, its intent (or purpose) was to identify a fetus that was undergoing acute hypoxia or asphyxial tissue damage during labor and delivery. The theory was based on the assumption that a fetus experiencing a hypoxic event would show characteristic patterns or decelerations on the fetal monitor, which would allow the clinician to treat or intervene before asphyxia and cerebral palsy (CP) occurred. Unfortunately, there has been no decrease in the rate of CP in the last 40 years with the use of EFM. Rather, CP rates have remained unchanged for the term fetus, and controversial and limited evidence suggests that the use of EFM in the preterm fetus may increase the number of infants with CP.

It is important to know that EFM does not accurately identify the fetus experiencing hypoxemia and subsequent metabolic derangements of acid-base balance. Interestingly, when nonreassuring features are seen on the EFM monitor, fewer than 50% of fetuses are hypoxemic or have acidemia. The strength of EFM is that it can identify the fetus that is well oxygenated and nonacidotic. When EFM tracings contain either variability (minimal, moderate within normal limits, or marked) or accelerations, the positive predictive value (or accuracy) in confirming the oxygenated and nonacidemic fetus is greater than 99%. Thus, when EFM tracings have one or both of these criteria, it is interpreted as "reassuring."

It also is important to consider that the interpretation of FHR tracings may be confounded by fetal prematurity. Interpreting preterm FHR tracings requires a knowledge of fetal development and underlying fetal and maternal physiologic changes. This section will also provide insight into the interpretation of the preterm FHR tracing.

Various physiologic events may affect uterine or uteroplacental blood flow to the fetus and reduce fetal oxygen (O_2) supply. The fetus may tolerate decreased uterine or umbilical blood flow for a time and even demonstrate a compensatory response as evidenced by a change in the fetal heart response. During such times, the FHR may indicate a physiologic stress; however, the fetus also may continue to demonstrate reassuring factors of fetal well-being, such as the presence of variability, accelerations, or both.

At other times, the O_2 delivery may fall below the critical level needed by the fetus and fetal reserves may be decreased. The FHR shows nonreassuring signs of fetal well-being in those situations. Sometimes, however, it is difficult to determine whether the onset of fetal compromise and nonreassuring pattern has occurred before or during labor.

Health care providers use clinical data about fetal status to plan interventions that promote or maintain fetal well-being or eliminate or lessen physiologic stressors to correct or improve nonreassuring FHR patterns. Recognizing the need for intervention becomes important because physiologic stressors on the mother, the fetus, or both may contribute to nonreassuring patterns.

Specific changes in physiology, especially during the dynamic intrapartum period, may precipitate characteristic FHR patterns. When those characteristic FHR patterns are observed, a related physiologic event is thought to be simultaneously present. With awareness of the event and its effect on the fetal system, health care providers may make more knowledgeable interpretations and clinical decisions. A systematic assessment of the fetal heart rate, with emphasis on the physiologic basis, can provide data to evaluate and confirm fetal well-being and to assist with overall maternal-fetal management (Figure 6-1). Baseline FHR characteristics of rate, variability, and rhythm will be addressed first. A discussion of fetal heart changes from the baseline, including accelerations and decelerations, will follow.

TABLE 6-1

Interpretation of Electronic Fetal Monitoring Data Using NICHD Terminology and Definitions

EFM TERMINOLOGY	DEFINITION
Baseline rate	Mean FHR rounded to increments of 5 bpm during a 10-min period excluding periodic or episodic changes, periods of marked variability, and segments of baseline that differ by > 25 bpm.
Bradycardia	Baseline rate < 110 bpm for > 10 min.
Tachycardia	Baseline rate > 160 bpm for > 10 min.

Variability
• Absent variability
• Minimal variability
• Moderate variablity
• Marked variability
	Fluctuations in the baseline FHR of 2 cycles/min or greater.
	    Amplitude from peak to trough undetectable.
	    Amplitude from peak to trough more than undetectable and < 5 bpm.
	    Amplitude from peak to trough 6–25 bpm.
	    Amplitude from peak to trough > 25 bpm.

Acceleration • Acceleration in preterm gestation < 32 weeks	Visually apparent abrupt increase (onset to peak < 30 sec) of FHR above the baseline. Peak is > 15 bpm. Duration is > 15 sec and < 2 min. Visually apparent abrupt increase (onset to peak < 30 sec) of FHR above the baseline. Peak of 10 bpm. Duration is 10 sec.
Prolonged acceleration	Acceleration > 2 min and < 10 min duration.
Early deceleration	Visually apparent gradual decrease (onset to nadir ≥ 30 sec) of FHR below the baseline. Nadir of deceleration occurs at peak of the contraction. Generally, the onset, nadir, and recovery of the deceleration occur at the same time as the onset, peak, and recovery of the contraction.
Late deceleration	Visually apparent gradual decrease (onset to nadir ≥ 30 sec) of FHR below the baseline. Generally, the onset, nadir, and recovery of the deceleration occur after the onset, peak, and recovery of the contraction.
Variable decelerations	Visually apparent abrupt decrease (onset to nadir < 30 sec) of the FHR below baseline. Decrease is ≥ 15 bpm. Duration is ≥ 15 sec < 2 min.
Prolonged deceleration	Visually apparent abrupt decrease (onset to nadir < 30 sec) in the FHR below the baseline. Decrease is ≥ 15 bpm. Duration is ≥ 2 min < 10 min.

Note: Adapted from "Fetal Assessment During Labor," by T. L. King & K. R. Simpson, 2001, in K. R. Simpson & P. Creehan (Eds.), *Perinatal Nursing* (pp. 378–416). Philadelphia: Lippincott, and from "Electronic Fetal Heart Rate Monitoring: Research Guidelines for Interpretation," National Institutes of Child Health and Human Development Research Planning Workshop, 1997, *Journal of Obstetric, Gynecologic, and Neonatal Nursing, 26*(6), 635–640. Copyright: AWHONN.

☞ FETAL HEART RATE

FHR Baseline Characteristics

Normal Range

The FHR baseline is the approximate mean rate assessed when the mother is not having a contraction and when the fetus is not having periodic or nonperiodic FHR changes. It is assessed for a minimum of 10 minutes. Although various ranges of normal baseline rates have been identified in the past, the currently accepted baseline rate of a term fetus is 110–160 bpm (King & Simpson, 2001; Murray, 1997; Parer, 1997; SOGC, 2002; Tucker, 2000). In the normal fetal heart, the FHR originates in the sinoatrial node (SA node) and sends electronic signals to other areas of the myocardium to coordinate contraction of the chambers and blood flow and, thus, cardiac output. The SA node has an "intrinsic" (or automatic) rate that causes the heart to beat at a normal rate (110–160 bpm at term). The SA node and other areas in the fetal conduction network can be influenced by various physiologic transmitters that produce an increase or decrease in the FHR. The identification of these changes and the knowledge of their individual physiologic bases are the foundation in the interpretation of baseline rates and characteristics. The intrinsic FHR in very early gestation (15–20 weeks) is significantly higher than it is at term (Garite, 2002). The heart rate of premature fetuses at gestations of 26–28 weeks may approach the upper range of normal but does not usually exceed 160 bpm. The health care provider may notice a slight but gradual decrease of the FHR baseline as gestational age increases.

The normal baseline FHR can be obtained by several different methods, the more common being auscultation, ultrasound/Doppler, or direct electrocardiogram (ECG) modalities. For a discussion of these methods, refer to Techniques of Fetal Heart Monitoring, in Chapter 5. In continuous EFM, the baseline FHR is measured by assessing the FHR tracing for a minimum of 10 minutes and observing a sustained average (mean) rate. Sustained (≥10 minutes) increases and decreases from the normal baseline rate are called tachycardia and bradycardia, respectively.

Tachycardia

Tachycardia is defined as a FHR above 160 bpm that lasts for at least 10 minutes. Tachycardia represents increased sympathetic and decreased parasympathetic autonomic tone and, therefore, is generally associated with a normal loss of FHR baseline variability (Freeman, Garite, & Nageotte, 1991). The fetus may or may not demonstrate variability for a period of time with mild tachycardia of 160–180 bpm.

It also is important to watch for gradual increases in the FHR that can occur over time, even when the FHR does not exceed 160 bpm, as this increase in rate may occur prior to a baseline tachycardia. Further assessment of the fetus with baseline tachycardia includes evaluating variability, identifying the presence or absence of accelerations and decelerations, and noting the duration of any observed pattern (Figure 6-2). Fortunately, tachycardia in a term fetus is usually benign (Freeman, et al., 1991).

The causes of tachycardia are most often related to maternal fever or to infection in the mother, fetus, or both. Other causes are hypoxemia, anemia, cardiac dysrhythmias, and congenital anomalies (King & Simpson, 2001). Maternal causes of FHR tachycardia are as follows:

◆ Fever

◆ Infection

◆ Dehydration

◆ Hyperthermia

◆ Hyperthyroidism

◆ Endogenous adrenaline or anxiety

◆ Medication or drug response
  • Ketamine, atropine, and phenothiazines
  • Hydroxyzine (Vistaril® and Atarax®)
  • Betasympathomimetics (terbutaline and ritodrine)
  • Sympathomimetic bronchodilators used in asthma patients: albuterol and so forth
  • Epinephrine
  • Selected positive inotropes (e.g., dobutamine and positive chronotropic drugs)
  • Over-the-counter medications (e.g., decongestants, appetite suppressants, and stimulants or caffeine)

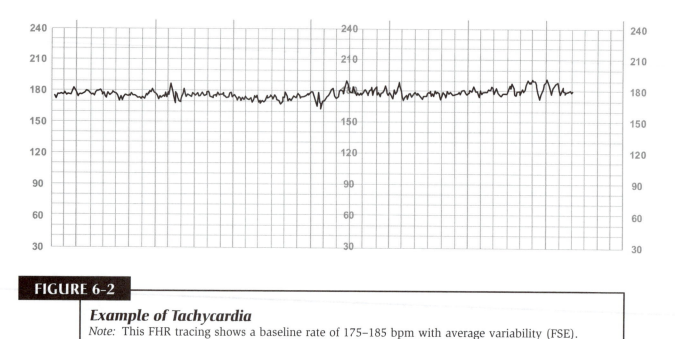

FIGURE 6-2

Example of Tachycardia
Note: This FHR tracing shows a baseline rate of 175–185 bpm with average variability (FSE).

◆ Illicit drugs (e.g., cocaine, amphetamines)

◆ Anemia

◆ Nicotine if inhaled (Nicotine is now thought to have a complex effect on FHR. If inhaled by smoking, nicotine may increase the FHR; however, if absorbed through a nicotine patch, it may decrease FHR) (Muller, Antunes, Behle, Teixeira, & Zielinsky, 2002; Oncken, Kranzler, O'Malley, Gendreau, & Campbell, 2002; Oncken et al., 1997)

Fetal causes include the following:

◆ Infection

◆ Activity or stimulation

◆ Compensatory effort following acute hypoxemia

◆ Chronic hypoxemia

◆ Fetal hyperthyroidism

◆ Fetal tachyarrhythmias (e.g., supraventricular tachycardia)

◆ Prematurity

◆ Congenital abnormalities

◆ Cardiac abnormalities or heart failure

◆ Anemia

Most importantly, tachycardia may be a sign of early fetal hypoxemia, especially when associated with decreasing variability and periodic changes such as variable and/or late decelerations. When tachycardia persists over 200–220 bpm (tachyarrhythmia) for an extended period of time, fetal hydrops or demise may occur. More information on these types of patterns is discussed in Chapter 13, Fetal Arrhythmias and Dysrhythmias.

Bradycardia

Bradycardia is defined as a FHR baseline less than 110 bpm that lasts for more than 10 minutes (Figure 6-3). Bradycardia accompanied by adequate variability may be a normal variant for the fetus. Fetuses that have physiologic bradycardia during labor are typically bradycardic in the nursery but are otherwise well oxygenated and normal (Garite, 2002). Average variability is less likely to be present when the FHR persists below 90 bpm for more than 10 minutes. If variability is present with bradycardia, the bradycardia can be considered

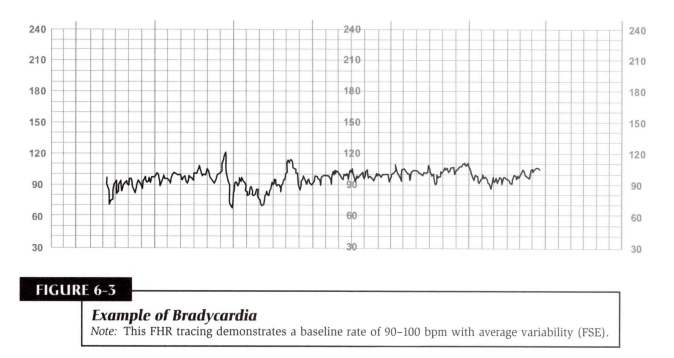

FIGURE 6-3

Example of Bradycardia
Note: This FHR tracing demonstrates a baseline rate of 90–100 bpm with average variability (FSE).

benign or reassuring (Freeman, et al., 1991). Conversely, bradycardia with loss of variability and late decelerations may be predictive of current or impending fetal hypoxia (NICHD Research Planning Workshop, 1997).

Fetal cardiac output (the amount of blood pumped out of both ventricles each minute) depends on the FHR because the immature fetal heart does not effectively alter stroke volume when additional cardiac output is needed. In the presence of bradycardia, the inability of the fetus to alter its cardiac output significantly increases the likelihood of inadequate O_2 delivery. It is important to understand that oxygenation and O_2 delivery are separate concepts. Oxygenation is the general term, and O_2 delivery is a specific variable in the overall process. The more the heart rate decreases, the lower the fetal cardiac output will be. Decreased cardiac output may ultimately decrease umbilical blood flow, which may result in insufficient O_2 transport and eventually fetal hypoxia (Parer, 1997). An exception to this physiologic process is congenital complete heart block (CCHB), which typically produces a fetal ventricular rate of approximately 60–70 bpm in the second trimester and approximately 50–60 bpm at term (Eronen, Heikkila, & Teramo, 2001). CCHB

may be associated with normal oxygenation although the physiologic mechanism is poorly understood. CCHB often is associated with maternal antiphospholipid antibody syndrome and clinical or serologic evidence of maternal collagen vascular disease, specifically systemic lupus erythematosus (Hohn & Stanton, 2002; Tucker, 2000). Fetuses that manifest CCHB in utero frequently require electrical cardiac pacing at birth and are at high risk for morbidity and mortality. Bradycardia is evaluated in conjunction with FHR variability and reactivity, as well as the severity and persistence of the bradycardia. Differentiating between a persistent bradycardic rate and a prolonged deceleration also helps to evaluate fetal status. It also is important to differentiate between fetal and maternal heart rates when assessing a persistent bradycardic rate. The maternal heart rate may be recorded rather than the fetal rate in both internal and external modes. To verify the FHR or to differentiate it from the maternal rate, real-time ultrasound may be used. Additionally, palpation of the maternal apical pulse and comparison to the FHR detected with EFM may be helpful to differentiate between the two if there is a significant difference in the rates. When there is not a significant difference between the two rates, an electronic fetal monitor that has the capability to continuously measure and record the maternal HR on the same channel as the FHR may be used to differentiate the two heart rates if available.

The etiology of bradycardia is frequently attributed to the fetal response to hypoxia. However, there are also nonhypoxic etiologies. The following maternal causes of fetal bradycardia have been identified:

◆ Supine position

◆ Hypotension

◆ Adrenergic-receptor blocking drugs (Propranolol)

◆ Connective tissue disease (systemic lupus erythematosus)

◆ Prolonged maternal hypoglycemia

◆ Anesthetics (e.g., epidural, spinal, pudendal, or paracervical)

◆ Conditions that cause acute maternal cardiopulmonary compromise (e.g., pulmonary embolus, amniotic fluid embolus, cerebral vascular events, uterine rupture, trauma)

Fetal causes of bradycardia include:

◆ Mature parasympathetic nervous system (PSNS)

◆ Umbilical cord occlusion (e.g., prolapsed cord)

◆ Acute hypoxemia

◆ Hypothermia

◆ CCHB

◆ Cardiac structural defect (caused by maternal cytomegolovirus infection interfering or damaging fetal heart formation)

◆ Excessive PSNS tone produced by chronic head compression in a vertex presentation, occiput posterior, or transverse position (vagal stimulation). The FHR usually does not decrease to less than 90–100 bpm in this instance.

◆ Late or profound hypoxemia

Variability

Variability includes the variations or fluctuations of the FHR during a steady state (in the absence of contractions, decelerations, and accelerations). The fetal heart produces an intrinsic (or automatic) rate that is influenced or controlled by the autonomic nervous system. The two divisions of the autonomic nervous system have opposite effects on the FHR; the sympathetic branch (cardioaccelerator) increases the heart rate, and the parasympathetic branch (cardiodecelerator or cardioinhibitor) decreases the heart rate. The constant "push-and-pull" effect on the FHR from sympathetic and parasympathetic neurotransmitters produces a moment-to-moment change in the FHR called variability. Because variability is in essence the combined result of autonomic nervous system branch function, its presence implies that both the sympathetic and parasympathetic branches are working and are oxygenated. Therefore, variability is one of the two most important characteristics of the FHR (accelerations are the other characteristic).

Physiology of Variability

Variability is derived from impulses of the medulla's sympathetic and parasympathetic nervous systems. Nerve fibers from these systems innervate (or connect) from the brain to the myocardium and SA and atrioventricular (AV) nodes, respectively (see Figure 3-3 in Chapter 3). The status of the brain stem's medulla oblongata, therefore, controls nerve fiber innervation to the heart and, thus, has a direct effect on variability. Influences that alter variability through the medulla are fetal oxygenation status, cardiac output regulation, fetal behavior during sleep and awake states, humoral regulation, and drug effects (Freeman, et al., 1991; Martin, 1982; Parer, 1997; Petrie, 1991). Normal variability of the FHR is a reflection of neurologic modulation of the FHR, normal cardiac responsiveness, and normal acid-base equilibrium (Freeman, et al., 1991; Rosen & Dickinson, 1993; Tucker, 2000). An anencephalic or hydrocephalic fetus without an intact medulla will exhibit minimal and absent variability regardless of fetal oxygenation state.

A transient fetal hypoxemia may stimulate chemoreceptors, which increase catecholamines, thereby circulating dopamine, and increase peripheral vascular resistance; cardiac output improves, thereby improving blood flow to the brain, heart, and adrenal glands. In this example, the presence of variability (LTV and STV) represents an intact neuromodulation of the FHR and normal cardiac responsiveness. Variability may increase with fetal breathing and hemodynamic changes; variability may increase or decrease with fetal sleep states. The quiet sleep state elicits fewer variability cycles, and the rapid eye movement (REM) sleep state elicits more variability (Martin, 1982). Additional fetal states may be integrated into the central nervous system (CNS) through the hypothalamus and sympathetic response exhibiting changes in variability oscillations, blood pressure, baroreflex, and heart rate (Parer, 1999).

Key points on variability include the following:

◆ Oxygenation of the CNS influences impulse transmission to the FHR.

◆ Adequate oxygenation and a mature and functioning autonomic nervous system contribute to the production of variability (LTV and STV).

◆ Absent or decreased variability may be due to a preterm gestation (< 28–32 weeks), alteration in the nervous system function, inadequate oxygenation, or by both.

◆ Alterations of fetal nervous system function are associated with normal fetal sleep and wake states; medications (especially CNS depressants such as magnesium sulfate $MgSO_4$), alcohol, and illicit drugs that cause fetal neurological damage thus affecting variability; morphine (Kopecky, et al., 2000); methadone (Anyaegbunam, Tran, Jadali, Randolph, & Mikhail, 1997); anomalies; and previous insults that have damaged the fetal brain (Wadhwa, Sandman, & Garite, 2001).

Identification and Measurement of Variability

Variability of the FHR is defined as the change in the heart rate over short and extended periods of time. The fetal heart has an automatic (intrinsic) rate that will be produced automatically at a rate of 110–160 bpm. If the heart does not receive any signals or transmissions from the fetal CNS, the FHR may remain in the "normal" baseline range, but it will appear flat or smooth on the tracing. Conversely, when the fetal heart is constantly being bombarded with messages and signals from the fetal CNS, the FHR will appear very irregular (jagged or rough). The sympathetic and parasympathetic branches of the fetal autonomic nervous system are primarily responsible for the irregular appearance; they work in a "push" and "pull" manner on the FHR by simultaneously telling the heart to speed up and slow down. The irregularities in the FHR baseline on both a second-to-second basis and on a longer minute-to-minute basis are called variability and are described as the fluctuations in the baseline FHR of 2 cycles/min or greater.

Clinically according to NICHD nomenclature, variability is described and communicated as a unit that is the summation of the fetal LTV and STV. When variability is described as one entity (i.e., variability versus LTV and STV), it still remains important to understand the physiologic basis of both LTV and STV.

Long-Term Variability

LTV is a characteristic of the baseline FHR and is characterized by fluctuations or oscillations in the FHR that are described as cycles per minute. The cycles portray the amplitude or rise and fall of the heart rate within its baseline range (Figures 6-4, 6-5, and 6-6). The frequency of the fluctuations of LTV can be determined by counting (a) the number of complete cycles per minute, (b) the number of turning points, or (c) the number of crossings over an imaginary line within 1 minute (Martin, 1982; Petrie, 1991). When LTV is measured for the amplitude and the number of cycles per minute, accelerations and decelerations are not included in the process.

LTV Categories

Different categories have been used to describe LTV. Each category defines a range of change in

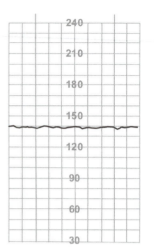 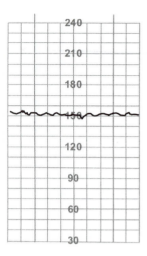

FIGURE 6-4A

Example of Decreased or Minimal LTV (Absent Variability) (External Ultrasound)

FIGURE 6-4B

Example of Decreased or Minimal LTV (Minimal Variability) (External Ultrasound)

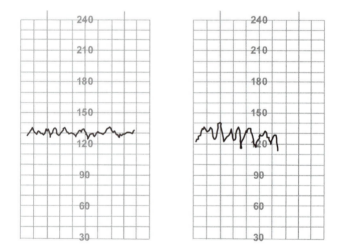

FIGURE 6-5

Two Examples Demonstrating Fetuses with Average or Within Normal Limits LTV (Moderate Variability) (External Ultrasound)

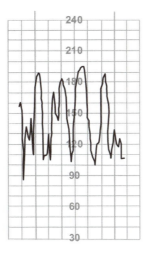

FIGURE 6-6

This Fetus is Exhibiting Marked or Saltatory LTV (Marked Variability) (External Ultrasound)

the heart rate from its baseline in bpm. Because this deviation from the baseline FHR is expressed in bpm, it is referred to as the amplitude. Consensus has yet to be achieved across the fetal monitoring community on categories of LTV. Fortunately, the LTV categories definitions presented in the FHMPP workshop correspond to the NICHD definitions for combined variability (Table 6-2).

Average or Moderate

Average or moderate LTV values of the FHR amplitude are described as 6–25 bpm, and the frequency of fluctuations or cycles as 3–6/min (Hammacher, 1969; Martin, 1982; Parer, 1997; King & Simpson, 2001). The fetal wake state, behavioral state, and responsiveness result in variations within this relatively wide average range. The presence of LTV indicates fetal oxygenation and the physiologic ability to compensate for stress (Tucker, 2000). Average LTV may indicate an awake, active fetus responding to the environment.

Decreased or Minimal

Decreased LTV may occur spontaneously or temporarily when the fetus is in a sleep cycle. When LTV is decreased or absent, it may also be signifi-

cant for presence of hypoxia or acidosis, which creates a challenge in interpretation for the health care provider. It is important for the health care provider to consider the entire clinical picture when determining the meaning of the findings (Menihan & Zottoli, 2001). In the presence of nonreassuring heart rate patterns, decreased FHR variability is associated with a high incidence of acidosis and low Apgar scores (Freeman, et al., 1991). In the absence of nonreassuring FHR patterns, decreased LTV is generally associated with an oxygenated fetus that has a benign decreased neurotransmission to the fetal heart. The fetus with associated depressed or reduced fetal brain function will most likely demonstrate decreased variability (Garite, 2002).

Interventions indicated for a persistent decrease in LTV, 0–2 bpm or 3–5 bpm range, are usually the same and will depend on individual maternal and fetal conditions. Therefore, it is clinically appropriate to consider 0–5 bpm change as a single category of LTV. When the duration of the pattern lasts longer than a fetal sleep cycle and the FHR remains nonreactive or does not react to stimulation, further nursing assessments and interventions may be considered. Fetal behavioral states alone can have a tremendous influence on

TABLE 6-2

Correlation of LTV Categories with NICHD Nomenclature

AMPLITUDE OF FHR CHANGE	DESCRIPTION	LTV CATEGORY	NICHD CATEGORY
< 3 bpm	Undetectable	Decreased or minimal	Absent variability
3–5 bpm	> Undetectable but ≤5 bpm	Decreased or minimal	Minimal variability
6–25 bpm	6–25 bpm	Average or within in normal limits	Moderate variability
> 25 bpm	> 25 bpm	Marked or saltatory	Marked variability

Note: Adapted from "Electronic Fetal Heart Rate Monitoring: Research Guidelines for Interpretation," National Institutes of Child Health and Human Development Research Planning Workshop, 1997, *Journal of Obstetric, Gynecologic, and Neonatal Nursing, 26*(6), 635–640. Copyright by Association of Women's Health, Obstetric, and Neonatal Nurses. Adapted with permission.

variability. Although more than 50% of fetal sleep cycles last fewer than 40 minutes, some fetuses will have sleep cycles lasting 80–90 minutes or more. Prior to initiating interventions with the onset of decreased variability, it is appropriate to review and evaluate the gestational age, fetal heart response, behavioral state, response to stimulation, and the total clinical picture (e.g., medications, narcotics, anomalies). The presence of decreased LTV alone does not predict a fetus experiencing hypoxemia or acidemia. When decreased LTV alone is present on admission and is not followed by any periods of average or normal LTV, the clinician may suspect a preexisting CNS event or prior fetal exposure to CNS-altering conditions. Refer to Chapter 3 for more detailed information on fetal behavioral states.

Marked or Saltatory

Marked or saltatory LTV is described as an amplitude range greater than 25 bpm. The pattern is often chaotic in appearance. The precise etiology of marked LTV etiology is uncertain even though it is noted to be primarily an intrapartum pattern (Parer, 1997; Petrie, 1991; Murray, 1997). Marked variability may be a compensatory mechanism and possibly an early sign of fetal hypoxia (Garite,

2002; Tucker, 2000). Conversely, clinical studies have shown that marked variability is associated with normal umbilical cord blood gases at an immediate delivery following the pattern. (O'Brien-Abel & Benedetti, 1992). Therefore, any interventions to resolve a marked or saltatory pattern should be patient specific (see Chapter 7).

Short-Term Variability

STV is defined as the moment-to-moment changes (reflecting R-to-R intervals) in the FHR that, when printed on the fetal monitor tracing, generally produce a small, irregular nature of the baseline. The presence of STV usually indicates a well-oxygenated, nonacidemic fetus. Within the autonomic nervous system, the parasympathetic nervous system (PSNS) has the greater influence on FHR variability when compared with the sympathetic branch. The parasympathetic influences occur much more rapidly than the sympathetic influences and are responsible for fine-tuning the fetal heart's STV or beat-to-beat intervals. The comparative sympathetic response time lag is 2–3 seconds, and the return to baseline is even slower (Martin, 1982). When stressed the fetal medulla will produce epinephrine and norepinephrine. These act on the fetal heart similar to sympathetic nervous system (SNS) stimulation, that is, the FHR increases, fetal heart contractility is stronger, and the arterial blood pressure increases (Parer, 1999). In the presence of hypoxia, impulse transmission is decreased, which results in decreased variability as the fetal compensatory mechanisms have failed to maintain fetal cerebral oxygenation (Parer, 1999). STV alone is believed to also be an important prognostic indicator of fetal outcome.

STV Assessment

With a spiral electrode placed on the fetus, the R-to-R interval of subsequent fetal cardiac cycles can be measured. This type of FHR measurement typically provides an accurate assessment of FHR and allows STV to be assessed (Garite, 2002). STV reflects changes in the FHR from one beat to the next beat. Time intervals between individual fetal heart beats are measured and computed, and the number value represents a calculated one-minute rate. When an external ultrasound transducer is placed on the maternal abdomen, the FHR is acquired by ultrasound or Doppler technology. Since the advent of the EFM, there have been great advances in the clinical and technical performance of the transducer. In the mid- to late-1980s, external FHR devices were produced with a type of software called *autocorrelation*. This advance in the measuring and recording of FHRs on the upper channel of the monitor paper significantly improved the visual recording by excluding erroneous information. In the late 1990s, continued improvement in the ultrasonography transducers included the addition of numerous transmitters and receivers on the USG device and of improved software, which better differentiated fetal gross body movements from FHR motion. This continued improvement in signal acquisition technology has prompted clinicians to use the information recorded with the USG as a representation of STV. It is important to remember, however, that when the external signal is incomplete or the absolute knowledge of STV is essential in the plan of care, the application of the spiral electrode will provide the more accurate measurement of STV. For most labors, the absolute verification of STV is not indicated, and clinical use of visual baseline variability is frequently adequate in interpreting the EFM data.

STV Characteristics

Fetal cardiac cycles are a continuing cycle of electrical impulses that produce and coordinate the individual chambers of the fetal heart to beat and pump blood to the body. These electrical impulses have individual features that can be identified on an ECG recording. Similar to the electrical conduction impulses of an adult, fetal electrical conduction impulses are labeled as the P wave, the QRS complex, and the T wave. When measuring a rate for the contracting heart, ECG technology uses the fetal R wave of the QRS complex. This wave is used because it is the easiest component of the cardiac cycle to identify and to measure the time from one R wave to the next R wave. This R-to-R interval is measured in milliseconds and is used in measuring and printing the FHR signal on the EFM tracing when a direct (spiral) electrode is used. Fetal heart cardiac cycles are influenced by internal and external stimuli that result in a constantly changing FHR. This constant change causes the recorded line of the FHR tracing to appear rough or squiggly, indicating the tiny increases and decreases in the rate over a period of time. Because this short-term interval is changing constantly in the healthy fetus, the numbers change continuously on the digital display of the monitor. It is difficult to numerically quantify these small changes visualized on the tracing into specific levels or categories. Because of the rapid and sometimes subtle nature of these changes, the more accurate method to assess STV is with internal, continuous fetal monitoring (ACOG, 1995b; May & Mahlmeister, 1994).

The most practical way to determine the presence or absence of STV is by direct visualization. Direct visualization is accomplished by examining the characteristics of the fetal heart tracing line and evaluating the tracing for roughness or smoothness (Figure 6-7). When the tracing appears rough, the term *present* may be used to describe STV. The term *absent* may be used to denote a smooth line (Figure 6-7).

Interpretation of FHR Variability

Variability (LTV and STV) provides useful information on the status of the fetus. The physiologic

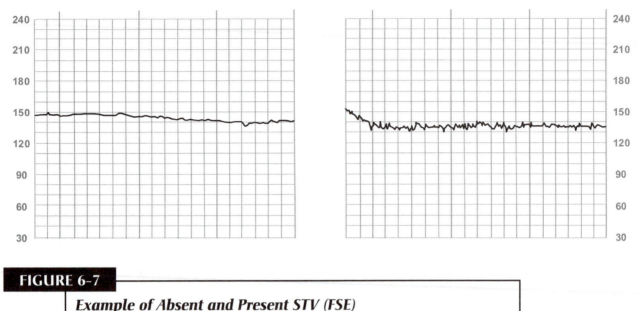

FIGURE 6-7

Example of Absent and Present STV (FSE)

Note: The first tracing depicts a fetus with absent STV. The second tracing depicts a fetus with present STV.

components of LTV and STV are interrelated and work in symphony to produce the appearance of the recorded tracing. Because of this relationship, LTV and STV can be interpreted and described as a single entity (see Table 6-3). This concept of "combined variability" makes no distinction between STV and LTV but rather encourages the visual interpretation of the visual amplitude of the complexes. Individual categories of variability are identified by visual recognition, which involves matching the pattern to a picture template of variability categories. Interestingly, visual recognition is more sensitive as an assessment parameter when compared with numerical data and rates and has significantly more reproducibility and agreement among different interpreters (Figure 6-8).

Factors to consider in analyzing variability may include the following:

◆ The presence of baseline variability is one of most reassuring findings in EFM because it confirms that the fetus is not in metabolic acidosis and is well oxygenated at the moment.

◆ Generally, LTV and STV change simultaneously, producing a uniform change in the combined or overall variability of the baseline. However, there are times when one may or may not be present with the other. There are times when STV is absent and LTV is present (e.g., sinusoidal or undulating patterns) and, conversely, there are times when LTV is decreased and STV is present (e.g., a sleeping fetus).

◆ A smooth FHR baseline (absent variability) that is present on admission and that does not change to a baseline with variability may be related to chronic fetal hypoxemia, a central nervous system anomaly, a cardiovascular anomaly, and/or a preexisting fetal brain injury or insult.

◆ The presence of FHR variability with deceleration patterns indicates the presence of fetal reserves and usually confirms that the fetus remains oxygenated and is not in a deteriorating metabolic acidemia.

◆ Absent variability of the FHR in combination with late or variable decelerations that persist over time and/or bradycardia may point toward impending acidemia or hypoxemia, which requires further assessment (as long as

TABLE 6-3

Baseline Variability Categories (When Described as One Entity)

CATEGORY	DEFINITION
Absent variability	Amplitude from peak to trough undetectable
Minimal variability	Amplitude from peak to trough more than undetectable and < 5 bpm
Moderate variability	Amplitude from peak to trough 6–25 bpm
Marked variability	Amplitude from peak to trough > 25 bpm

Note: From "Electronic Fetal Heart Rate Monitoring: Research Guidelines for Interpretation," National Institutes of Child Health and Human Development Research Planning Workshop, 1997, *Journal of Obstetric, Gynecologic, and Neonatal Nursing, 26*(6), 635–640. Copyright: AWHONN.

variability is visually apparent— > 3 bpm—the fetus usually is not in metabolic acidemia and remains centrally oxygenated).

When there is a change in the variability, the following questions may assist with the interpretations:

◆ Was the fetus previously active and was LTV within normal limits?

◆ Could the fetus be in a temporary sleep pattern?

◆ If variability can be evaluated, is it present?

◆ Does the fetus respond to stimuli?

Undulating Patterns

Undulating variations in the FHR baseline are defined as repeating cycles or changes in the FHR that result in an upward increase in the rate followed by a decrease in the rate. These increases and decreases from an imaginary baseline are equal and resemble a sine or radio wave. The pattern is distinctive, with a baseline rate that usually is stable within normal range, a frequency of 2–5 cycles/minute and an amplitude of the undulations being 5–15 bpm above and below the baseline. This pattern is often described as either *sinusoidal* or *pseudosinusoidal.* It is sometimes difficult to differentiate one from the other. Hence,

the word *undulating* describes the characteristic shape of the wave and may be used when sinusoidal waves cannot be visually distinguished from pseudosinusoidal waves. In a true sinusoidal pattern, the undulating nature of the pattern does not represent normal variability.

This pattern has been associated with hypoxia and is most often seen in the presence of severe fetal anemia (Garite, 2002) (Figure 6-9). The specific physiologic mechanism that produces the sinusoidal baseline is unknown, but several maternal-fetal conditions have been associated with this pattern, including fetal-maternal hemorrhage, placental abruption, and fetal anemia associated with Rh isoimmunization (King & Simpson, 2001; Parer, 1997).

The less smooth and less constant type of undulating pattern, which appears following maternal analgesic administration, is thought to be benign and is often called pseudosinusoidal or false sinusoidal. In contrast to true sinusoidal baselines, oscillations above and below the baseline are typically unequal, and normal variability and fetal reactivity may be present (Figure 6-10). This pattern has been described as appearing "sawtoothed" and has been noted to occur following maternal administration of narcotics such as Stadol® and Demerol®. In addition to CNS depressants, fetal behaviors such as thumb sucking may produce this pattern.

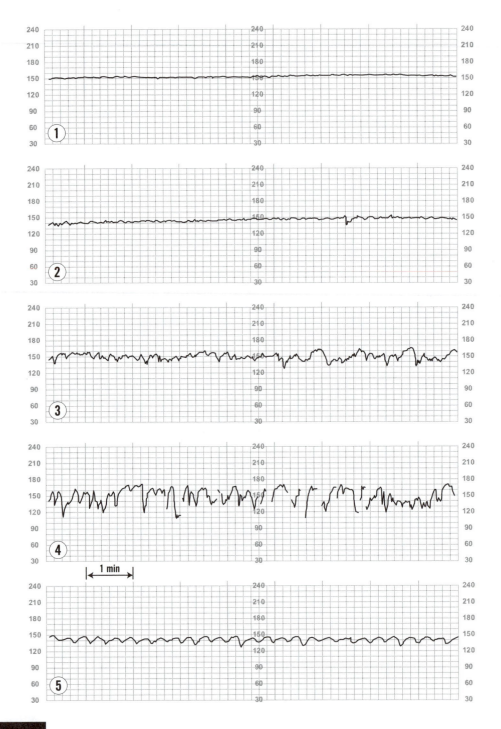

FIGURE 6-8

Visual Variability Scale

From "Electronic Fetal Heart Rate Monitoring: Research Guidelines for Interpretation," National Institutes of Child Health and Human Development Research Planning Workshop, 1997, *Journal of Obstetric, Gynecologic, and Neonatal Nursing, 26*(6), 635–640. Copyright: AWHONN.

Note: Varying degress of FHR variability. 1, Undetectable; 2, minimal; 3, moderate; 4, marked; and 5, the sinusoidal pattern. Original scaling, 30 bmp per cm vertical axis, and paper speed 3 cm-min^{-1} horizontal axis.

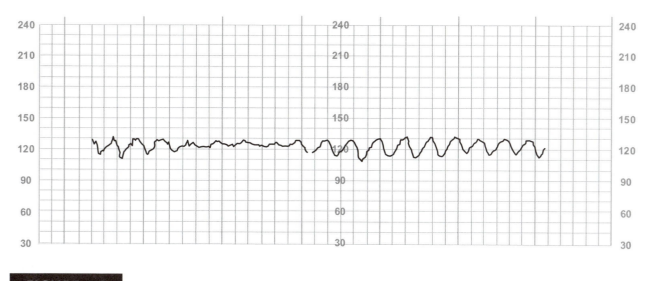

FIGURE 6-9

Example of Sinusoidal Pattern Associated with Fetal-Maternal Hemorrhage (FSE)

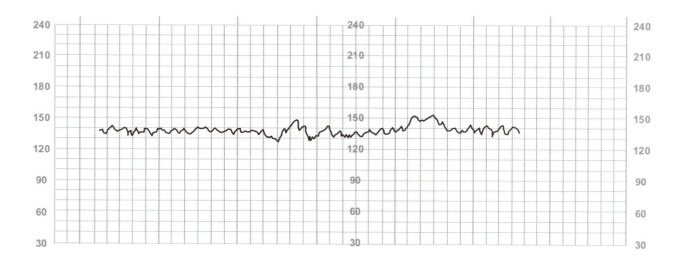

FIGURE 6-10

Example of an Undulating, Pseudosinusoidal Pattern with Normal Periods of Variability and Reactivity (FSE)

Characteristics of Sinusoidal Patterns

Sinusoidal patterns have the following characteristics:

1. Oscillating pattern is persistent: 110–160 bpm (in the shape of a sine wave).
2. Amplitude of undulations is usually 5–15 bpm above and below the baseline.
3. Frequency of undulations is usually 2–5 cycles/minute.
4. STV is absent.
5. There are no fetal accelerations, even in response to fetal movement or stimulation.

Events Associated with a Sinusoidal Pattern

Events associated with a sinusoidal pattern include the following:

1. Severe fetal anemia
   - Rh isoimmunization
   - Abruptio placentae
   - Fetal-maternal hemorrhage
   - Severe fetal acidosis
2. Unknown etiology

Characteristics of Pseudosinusoidal Patterns

1. "Saw-toothed" appearances: 110–160 bpm
2. Less uniform oscillations
3. Periods of normal variability (LTV, STV).
4. Accelerations may be present

Events Associated with Pseudosinusoidal Patterns

1. Narcotic administration or ingestion
2. Analgesic administration
3. Fetal thumb sucking
4. Unknown etiology

Further Considerations for Undulating Fetal Patterns

Actions and interventions are most commonly based on the patient's history and/or clinical suspicion. The following is a list of interventions that can individually be implemented based on the patient's status:

1. Assess current and previous EFM data for area of normal baseline.
2. Assess maternal-fetal history to identify and rule out the fetus at risk (e.g., Rh-negative mother with Rh sensitization).
3. Continue to monitor the pseudosinusoidal pattern.
4. Consider ultrasonography to evaluate for fetal cardiac failure (e.g., hydropic appearance).
5. Perform Kleihauer-Betke test on maternal serum or alpha-fetoprotein test of vaginal blood to detect fetal red blood cells.
6. Prepare for additional testing, possible intrauterine transfusion of the fetus, surgical delivery, and intensive neonatal care or transport to level-III facility.

The literature reports that sinusoidal patterns due to anemia have been reversed following fetal transfusion or postdelivery neonatal exchange transfusions (Modanlou & Freeman, 1982; Murray, 1997; Parer, 1997).

Although undulating patterns have been discussed under variability, the sinusoidal pattern is excluded from the definition of FHR variability (Parer, 1997). Undulating patterns are included here because they are evaluated when assessing baseline rate and variability.

☞ RHYTHM

Rhythm describes the regularity or irregularity of the FHR. The rhythm may be auscultated by the care provider or recorded on the EFM tracing when the spiral electrode is used. It is annotated as regular or irregular.

As more sophisticated technology is used to assess the fetal heart rhythm, more information can be obtained about the presence and nature of an irregular heartbeat or dysrhythmia. The irregular heartbeat may be differentiated from possible artifact or electronic interference by verification using a technique such as auscultation, ultrasound scan, echocardiogram, or ECG. This will determine the type of dysrhythmia present or rule out artifact (Feinstein, Sprague, & Trepanier, 2000).

With an auscultation device such as a fetoscope or Pinard stethoscope, the caregiver can hear the actual heart sounds to determine if the rate is regular or irregular. If the fetal spiral electrode (FSE) is used, actual cardiac electrical impulses are detected. An irregular rhythm can be heard with a Doppler device, but the sound generated is not the actual heart sound. Instead, the sound is a mechanical representation of the heart rate, which is based on heart movement as sound waves from the fetal heart valves and walls are reflected back to the ultrasound device (Tucker, 2000; Feinstein, et al., 2000).

Information transmitted by the spiral electrode mode often will illustrate a distinctive irregularity on the tracing, particularly if the logic button (signal filter) is disabled, depending on the machine. The FSE mode will graph an irregularity that must first be differentiated from possible artifact or electronic interference by verification with some other technique, such as auscultation, ultrasound scan, or echocardiogram. Some manufacturers have placed the option of obtaining a printed recording of the fetal ECG directly onto the tracing when an internal electrode is being used. This feature may be useful in evaluating an irregular fetal rhythm. Most irregularities in the FHR display an organized pattern that distinguishes them from the chaotic appearance of artifact.

🖥 PERIODIC AND NONPERIODIC PATTERNS

As the FHR accelerates and decelerates away from the baseline rate in direct relation to uterine contractions and persists over a period of time, the response is classified as a periodic pattern or a periodic change. The pattern may receive a descriptive label and a presumed underlying physiology on the basis of its appearance. For example, alterations of fetal blood flow through the umbilical cord or alterations of the uteroplacental unit are presumed on the basis of their characteristic pattern appearances. Periodic changes include accelerations and the three types of decelerations: early, late, and variable.

Deceleration and acceleration patterns may appear to be unassociated with uterine contractions. When this transpires, the event or pattern is described as nonperiodic. Accelerations are

the most common nonperiodic FHR event (Figure 6-11).

Accelerations

Acceleration Definition

Accelerations are abrupt, transient increases in the FHR above the baseline. The NICHD defines accelerations as a visually abrupt increase (onset to peak < 30 seconds) above the baseline FHR (NICHD Research Planning Workshop, 1997). They can be periodic or nonperiodic. The amplitude, or peak of the increase, is 15 beats or greater above the baseline and continues for a minimum of 15 seconds but not longer than 2 minutes (King & Simpson, 2001; NICHD Research Planning Workshop, 1997; Parer, 1997). Earlier gestations, usually before 32 weeks, have less frequent accelerations with lower amplitude because of the immature autonomic nervous system. Before 32 weeks, the acceleration is defined as having amplitude of 10 bpm above the baseline with duration of at least 10 seconds (Garite, 2002; King & Simpson, 2001; NICHD Research Planning Workshop, 1997; Tucker, 2000). Note that once accelerations are demonstrated, the fetus should be able to maintain this ability to accelerate its heart rate for the remainder of the gestation. Accelerations are benign patterns, identify a well-oxygenated fetus, and require no interventions. Although accelerations usually do not last longer than 2 minutes, multiple accelerations may coalesce and appear as though there has been a change in FHR baseline.

Periodic accelerations may occur simultaneously with the uterine contraction and are usually smooth in configuration. A periodic acceleration may be biphasic or triphasic and may be the forerunner of a variable deceleration pattern. Nonperiodic accelerations do not occur in a consistent pattern but rather occur in response to environmental stimuli or fetal activity. This type of acceleration is often peaked or abrupt and is associated with the active fetus that is nonacidotic and oxygenated. Regardless of when they occur, accelerations are one of the most reassuring findings in EFM because their presence confirms that the fetus is well oxygenated and is not in metabolic acidemia.

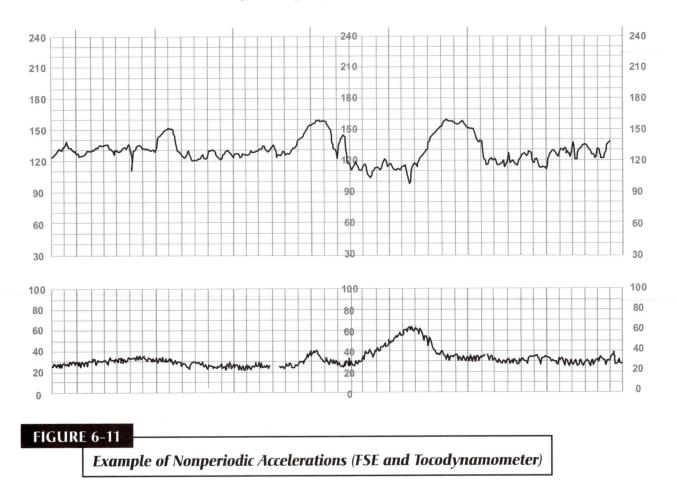

FIGURE 6-11

Example of Nonperiodic Accelerations (FSE and Tocodynamometer)

Acceleration Physiology

Periodic accelerations are accelerations that occur with contractions. There are currently several theories that explain the etiology. One explanation is that a mild compression of the umbilical cord with the contraction may occlude only the umbilical vein. The decrease in blood flow to the fetus decreases systemic blood pressure, which triggers a compensatory acceleration of the FHR. A second explanation is direct sympathetic stimulation of the fetus. Some researchers hypothesize that fundal pressure exerted on the vertex of a breech presentation may elicit a sympathetic response and acceleration. A third explanation for periodic accelerations may be repetitive fetal movement during a series of contractions.

Nonperiodic accelerations occur spontaneously, with or without contractions. They are often associated with environmental stimuli (e.g., vibroacoustic stimulation) and fetal movement. Other causes that may stimulate the sympathetic nervous system include scalp stimulation, occiput posterior presentation, or application of the FSE. The most important point to remember is that accelerations of the FHR, whether periodic or nonperiodic, are associated with the functioning of the fetal medulla oblongata and fetal well-being. When accelerations are associated with a normal baseline, average variability, and no periodic changes, the pattern can be highly predictive of a well-oxygenated fetus (King & Simpson, 2001).

Decelerations

Decelerations are described as a decrease in the baseline FHR. There are a variety of decelerations commonly referred to as early, variable, late, prolonged, or combined patterns. They are also described as periodic or nonperiodic changes in the FHR baseline on the basis of their relationship to uterine activity. Periodic decelerations are decelerations that have an associated relationship with uterine activity, whereas nonperiodic decelerations have no associated relationship with uterine activity. In 1997, the NICHD Research Planning Workshop described decelerations as a "visually apparent" decrease in the FHR from the baseline of at least 15 bpm that lasts for duration of 15 seconds or more (NICHD Research Planning Workshop, 1997). Decelerations can be classified as abrupt (or rapid) onset or gradual onset. In abrupt or rapid decelerations, the time from the onset of the deceleration to its nadir (lowest point) is less than 30 seconds. If the time from the onset of the deceleration to the nadir is greater than 30, the deceleration is classified as a gradual onset. When decelerations meet the criteria for rapid or abrupt onset, they are most likely variable decelerations. More than 90% of all abrupt or rapid onset decelerations are caused by cord compression and are classified as variables (Cusick, Smulian, & Vintzileos, 1995). Decelerations that meet the criteria for gradual onset are either early decelerations or late decelerations. To differentiate the two types, the nadir of the deceleration is compared with the apex (strongest point) of the contraction.

If they occur at the same time, the deceleration is classified as an early deceleration. When the nadir of the deceleration occurs after the apex or peak of the contraction, the deceleration is classified as a late deceleration.

Variable Deceleration

Variable Deceleration Definition

Variable decelerations are abrupt decelerations of the FHR most commonly in response to cord compression. They can be periodic or nonperiodic and may vary in duration, depth or nadir, and timing. Nonperiodic variable decelerations may occur before labor. Additionally, nonperiodic variable decelerations that decrease 15 bpm or more with duration of at least 15 seconds should receive further evaluation (ACOG, 1995b).

The shape of a variable deceleration may be U, V, or W, or it may mimic other patterns (Figure 6-12). When variable decelerations become a persistent pattern over time, fetal tolerance is confirmed by the presence of variability or accelerations of the FHR. Progression of variable decelerations is more important than absolute parameters in distinguishing those patterns that

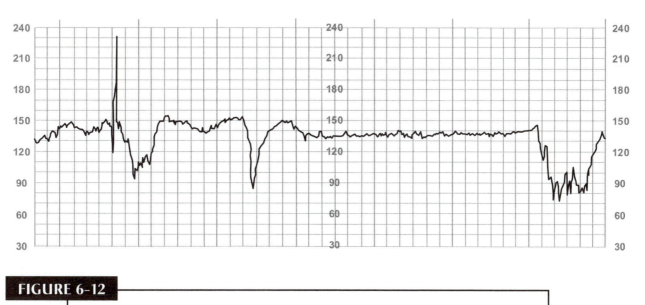

FIGURE 6-12

Example of Variable Decelerations That Exhibit a Variety of Possible Shapes, Including U, V, and W (FSE)

are reassuring from those that are nonreassuring (ACOG, 1995b). Classification systems for variable decelerations have been described but have not been agreed on. Despite the lack of consensus on specific names for variable decelerations, experts agree that presence or absence of FHR variability is the primary indicator of fetal response to the deceleration (Parer, 1997).

Variable decelerations are usually abrupt and decelerate quickly. Recent recommendations for the definition of variable decelerations identify that onset to nadir usually occurs in less than 30 seconds (NICHD Research Planning Workshop, 1997). Changing the maternal position may alter its shape, depth, and duration to improve or worsen the pattern. Variable decelerations may resemble or be in combination with other pattern types. They are the most common deceleration found in the laboring patient and are usually transient and correctable phenomena (Garite, 2002; Tucker, 2000).

Variable Deceleration Physiology

In general, variable decelerations result from decreased umbilical cord perfusion, usually caused by umbilical cord compression. The umbilical vessels may be partially compressed so that the thinner walled umbilical vein is compressed first followed by compression of the umbilical artery. Umbilical vein compression is thought to stimulate acceleration phases due to the drop in the fetal blood pressure and the initiation of baroreceptor compensatory mechanism of the fetus. The baroreceptor response originates in the carotid bodies and aortic arch and is transmitted to the midbrain and then to the SNS. This initial increase in FHR is the acceleration, which precedes variable decelerations. As the umbilical cord continues to be compressed, the umbilical artery is compressed and the fetal baroreceptors detect an increase in systemic vascular resistance. As the contraction strengthens and both the umbilical vein and artery are compressed, the resulting hemodynamic changes are presumed to trigger the vagal (parasympathetic) response, slowing the FHR via the sinus node and resulting in an abrupt drop in FHR, which is commonly recognized as a variable deceleration. As perfusion to the umbilical cord

is restored, the cord vessels gradually open and the FHR returns to the baseline. The umbilical arteries usually open first, but if the flow in the umbilical vein is still blocked, then an acceleration of the same mechanism preceding the deceleration occurs (Garite, 2002; Parer, 1997). It is important to note that the depth of the deceleration depends on fetal baroreceptor stimulation that produces a reflex mediated response in heart rate. The depth of the variable decelerations is reflex mediated and is not related to the degree of fetal hypoxemia or fetal acid-base status. Therefore, in the evaluation of fetal tolerance to the decelerations, it is most important to assess baseline rate, variability, and the presence of accelerations.

The acceleration that precedes or follows the deceleration is a physiologic compensatory response to hypoxemia (O_2 deprivation). Shoulders are not associated with poor outcome (Schifrin & Clement, 1990). The term *shoulder* describes a compensatory acceleration that may precede or follow the deceleration, with an increase in rate generally less than 20 bpm and lasting less than 20 seconds s (Figure 6-13). When short-term variability is present, the pattern is reassuring.

The term *overshoot* or *rebound overshoot* describes a blunt acceleration that follows the deceleration. An overshoot is a gradual, smooth acceleration that lasts more than 60 to 90 seconds with an increase in rate of 10 to 20 bpm; it has no variability, has no abruptness, and returns to baseline gradually. When overshoots are repetitive and short-term variability is absent, the pattern is nonreassuring.

Nonperiodic variable decelerations may occur prior to labor, indicating cord compression (Figure 6-14). During antepartum nonstress testing, variable decelerations that decrease 15 bpm or more with duration of at least 15 seconds require further evaluation in the pregnancy at risk for fetal compromise. In such cases, either oligohydramnios or umbilical cord entanglement may be present. Cases exist in which variable decelerations have been documented in conjunction with fetal movement. However, there is little data on the outcome of such pregnancies. A variety of factors interrupt umbilical cord blood flow or inhibit the cord from floating freely (Garite, 2002; Menihan & Zottoli, 2001; Tucker, 2000):

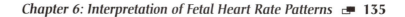

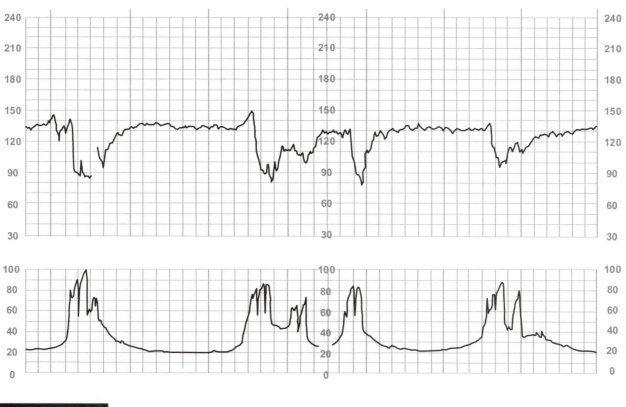

FIGURE 6-13

Example of Variable Decelerations with and without "Shoulders"
(External Ultrasound)

◆ Occult or overt prolapsed cord

◆ Oligohydramnios or thick meconium

◆ Knot in the cord or short cord

◆ Unspiraled cord

◆ Cord around fetal neck (nuchal cord) or other body part

◆ Decreased Wharton's jelly

◆ Thin cord

◆ Second stage of labor or descent of fetus

◆ Maternal position (cord between fetus and maternal pelvis)

◆ Fetal position (cord between fetus and uterine wall, cord wrapped around fetal parts)

◆ Monoamniotic multiple gestation (cord entanglement)

Reassuring Variable Deceleration Characteristics

Characteristics of variable decelerations that are reassuring may include:

◆ Duration of less than 60 seconds

◆ Rapid return to baseline

◆ Accompanied by normal baseline rate and variability (Freeman, et al., 1991).

Nonreassuring Variable Deceleration Characteristics

Characteristics of variable decelerations that are nonreassuring may include:

◆ Prolonged return to baseline

◆ Presence of overshoots

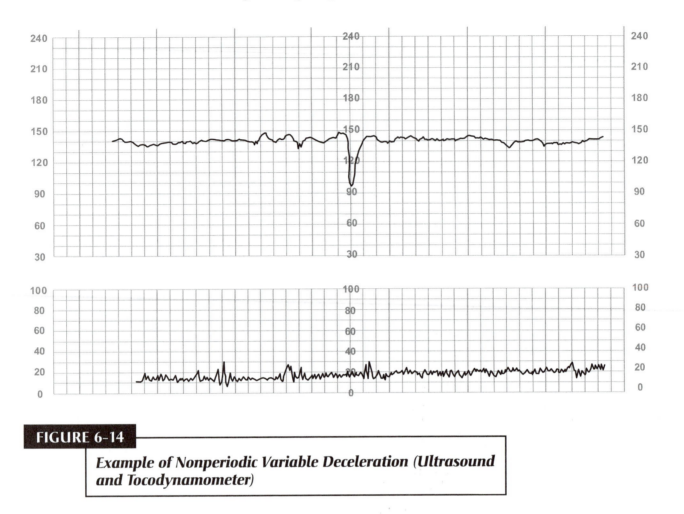

FIGURE 6-14

Example of Nonperiodic Variable Deceleration (Ultrasound and Tocodynamometer)

◆ Tachycardia

◆ Absence or loss of STV and/or LTV

◆ Persistent to less than 60 bpm and greater than 60 seconds (ACOG, 1995b).

Late Decelerations

Late Deceleration Definition

Late decelerations are a gradual decrease and return to the FHR baseline associated with uterine contractions (Figure 6-15). Late decelerations are classified or identified based on the onset and timing of the deceleration in relation to the contraction cycle. Late decelerations are gradual in onset, requiring more than 30 seconds from the beginning to nadir. The nadir (bottom) of the deceleration is offset or occurs after the acme (peak) of the contraction. The nadir commonly decreases 5–30 bpm and rarely 30–40 bpm below the baseline.

According to NICHD definitions (1997), if decelerations do not decrease below the baseline for a minimum of 15 bpm and last for a minimum of 15 seconds, they are not classified as late deceleration or as any other type of deceleration. The baseline rate may increase with repetitive late decelerations. The key point is that fetal tolerance of late decelerations is assessed by evaluating the baseline rate, the presence of variability, and the presence of accelerations.

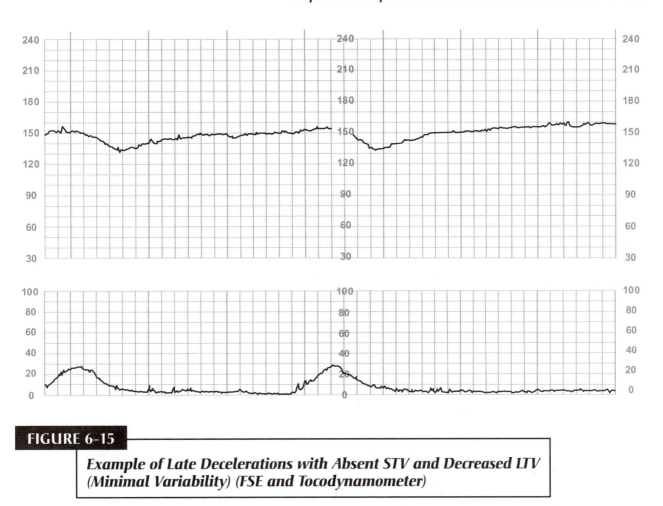

FIGURE 6-15

Example of Late Decelerations with Absent STV and Decreased LTV (Minimal Variability) (FSE and Tocodynamometer)

Late Deceleration Pathophysiology

The mechanism of late decelerations is complex and is not completely understood. They are thought to be a FHR response to transient alterations in O_2 transport produced or attenuated by uterine contractions. When the normal exchange of volatile and nonvolatile gases occurs through diffusion gradients across the placental surface area, O_2 passively moves from the maternal circulation to the fetal circulation. Because the process is passive and depends on environmental, maternal, fetal, and placental variables, it is not unusual for the fetus to experience alterations in O_2 availability. During instances of decreased O_2 transport in the presence of uterine activity, the fetus may demonstrate a late FHR deceleration. The gradual decrease in the FHR may be related to the time it takes for intervillous blood to reach the fetal heart and brain in the presence of uterine activity. When O_2 content of intervillous blood is lower than the fetal circulating blood, chemoreceptors are stimulated resulting in a transient decrease in FHR. This type of deceleration is also called a reflex late deceleration because the lateness is reflex mediated and not myocardial mediated. Reflex late decelerations will be accompanied by normal baseline FHR and average variability.

Late decelerations also can be produced by direct myocardial suppression of the fetal conduction system. Electrical conduction and performance of the human heart can be significantly altered in the presence of metabolic acidosis. Late decelerations may occur in the fetus that is in metabolic acidemia and experiences a decrease in O_2 availability as a result of uterine activity. In such a fetus, late decelerations may be produced by myocardial depression. When late decelerations occur in a metabolically acidemic fetus, it would be reasonable to anticipate absent variability and the absence of accelerations.

A pattern of persistent late decelerations requires attention. Maternal factors that may decrease O_2 availability (uteroplacental insufficiency) to the fetus are listed in Table 6-4.

Early Decelerations

Early Deceleration Definition

An *early deceleration* is defined as a gradual decrease in the FHR in which the nadir occurs at the peak of the contraction. The NICHD further describes the gradual decrease as more than 30 seconds from onset to nadir (NICHD Research Planning Workshop, 1997). Early decelerations are thought to be associated with compression of the fetal head during uterine contractions. They rarely go more than 30–40 bpm below the baseline FHR (Garite, 2002; NICHD Research Planning Workshop, 1997) and baseline variability is frequently present. Maternal position changes do not usually alter the pattern.

Early Deceleration Physiology

Early decelerations are thought to be caused by fetal head compression that results in a reflex vagal response. Compression of the fetal head can occur during labor from cervical resistance to the fetal head, compression of the head during pushing, crowning, forceps application, and vacuum extraction. Fetal head compression may result in altered cerebral blood flow, which precipitates vagal nerve stimulation with the resultant slowing of the FHR (Garite, 2002; King & Simpson, 2001). Early decelerations are benign, and no intervention is needed.

Factors Associated with Early Decelerations

A number of factors are associated with early decelerations (See Figure 6-16). For example, they occur more frequently in primigravidas and happen more often during early active labor, usually at 4–7 cm. In addition, the following factors are associated with early decelerations:

◆ Cephalopelvic disproportion

◆ Unengaged presenting part

◆ Persistent occiput posterior presentation

Combined Deceleration Patterns

Fetal monitoring instruction defines each pattern type separately, often omitting the fact that various types of patterns may appear consecutively or simultaneously (Figures 6-17 and 6-18). The terminology used, such as late, variable, and early deceleration, suggests that only a single deceleration pattern may exist for a given patient. Considering the physiology of deceleration patterns and the complexity of pregnancy, it is possible to have complex patterns that cannot be classified as early, late, or variable deceleration patterns. These patterns may result when more than one mechanism causes a combination of deceleration patterns, which contain characteristics of both of the "single" patterns with regard to shape and timing. There are not enough data on the relevance of complex and combined FHR patterns and pregnancy outcome. Therefore, interpretation and subsequent interventions are commonly based on the presumed primary cause of the pattern.

Interpretation of complex and combined deceleration patterns may be enhanced by assessment of onset (gradual versus abrupt), timing, FHR variability, and the presence of accelerations.

Although there is no agreed-upon terminology for the identification of complex FHR patterns, the recognition that more than one FHR patterns can occur simultaneously is important. When challenging FHR findings are identified, further assessment of FHR baseline rate, the presence of variability, and the presence of accelerations can provide methods to confirm fetal tolerance to the labor.

Prolonged Decelerations

Prolonged Deceleration Definition

Prolonged decelerations are decelerations of the FHR that last longer than 2 minutes but less than 10 minutes. A deceleration that lasts longer than 10 minutes is considered a baseline change

TABLE 6-4

Maternal Factors That May Decrease Uteroplacental Circulation

FACTOR	RELATED CAUSES OR CHARACTERISTICS
Hypotension[a]	• Supine position[a] • Maternal trauma or blood loss[a] • Regional anesthesia[a]
Hypertension	• Gestational hypertension or chronic hypertension • Medications (e.g., illicit drugs such as cocaine and amphetamines)
Placental changes that may affect uteroplacental gas exchange	• Postmaturity • Premature aging, including calcification and necrosis • Old and new abruptio sites • Placenta previa • Placental malformation
Physiologic conditions that may be associated with decreased maternal arterial hemoglobin/O_2 saturation	• Hyperventilation[a] • Hypoventilation[a] • Cardiopulmonary disease
Uterine hyperstimulation or hypertonus	• With or without oxytocin, misoprostol, or prostaglandin administration
Increased association with other high-risk conditions of pregnancy	• Chronic maternal diseases, such as diabetes and collagen disease • Maternal smoking • Poor maternal nutrition • Multiple gestation (especially monochorionic) • Anemia

[a] May be associated with reflex late decelerations or those that occur in the fetus that remains oxygenated and is not in metabolic acidemia, which are more likely to be reversed with interventions (Parer, 1999; Petrie, 1991).

(NICHD Research Planning Workshop, 1997; Parer, 1997; Tucker, 2000). Prolonged decelerations are considered nonperiodic because they occur in response to nonrepetitive stimuli (Figure 6-19). Although prolonged decelerations may appear dramatic, most can be modified with simple interventions such as position change. Prolonged deceleration assessment may include the duration, depth, return to baseline, baseline FHR variability after deceleration, and response to interventions.

Prolonged Deceleration Physiology

Unlike other types of decelerations (early, late, and variable), prolonged decelerations may be caused by any of the mechanisms previously described as causing a deceleration. Such mechanisms include cord compression, head compression, and uteroplacental insufficiency (Garite, 2002). In general, prolonged deceleration physiology is dependent on the precipitating cause. If prolonged decelerations do not recur, the fetus generally recovers to its predeceleration phase.

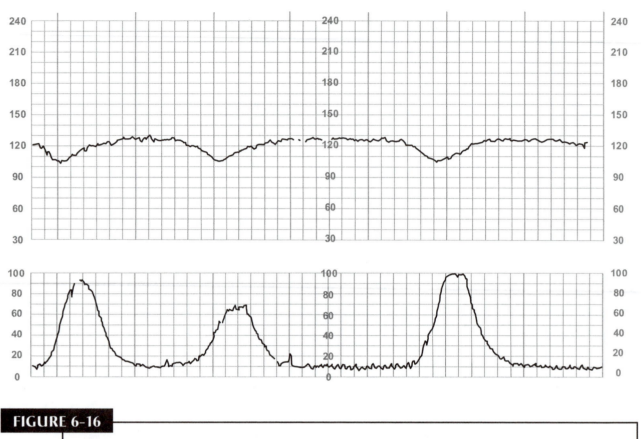

FIGURE 6-16

Example of Early Decelerations in a Pattern with Active Labor and Cephalopelvic Disproportion (External Ultrasound and Tocodynamometer)

Factors Associated with Prolonged Decelerations

Many factors are associated with prolonged decelerations:

◆ Profound changes in the fetal environment:
  • Abruptio placentae
  • Uterine hypertonus
  • Uterine hyperstimulus
  • Terminal fetal conditions
  • Maternal death
  • Cord accidents

◆ Hypotension associated with drug responses or maternal positioning:
  • Sympathetic blockade with anesthesia (epidural or spinal)
  • Paracervical block

◆ Vagal stimulation with a vaginal examination or the Valsalva maneuver

◆ Cord impingement (short cord, true knot in the cord, or umbilical cord thrombosis)

◆ Cord prolapse

◆ Uterine rupture

◆ Maternal seizures, status asthmaticus, or maternal cardiorespiratory collapse

◆ Cord compression for substantial periods of time (i.e., maternal position change or fetal movement)

◆ Rapid fetal descent

◆ Oligohydramnios with decreased Wharton's jelly

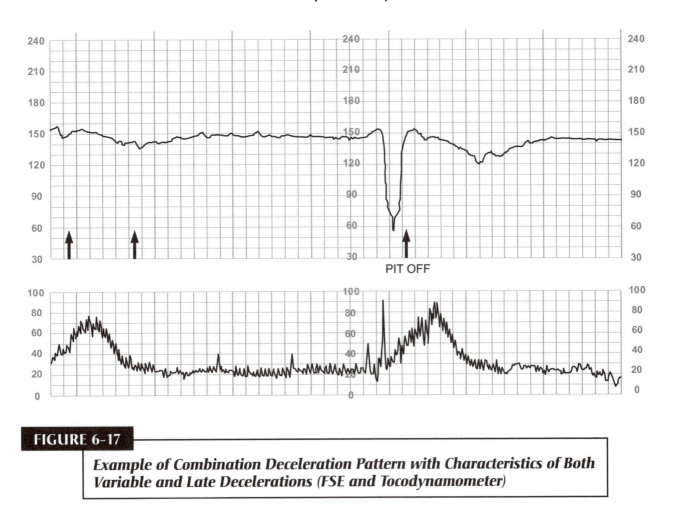

PIT OFF

FIGURE 6-17

Example of Combination Deceleration Pattern with Characteristics of Both Variable and Late Decelerations (FSE and Tocodynamometer)

◆ Procedures such as vaginal examination, fetal blood sampling, or application of internal fetal monitor

The degree to which such decelerations are nonreassuring depends on the status and response of fetus after the deceleration has ended.

🖙 UTERINE ACTIVITY

Although different terms are used to describe aspects of normal and abnormal labor, for the purpose of this manual, the terms listed in Table 6-5 will be used. However, the ultimate definition of adequate labor is based on clinical data, that is, cervical effacement and dilatation and fetal descent (Norwitz, Robinson, & Repke, 2002).

Identifying inadequate labor (subnormal or abnormal uterine activity) entails assessing the "3 Ps" of labor—power, passenger, and passage (pelvis)—for correctable causes. There is no one definition of *adequate labor* because it is the strength and frequency of uterine contractions that result in progressive cervical dilation. A wide range of contraction strength, frequency, and resting tone exists during adequate labor with spontaneous contractions every 2–4.5 minutes, with an intensity of 25–80 mm of mercury (mm Hg), and 95–395 Montevideo units.

Montevideo units are a quantitative measurement of the uterine contraction intensity over a 10-minute period. Montevideo units are derived by subtracting the resting tone of the uterus from the peak pressure of the contraction (in mm Hg) for each contraction that occurs in a 10-minute

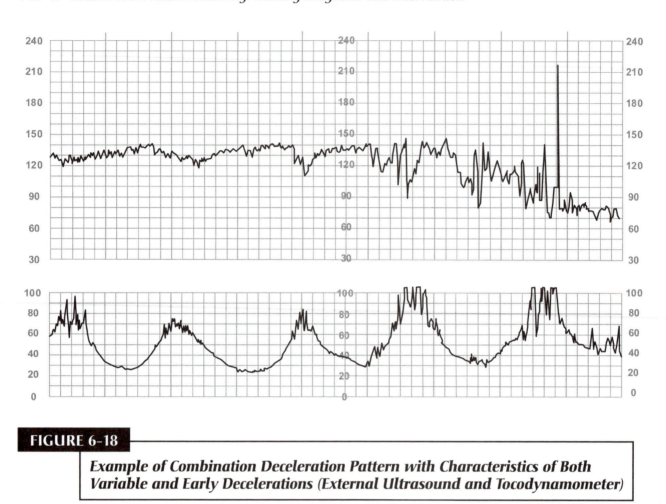

FIGURE 6-18

Example of Combination Deceleration Pattern with Characteristics of Both Variable and Early Decelerations (External Ultrasound and Tocodynamometer)

period. The calculated numbers are then added together for the total number of Montevideo units in that 10-minute period. When intrauterine pressure monitoring is used, it is appropriate to describe the uterine contractions and the baseline tonus in actual mm Hg.

Uterine activity is an integral part of fetal monitoring interpretation. To understand the significance of the FHR tracing, one must interpret the data in concurrence with uterine activity and characteristics. *Contraction of the uterus* is the shortening of the uterine muscle in response to a stimulant (i.e., endogenous oxytocin). Once the contraction subsides, the muscle fibers return to their original length (Oxorn, 1986). Uterine activity can be assessed by maternal report and observation, palpation, use of a tocodynamometer, and use of intrauterine pressure monitoring. Interpretation of uterine activity includes the assessment of four components: frequency, duration, inten-

sity of the contractions, and uterine resting tone. *Labor* is defined as the progressive dilation and effacement of the maternal cervix. It typically occurs when rhythmic uterine contractions of adequate frequency, intensity, and duration produce pressure on the maternal cervix through the fetal presenting part that ultimately acts as a mechanical dilator. The result of the contractions is usually progressive cervical effacement and dilatation with descent of the presenting part.

The *frequency of contractions* is defined as the beginning of one contraction to the beginning of the next contraction. The frequency is described in minutes and may include a range. *Contraction duration* is the time from the beginning of the contraction to the end of the contraction and is measured in seconds or minutes. *Intensity* is the strength of the contraction. The intensity is measured externally by palpation (mild, moderate, or strong) or internally by an intrauterine pressure

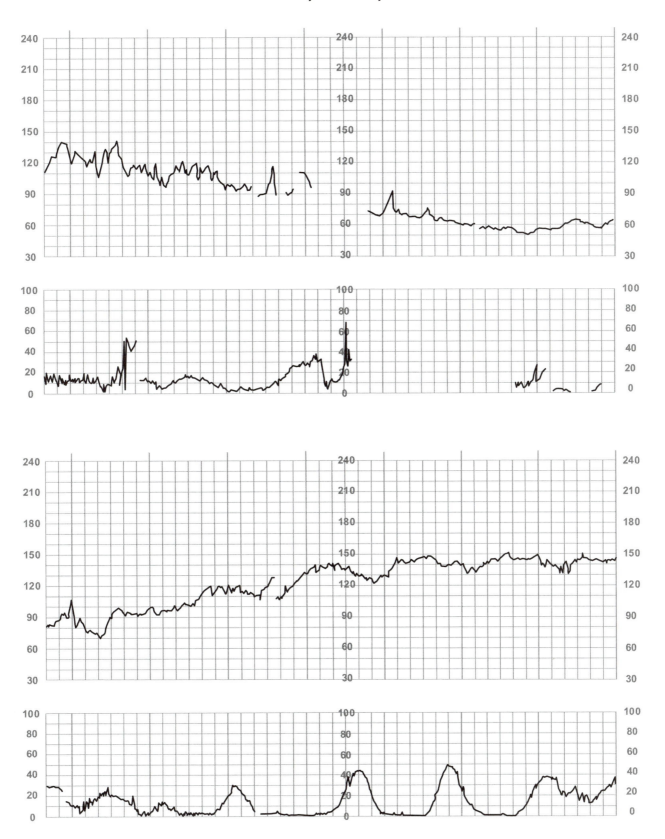

FIGURE 6-19

Example of Nonperiodic Prolonged Deceleration (External Ultrasound and Tocodynamometer)

TABLE 6-5

Abnormal Labor Patterns

STAGE OF LABOR	ABNORMAL PATTERN
First stage (active or latent phase):	Protraction or arrest of cervical dilatation
Latent phase arrest	Labor not begun
Prolonged latent phase	Latent phase: ≥20 hr (nulliparous) ≥14 hr (multiparous)
Primary dysfunctional labor	Rate of cervical dilatation in active phase: ≤1.2 cm/hr (nulliparous) ≤1.5 cm/hr (multiparous)
Secondary arrest	Cessation of previous normal uterine contractions (UC) (in active phase) > 2 hr
Combined	Arrest of dilatation when the patient had previously demonstrated primary dysfunctional labor
Second stage:	
Protraction of descent	Descent of presenting part: < 1 cm/hr (nulliparous) < 2 cm/hr (multiparous)
Arrest of descent	Failure of descent of presenting part to descend
Uterine hyperstimulation	Excessive frequency of UC (polysystole) or increased uterine tone (hypertonia)
Dystocia	Indications for cesarean delivery in which one or more of the "3 Ps" do not work appropriately; includes failure to progress, relative cephalopelvic disproportion, and absolute cephalopelvic disproportion

catheter (IUPC) in mm Hg. *Resting tone* or *baseline tonus* is the pressure in the uterus between contractions that originates from the tension in the uterine wall. The tension is measured by palpation (soft or firm) or with an IUPC in mm Hg.

Factors That Affect Labor

Once the contraction frequency, duration, and intensity and the uterine resting tone have been interpreted, uterine activity is evaluated as adequate or inadequate to cause cervical change. *Dystocia* is defined as difficult childbirth and most commonly includes arrest of the active phase, arrest of the descent, or both. If the uterine contraction pattern does not produce progressive cervical dilatation, effacement, and decent of the presenting part, the labor may be called *dysfunctional*, with dystocia being the cause. A number of factors may contribute to dystocia, including abnormal uterine musculature, abnormal nerve innervation, structural abnormalities of the uterus, excessive analgesia, maternal fatigue, and altered humoral effects (ACOG, 1995a; Garfield, 1987; Huszar & Roberts, 1982; May & Mahlmeister, 1994).

Dysfunctional contractions may be physiologically described as subnormal (or hypotonic), hypertonic, or abnormal. These dysfunctional contractions can be more frequent in occurrence and less effective. During spontaneous and induced labor, frequency also may be mistaken for effectiveness, especially if the intensity and duration of contractions are not assessed (ACOG, 1995a). The uterus may be unable to contract effectively, as seen by hypotonus and hypertonus. It is important to identify an abnormal contraction pattern so that appropriate interventions may be instituted.

Factors affecting labor include those that are fixed and cannot be changed, as well as those that are dynamic or changeable. Factors that cannot be changed include maternal age, parity, relative health status, pelvic size and shape, fetal size, presentation (that did not convert with external version), and gestational age. Fetal situations also may contribute to labor dystocia, including abnormalities in size, position, or anatomy. Factors that may be changed to some degree are hydration, maternal psychological status and anxiety, intensity and duration of contractions, maternal position, pushing efforts, drugs, and medications.

Hydration

Hydration often is overlooked as an influence on labor because the onset of dehydration may be gradual. Patients involved in sustained exercise such as labor do not voluntarily ingest adequate amounts of fluid, which can result in a phenomenon called autodehydration (Garite, 2002). Maternal fluid loss also occurs with perspiration, rapid and heavy breathing, vomiting, and body maintenance needs. This situation is compounded when fluid intake before admission to labor and delivery is restricted, thereby creating the potential for fluid volume deficit.

The administration of fluids promotes adequate maternal intravascular volume, which can protect against decreased uteroplacental perfusion (King & Simpson, 2001). Hydrated patients respond to induction or augmentation with fewer complications and less need for interventions than a dehydrated patient (Garite, Weeks, Peters-Phair, Pattillo, & Brewster, 2000). An intravenous infusion and/or P.O. clear fluids may improve labor progress, as well as endurance, thereby preventing or lessening the need for augmentation. Recently, maternal oral hydration with water (women were asked to drink 2 liters of water before an ultrasound) was shown to increase amniotic fluid volume in both women with normal amniotic fluid volume and those with oligohydramnios. Interestingly, intravenous infusion of a hypotonic solution increased amniotic fluid volume in women with oligohydramnios, but an infusion with an isotonic solution did not increase the fluid (Hofmeyr & Kulier, 2002). For the clinician, it is important to know that the intravenous administration of fluids for the treatment of fetal distress and fetal oligohydramnios may increase amniotic fluid volume, which may protect the fetus during labor.

Caution should be used to avoid overloading the patient with high dextrose or hypotonic intravenous fluids. Infusion of solutions that are greater than 5% dextrose or are hypotonic can lead to maternal glycosuria, osmotic diuresis, and/or maternal and neonatal hyponatremia (Davis & Riedmann, 1991; Garite, et al., 2000; Grylack, Chu, & Scanlon, 1984; Morton, Jackson, & Gillmer, 1985; Omigbodun, Fajimi, & Adeleye, 1991; Silverton, 1989; Singhi & Chookang, 1984).

Oral hydration also can be used as a means to expand a patient's intravascular volume. Oral hydration in labor remains a controversial issue because of the longstanding concern that it may cause or contribute to maternal aspiration syndrome if general anesthesia is required. There is neither evidence suggesting any benefit of withholding oral fluids nor evidence suggesting any additional risk in allowing oral fluids during labor. If oral hydration is used, it is recommended that it be restricted to nonparticulate fluids (Elkington, 1991; Enkin, et al., 2000).

The traditional role of intravenous fluid hydration in the preterm labor patient was recently challenged. In a 2002 Cochrane Database analysis (Stan, Boulvain, Hirsbrunner-Amagbaly, & Pfister, 2002), hydration was determined to play no role in reducing preterm labor and/or preterm delivery. Thus, the practice of using fluid boluses in the management of preterm labor should be reconsidered.

Maternal Anxiety

Maternal anxiety can influence labor progress by stimulating the adrenal glands to secrete catecholamines (e.g., adrenaline, epinephrine, norepinephrine) that bind with uterine B receptors. The increase in maternal catecholamines may increase the patient's heart rate, blood pressure, respirations, and blood flow to major organs such as the brain, heart, and adrenal glands. In turn, blood flow to the uterus may decrease, which can result in ineffective uterine activity. Increased maternal catecholamine levels also may increase the duration of the first stage of labor and decrease Montevideo units (Arnold-Aldea & Parer, 1990; Lederman, Lederman, Work, & McCann, 1978; Murray, 1997; Simkin, 1986).

In addition, maternal anxiety can influence the FHR. The epinephrine produced when anxiety is present constricts vessels. As a result, O_2 delivery to the fetus decreases, which may decrease fetal O_2 and pH levels and increase fetal carbon dioxide (CO_2) levels. As a result, fetal blood pressure falls, causing decelerations, bradycardia, or both (Arnold-Aldea & Parer, 1990; Murray, 1997; Myers, 1975). Researchers have noted that when pregnant monkeys become frightened, the fetus demonstrates bradycardia.

Because maternal anxiety may contribute to the progress of labor, it is important to use anxiety-relieving measures, such as coaching support and pain management, for the laboring patient. A Cochrane review completed in 1997 (14 trials of more than 5,000 women in a wide-range of settings in 10 countries) showed that continuous labor support provided by midwives, student midwives, nurses, doulas, lay women, or female relatives was associated with significant reductions in the likelihood of cesarean delivery, operative vaginal delivery, use of intrapartum analgesia or anesthesia, and a 5-minute Apgar score of below 7 (Hodnett, 2002). In addition to the benefits found by the Cochrane review, such support can lead to shorter labors, decreased need for oxytocin, and increased satisfaction with the childbirth experience (AWHONN, 2000b). In a study recently completed in North America that compared the outcomes of women cared for by nurses trained in labor support versus those women who received usual care, Hodnett and associates found that there were no significant difference in cesarean delivery and other birth outcomes. The investigators suggested that the benefits of continuous labor support were likely overpowered by the effects of birth environments characterized by high rates of routine medical interventions (Hodnett et al., 2002). Although there were no major clinical differences found, women indicated that they would choose to have the continous labor support in future labors (Hodnett et al., 2002).

Duration of Labor

The duration of each stage and phase of labor is different for each patient and depends on numerous factors. The average hours of duration for each stage and phase of labor are different for the primiparous woman when compared to a multiparous one (see Table 6-6).

Although average times have been established for the anticipated length of labor, no two labors are identical. Therefore, the clinician monitoring a patient's progress of labor should individualize assessments (see Table 6-7) and plans of care for the individual.

The duration of second stage of labor has historically been scrutinized. Over the past three decades, the second stage of labor has been medically permitted to continue for increasing lengths of time. Today there is no longer a need to automatically proceed to cesarean section (c-section) when a limit of 2 hours has been reached. As long as progress in the descent of the vertex (without significant molding or caput) is noted, and fetal surveillance demonstrates fetal well-being and the absence of unfavorable physiologic response or nonreassuring patterns, the duration of the second stage of labor is unrelated to outcome. Thus, allowing the second stage to continue for greater than 2 hours may be reasonable and may be the most appropriate decision (Cohen, Acker, & Friedman, 1989; Schifrin & Cohen, 1989; Rouse, Owen, & Hauth, 1999).

TABLE 6-6		
Duration of Labor		
	PRIMIPAROUS	**MULTIPAROUS**
Total duration of labor	10.1 hr	6.2 hr
Stage of labor:		
Duration of latent phase	6.4 hr	4.8 hr
Duration of first stage	9.7 hr	8.0 hr
Duration of second stage	33.0 hr	8.5 hr
Rate of cervical dilatation in active phase	3.0 cm/hr	5.7 cm/hr
Duration of third stage	5.0 min	5.0 min

Note: Adapted from *Labor: Clinical Evaluation and Management* (2nd ed.), by E. A. Friedman, 1978, Norwalk: Appleton-Century-Crofts.

Maternal Position and Pushing

Maternal position during labor affects uterine blood flow and placental perfusion. The supine position causes compression of the vena cava and aortoiliac vessels by the weight of the gravid uterus, which results in decreased blood flow returning to the maternal heart and causes a fall in cardiac output, blood pressure, and uterine blood flow (ACOG, 1995b). This condition is referred to as the "vena caval" syndrome. Because of the risk of the vena caval syndrome, the supine position may cause the appearance of late decelerations and a decrease in fetal scalp pH (Abitbol, 1985). Compression of the vena cava and thoracic vessels can be remedied by positioning the patient in a lateral, sitting, standing, or Fowler's position.

Repeated clinical studies have shown that the upright position has a favorable effect on uterine contractility (Caldeyro-Barcia, 1979; Flynn, Kelly, Hollins, & Lynch, 1978; Read, Miller, & Paul, 1981; Roberts, Mendez-Bauer, & Wodell, 1983). In one randomized, controlled trial, women who assumed the upright position, which included squatting, experienced less pain and perineal trauma and received fewer episiotomies than those in supine positions (de Jong et al., 1997). Additionally, women who labored in the upright position gave birth to fetuses whose O_2 saturations were higher during labor (Gupta, Brayshaw, & Lilford, 1989; Mayberry, Hammer, Kelly, True-Driver, & De, 1999; Sampselle & Hines, 1999).

Once the second stage of labor begins, the squatting position for pushing may be one of the most effective. However, women from western countries such as the United States and Canada have difficulty maintaining this position. If squatting is difficult for the woman, it can be simulated by having the patient sit on a birthing ball or on a toilet (Mayberry, et al., 1999; Mayberry, et al., 2000). A woman may also sit in bed and maintain a forward thrust of her upper body as an alternative to squatting (Shermer & Raines, 1997).

If possible and indicated, pushing should be initiated in response to Ferguson's reflex, which is the stimulation of nerve receptors in the pelvic floor in response to pressure of the fetal head as it descends past the ischial spines (Mayberry, et al., 1999, Mayberry, et al., 2000). Pushing should be encouraged when there is a spontaneous urge to bear down rather than using cervical dilatation as the sole indicator for the onset of pushing (Roberts & Woolley, 1996). A recent study reported that women who used spontaneous pushing efforts were less likely to require episiotomies and to experience second- or third-degree perineal lacerations (Sampselle & Hines, 1999).

TABLE 6-7

Characteristics of Uterine Contractions Associated with Normal Labor and Variations in Labor

NORMAL LABOR	SUBNORMAL LABOR	ABNORMAL (HYPOTONIC) LABOR
Fundal origin and dominance	Fundal dominance	No fundal dominance
Coordinated	Less coordinated	Even less coordinated; may have different pacemakers in charge (usually)
2–5 per 10-min frequency	Less than 2–5 per 10-min frequency	Irregular (usually); mixed with subnormal and normal uterine patterns
45–90 s duration	Less than 30 s duration	Ineffective dilatation and effacement/fetal descent
40–60 mm Hg first stage intensity	Irregular	Irregular; ineffective dilatation and effacement/fetal descent
70–80 mm Hg late first stage and second stage	Irregular; ineffective or prolonged dilatation and effacement/fetal descent	Irregular; ineffective dilatation and effacement/fetal descent
Tonus • 5–12 mm Hg without stimulation • 20 mm Hg possibly reached when oxytocin is used	Irregular; usually relaxed for longer periods of time; responds well to oxytocin augmentation	Irregular; can be relaxed with little uterine activity; can also have limited relaxation between contractions because of frequent but less effective contractions
Fundus at peak not indentable	Fundus at peak indentable	Fundus at peak either indentable or not indentable
Presenting part tightly applied to cervix	Cervix at peak not tightly applied to presenting part; usually responds well to oxytocin augmentation	Cervix at peak loosely applied to presenting part; room for examining finger to slip between presenting part and cervix

Note: Information in this table can be found in Klavin, Laver, & Boscola (1977); Turley (2000); May & Mahlmeister (1994); and Norwitz, et al. (2002).

Traditional pushing techniques use directed, strong, and sustained pushing with contractions. Pushing that includes breath holding against a closed glottis or Valsalva maneuver has negative hemodynamic effects on the mother. It results in an increase in intrathoracic and abdominal pressure, which creates vasoconstriction and a decrease in cardiac output and affects blood flow in the intervillous space. This result can cause compromised perfusion and nonreassuring FHR tracings, thereby leading to changes in fetal acid-base status (Barnett & Humenick, 1982; Holland & Smith, 2000; Sleep, et al., 2000; Caldeyro-Barcia, 1979). Research indicates that the exhalatory or "open glottis" pushing technique is more physiologic. Open glottis pushing is the spontaneous involuntary bearing down with each contraction. It usually involves 5 to 6 pushes of 4 to 6 seconds with each contraction (Roberts & Woolley, 1996). After the cervix is completely dilated, the woman begins the open glottis pushing technique when she feels the urge to push (Ferguson's reflex). She then bears down while at the same time vocalizing expiratory grunts. She does not hold her breath during the open glottis pushing.

Traditionally, women have been taught to begin pushing before she feels the urge to push (Ferguson reflex) during the second stage of labor (Aderhold & Roberts, 1991). However, that practice has been found to be a difficult task to accomplish with women receiving epidural anesthesia and to be associated with increased use of forceps (to rotate the fetus), increased maternal fatigue, increased second- and third-degree lacerations, need for episiotomies, interference with fetal rotation and descent, and increased intrathoracic and abdominal pressures resulting in less-than-optimal FHR patterns (AWHONN, 2000a).

Delayed pushing means waiting for fetal descent to occur or for the interaction of the Ferguson's reflex before actually pushing in the second stage of labor, despite complete dilatation. Delayed pushing is also referred to as *laboring down, passive pushing,* and *rest and descend* (AWHONN, 2000a). Research has shown that delayed pushing has been successful in preventing negative fetal effects, decreasing the use of instrumental delivery, decreasing the duration of second stage of labor, decreasing maternal fatigue, and decreasing

second- and third-degree lacerations and episiotomies (AWHONN, 2000a). U.S. and Canadian strategies for second stage management are continuing to evolve as more clinical evidence is integrated into clinical practice.

Drugs and Medications

Agents that alter uterine contractions and that have potential fetal effects include oxytocin prostaglandin, misoprostol, MgSO₄, beta sympathomimetics, antiprostaglandins (indomethacin), and illicit drugs (cocaine, amphetamine) (Baxi & Petrie, 1987). Medication administered for induction or augmentation, such as oxytocin, necessitates maternal-fetal evaluation or monitoring because individual sensitivity and clearance rates vary. ACOG/AWHONN guidelines discuss administration of oxytocin for the induction and augmentation of labor (ACOG, 1999; Simpson, 2002). Administration of prostaglandin and misoprostol for ripening the cervix or inducing labor also necessitates maternal-fetal observation, especially during the first 4 hours following administration (ACOG, 1999; Simpson, 2002).

Beta sympathomimetics, prostaglandin synthetase inhibitors, MgSO₄, and calcium channel blockers frequently are used to treat preterm labor. Assessment and interpretation of the uterine pattern and fetal response are indicated when those drugs are used.

Hyperstimulus and Hypertonus

Hyperstimulus is usually defined as uterine contractions that occur more frequently than every 2 minutes; uterine relaxation less than 30 seconds between contractions; or uterine contractions that continue longer than 90–120 seconds. Hypertonus usually is defined as elevated resting tone greater than 20 to 25 mm Hg, depending on the type of IUPC used (Tucker, 2000), or peak pressure of the uterine contraction greater than 80 mm Hg (in the absence of pushing), or Montevideo units greater than 400. Because types of IUPCs differ in the techniques for zeroing to atmospheric pressure, palpation of both contraction intensity and resting tonus can help affirm the data. It is important to review all information provided by the IUPC manufacturer to ensure proper placement and calibration or zeroing of the catheter. The catheter frequently may need adjusting (Menihan & Zottoli, 2001).

Uterine hypertonus and hyperstimulation may be treated if there is concern about fetal well-being. Reducing uterine activity, a physiologic goal, may be accomplished through a variety of practices; these practices are frequently termed *intrauterine resuscitation* (King & Simpson, 2001; Tucker, 2000). Initial interventions include those that promote normal or physiologic labor such as ensuring adequate intravascular volume by changing position, providing hydration or intravenous fluids, and reducing maternal anxiety or pain. The benefits of maternal tocolysis in the presence of excessive uterine activity warrant consideration. Individual studies have recommended the use of a beta sympathomimetic drug (such as terbutaline hydrochloride) in treating sustained hyperstimulation when there are no contraindications present and when the mother appears hemodynamically stable. There is not enough evidence based on fetal outcomes to evaluate the use of betamimetics for suspected fetal compromise (Hofmeyr & Kulier, 2002). However, available research does suggest that betamimetic therapy is useful in buying time when fetal compromise is diagnosed during labor (Hofmeyr & Kulier, 2002). In addition, betamimetic therapy is found to be more successful as a tocolytic than MgSO$_4$ (Magann, et al., 1993).

Other techniques used for intrauterine resuscitation include changing the maternal position and decreasing or discontinuing the contraction-stimulating medication. Although additional interventions for fetal resuscitation have been previously recommended (e.g., maternal O$_2$ administration, repetitive fluid boluses) there is no evidence that these actions have an effect on fetal outcome (Hofmeyr & Kulier, 2002).

Assessment of Uterine Activity

Assessment of uterine activity (See Figure 6-20) should take into account the following:

◆ Resting tone

◆ Duration of contractions

◆ Intensity of contractions

◆ Frequency of contractions

◆ Cervical changes as appropriate

◆ Presence of factors affecting uterine contractions

◆ Changes in uterine activity in response to interventions

◻ INTERPRETATION ISSUES FOR SELECTED POPULATIONS

The 21st century has brought a new generation of obstetric patients. Pregnancies that were once considered risky or dangerous are now becoming more common in our everyday practice. These patients include preterm labor patients, those with multiple gestations, and prior c-section patients. Such patients often are identified as high risk and may require special care, which includes close observation of both mother and fetus, regardless of the method of monitoring.

Monitoring the Preterm Pregnant Patient

"Interpreting FHR tracings from preterm fetuses requires knowledge of the underlying physiological changes related to fetal development" (Eganhouse & Burnside, 1992). A preterm fetus, compared with a term fetus, generally will possess different characteristics: a higher baseline FHR without evidence of fetal compromise, decreased variability, decrease in the number and amplitude of accelerations, and limited pronounced changes in the appearance of the FHR tracing with fetal rest and state changes (Castillo, et al., 1989; Eganhouse & Burnside, 1992; Murray, 1997; Naef, et al., 1994; Pillai & James, 1990; Schifrin & Clement, 1990).

Physiology

The SNS dominates the FHR response until approximately 28 weeks of gestation, when the PSNS overtakes the sympathetic control. Thus, a base-

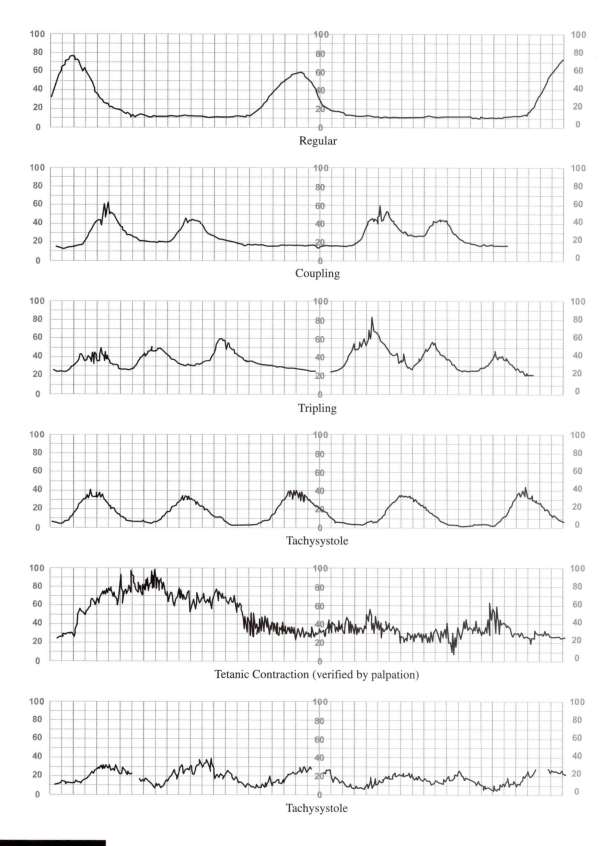

FIGURE 6-20

Samples of Uterine Activity That Represents a Regular Uterine Contraction Pattern and Variations (Tocodynamometer)

line FHR of 150–160 bpm is considered normal in a preterm fetus. The dominance of the FHR control by the PSNS slows the baseline FHR with increased gestational age. FHR accelerations can be seen as early as 24 weeks, yet those accelerations may increase only 10 bpm above the FHR baseline and may be sustained for 10 seconds. These "preterm" accelerations (Ikuo, Akio, & Taro, 1992; Pillai & James, 1990), are seen more frequently than the typical acceleration of 15 bpm above the FHR baseline sustained for 15 seconds.

FHR reactivity increases dramatically after 32 weeks of gestation. Current guidelines state that a term FHR demonstrates reactivity by accelerating 15 bpm above the baseline for a minimum of 15 seconds (Castillo, et al., 1989; Eganhouse & Burnside, 1992; Murray, 1997). Exclusive use of these criteria for fetuses of less than 32 weeks gestation increases the likelihood of false nonreactive nonstress tests; some studies show a rate as high as 31.9% (Patkos, Boucher, Broussard, Phelan, & Platt, 1986). Modifying the criteria for nonstress tests to accelerations of 10 bpm above baseline sustained for 10 seconds may be adequate as a reactive strip for the preterm fetus. In addition to modifying the baseline parameters, the time element is extended to 60–90 minutes instead of the routine 20 minutes (Brown & Patrick, 1981; Castillo, et al., 1989; Ikuo, et al., 1992). In addition, abrupt variable shaped decelerations lasting 10–20 seconds are common in low-risk fetuses between 20–30 weeks of gestation (Pillai & James, 1990). There is no evidence to suggest that such decelerations require interventions; rather, they are thought to be a normal finding. Fetal movement in these preterm fetuses may even elicit small decelerations instead of accelerations (Schifrin & Clement, 1990).

Uterine Activity

When assessing the preterm pregnancy, care providers also need to look at uterine activity (UA). Because of the decreased sensitivity of tocodynamometers when used on a preterm uterus when compared with a term uterus, detecting UA can be challenging for the perinatal professional. Therefore, it may be beneficial to incorporate the skill of uterine palpation when there are questions regarding UA. UA may escalate in the 24 hours prior to the onset of preterm labor (Eganhouse & Burnside, 1992; Morrison, 1992; Newman, Campbell, & Stramm, 1990). Nurses need to understand key concepts regarding the assessment of preterm UA:

◆ Preterm contractions are often painless.

◆ Low-amplitude/high-frequency contractions may be an early sign of increasing UA (Eganhouse & Burnside, 1992).

◆ Perceived UA has been reported to increases 24 hours before the onset of preterm labor.

◆ Standard tocodynamometers may not be sensitive enough to detect or record UA in preterm gestation (Eganhouse & Burnside, 1992; Naef, et al., 1994).

Preterm labor and birth affects 8 to 10 pregnancies per 100 and accounts for the majority of morbidity and mortality in neonatal care units across North America. In the United States, the cost of caring for premature infants on an annual basis exceeds $4 billion and shows no sign of decreasing. Because preterm delivery is associated with potentially poor outcomes, research on methods not only to treat preterm labor but also to predict preterm labor and birth is ongoing. One such method is home uterine activity monitoring. The monitoring system is based on the premise that pregnancies that will end in a preterm birth have an increased number of contractions compared with a normal pregnancy. Early intervention can take place if a contraction episode precedes cervical dilation and delivery. Unfortunately, the method is of little to no benefit in predicting preterm labor. Even though studies have found that women who give birth prematurely do have slightly more contractions throughout their pregnancy when compared with women who give birth at term, there is no predictable pattern that can predict premature birth (NIH, 2002).

In January 2002, NICHD released the findings of a multicenter study conducted at the 11 centers participating in the NICHD Network of Maternal-Fetal Medicine Units. The study encompassed 306 women, and more than 34,908 hours of EFM recordings were analyzed. The researchers concluded that the ambulatory or home monitoring of uterine contractions does not identify women destined to have preterm delivery (Iams, et al., 2002; NIH, 2002).

In addition, the researchers also evaluated the use of fetal fibronectin in the identification of preterm labor and found that is was not predictive of preterm labor and birth (Moawad, et al., 2002).

Maternally administered corticosteroids, such as betamethasone, have been widely used for fetal pulmonary maturity in preterm singleton pregnancies and multiple gestations. This is one of the most effective obstetric interventions for reducing infant morbidity and mortality associated with a preterm birth (Mercer & Lewis, 1997). In 1994 and 2000, the National Institutes of Health (NIH) sponsored multidisciplinary conferences to assess the effectiveness of antenatal corticosteroid therapy on fetal lung maturation. The 2000 consensus statement recommends that corticosteroids be given if fetal pulmonary immaturity is suspected or documented in those patients who are at risk for preterm delivery between 24–34 weeks gestation. Data from currently available research studies that assessed the risks and benefits of repeat (rescue) courses of antenatal steroids are inadequate. The NIH recommend that repeat courses of corticosteroids not be used routinely (NIH, 2000). Health care providers can refer to the NIH Consensus Statement *Antenatal Corticosteroids Revisited: Repeat Courses* for the complete consensus statement on clinical recommendations (NIH, 2000).

Corticosteroid administration may have an effect on antenatal testing for fetal well-being. Administration of either betamethasone or dexamethasone may suppress FHR characteristics and biophysical activities. Specifically, the FHR tracing may show a reduction in FHR accelerations, STV, and LTV.

Biophysical activities such as fetal movement and breathing activity have also been shown to be reduced on ultrasound evaluation. The effects of the steroids can be seen for as long as 96 hours after administration. (Rotmensch, et al., 1999). It is important to remember that these effects are transient. Increased awareness of the FHR and activity characteristics associated with maternal corticosteroid administration may prevent unwarranted deliveries of the preterm fetus.

Monitoring the Multiple Gestation Patient

The number of multiple gestation pregnancies, which include twins, triplets, and higher-order multiples, has significantly increased in the United States over the past decade. Those pregnancies are at increased risk for fetal and neonatal morbidity and mortality as well as maternal morbidity and mortality.

Because multiple gestations have the inherent risks of preterm birth and increased fetal and neonatal morbidity and mortality, antepartum surveillance often begins by 24–28 weeks gestation. Agreed-upon protocols for the acquisition and interpretation of antepartum data in the preterm multiple gestation do not exist because limited information exists on the meaning of specific physiologic findings. Monitoring of multiple gestation patients, however, poses significant challenges related to the limitations of instrumentation, size, number and/or positions of fetuses, and complications related to preterm labor as well as other pregnancy complications such as gestational hypertension, polyhydramnios, premature rupture of membranes, and intrauterine fetal demise of one or more fetuses. Because preterm labor is a potential complication of a multiple pregnancy, it is important to teach the mother about the early and subtle signs of preterm labor and to instruct her to report any occurrence.

Many commercially available monitors have the capability to monitor two fetuses simultaneously and to print two separate recordings on the same tracing. Twin monitoring is typically accomplished with two separate ultrasound transducers or an ultrasound transducer and a direct ECG electrode (spiral electrode). Familiarity with the manufacturer's instructions on using dual-mode monitoring as well as troubleshooting the system may be helpful to the caregiver.

In addition to providing the benefits of monitoring and recording two fetuses on one tracing, some EFM monitors will alert the clinician to duplicate monitoring of the same fetus by printing special marks on the tracing. That type of technology may be helpful because synchrony of fetal movement and the FHR are common with twins. If two separate monitors are used to monitor a twin pregnancy, it is important to compare the two printouts to ensure that both fetuses are actually being monitored (Murray, 1997). Real-time ultrasonography may be needed to visualize cardiac movement of each fetus when there is a question regarding FHR. For further information on the nurse's role in limited obstetric ultrasound, refer to AWHONN's *Clinical Competencies and Education Guide: Limited Ultrasound Examinations In Obstetric And Gynecologic/Infertility Settings* (AWHONN, 1998b).

However, very few monitors are capable of monitoring triplet or greater gestations. When such a monitor is used, there is little certainty that individual fetuses can be identified from one monitoring session to the next as well as during the full length of labor. In gestations of triplets or greater, antepartum and intrapartum monitoring may have to be accomplished with ultrasound only, performed at the timing and discretion of the physician or other ultrasound credentialed provider.

An important aspect of monitoring multiple gestations is ensuring that each fetus is properly identified and monitored appropriately. When the patient with twins is monitored, each fetus can be identified (i.e., "A" and "B") depending on its location in the maternal abdomen. The fetus that is presenting first or that is closest to the maternal cervix is labeled "A"; the second fetus is labeled "B." (In a triplet gestation fetus "B" is the second one closest to the maternal cervix, and fetus "C" is in the most distant position from the maternal cervix.) The position of each fetus in the uterus as well as which fetus corresponds to the dark and light lines on the tracing should also be recorded. This documentation should be recorded in the patient record as well as on each tracing obtained (Murray, 1997).

Every effort should be made to keep each labeled fetus on its assigned ultrasound transducer for subsequent monitoring sessions. If monitoring is performed using this procedure, there is greater likelihood that fetus "A" will be the dark line on the current tracing and the prior tracings and that fetus "B" will be the light line on the current and prior tracings. This consistency in labeling will assist in the assessment of fetal well-being over time.

Complications of Pregnancy and Labor

A number of maternal conditions may alter the EFM information observed. The EFM technology may give reliable information, yet it has limitations as discussed in Chapters 5 and 8. The use of drugs in labor such as $MgSO_4$, tocolytics, and analgesia or anesthesia and altered maternal conditions, some of which are listed below, may alter EFM data and make interpretation difficult, even for the most skilled practitioner:

◆ Hypoglycemia

◆ Hyperglycemia

◆ Diabetic ketoacidosis

◆ Hypertensive disorders of pregnancy

◆ Eclamptic seizures

◆ Placenta previa

◆ Placental abruption

◆ Uterine rupture

◆ Anaphylactoid syndrome of pregnancy (amniotic fluid embolism)

◆ Multiorgan Dysfunction Syndrome

◆ Myocardial infarction

◆ Multiple sclerosis

◆ Trauma

Examples of selected pregnancy complications with associated FHR patterns are presented in Chapters 11 and 14.

☞ SUMMARY

Although EFM has limited use in identifying the fetus undergoing compromise, it has proven very valuable in identifying the fetus that is not in metabolic acidosis and that is well-oxygenated. Interpretation requires a knowledge of the physiologic basis for monitoring, the baseline characteristics, and pattern interpretation; experience with UA monitoring, and an understanding of the monitoring of special populations to better comprehend the fetal and maternal findings. Chapter 7 will discuss collaborative diagnosis and interventions based on these interpretation skills.

⌨ REFERENCES

Abitbol, M. (1985). Supine position in labor and associated fetal heart rate changes. *Obstetrics and Gynecology, 65*(4), 481–486.

Aderhold, K. J., & Roberts, J. E. (1991). Phases of second stage labor: Four descriptive case studies. *Journal of Nurse-Midwifery, 36*, 267–275.

Albers, L. L. (1994). Clinical issues in electronic fetal monitoring. *Birth, 21*(2), 108–110.

American College of Obstetricians and Gynecologists (ACOG). (1995a). *Dystocia and the augmentation of labor* (Technical Bulletin No. 218). Washington, D.C.: Author.

ACOG. (1995b). *Fetal heart rate patterns: Monitoring, interpretation, and management* (Technical Bulletin No. 207). Washington, D.C.: Author.

ACOG. (1998). *Inappropriate use of the terms fetal distress and birth asphyxia* (Committee Opinion No. 197). Washington, D.C.: Author.

ACOG. (1999). *Induction of labor* (Practice Bulletin No. 10). Washington, D.C.: Author.

Anyaegbunam, A., Tran, T., Jadali, D., Randolph, G., & Mikhail, M. S. (1997). Assessment of fetal well-being in methadone-maintained pregnancies: Abnormal nonstress tests. *Gynecologic and Obstetric Investigations, 43*(1), 25–28.

Arnold-Aldea, S. A., & Parer, J. (1990). Fetal cardiovascular physiology. In R. D. Eden & F. H. Boehm (Eds.), *Assessment and care of the fetus: Physiological, clinical and medicolegal principles* (pp. 29–42). Norwalk, CT: Appleton & Lange.

AWHONN. (1998a). *Clinical competencies and education guide: Antepartum and intrapartum fetal heart rate monitoring.* Washington, D.C.: Author.

AWHONN. (1998b). *Clinical competencies and education guide: Limited ultrasound examinations in obstetric and gynecologic/infertility settings.* Washington, D.C.: Author.

AWHONN. (2000a.) *Nursing management of the second stage of labor: Evidence-based clinical practice guidelines.* Washington, D.C.: Author.

AWHONN. (2000b). *Professional nursing support of laboring women* (Clinical position statement). Washington, D.C.: Author.

Barnett, M. M., & Humenick, S. S. (1982). Infant outcome in relation to second stage labor pushing method. *Birth, 9*, 221–229.

Baxi, L. V., & Petrie, R. H. (1987). Pharmacologic effects of labor: Effects of drugs on dystocia, labor, and uterine activity. *Clinical Obstetrics and Gynecology, 30*(1), 19–32.

Beckmann, C. A., Van Mullem, C., Beckmann, C. R., & Broekhuizen, F. F. (1997). Interpreting fetal heart rate tracings. Is there a difference between labor and delivery nurses and obstetricians? *Journal of Reproductive Medicine, 42*(10), 647–650.

Brown, R., & Patrick, J. (1981). The nonstress test: How long is enough? *American Journal of Obstetrics and Gynecology, 141*(6), 646–651.

Caldeyro-Barcia, R. (1979). The influence of maternal bearing-down efforts during second stage on fetal well-being. *Birth and the Family Journal, 6*, 17–21.

Castillo, R. A., Devoe, L. D., Arthur, M., Searle, N., Metheny, W. P., & Ruedrich, D. A. (1989). The preterm nonstress test: Effects of gestational age and length of study. *American Journal of Obstetrics and Gynecology, 160*(1), 172–175.

Cohen, W. R., Acker, D. B., & Friedman, E. A. (Eds.) (1989). *Management of labor* (2nd ed.). Rockville, MD: Aspen.

Cusick, W., Smulian, J. C., & Vintzileos, A. M. (1995). Intrapartum use of fetal heart rate monitoring, contraction monitoring, and amnioinfusion. *Clinics of Perinatology, 22*(4), 875–906.

Davis, L., & Riedmann, G. (1991). Recommendation for the management of low risk obstetric patients. *International Journal of Gynaecology and Obstetrics, 35*(2), 107–115.

de Jong, P. R., Johanson, R. B. Baxen, P., Adrians, V. D., van der Westhuisen, S., & Jones, P. W. (1997). Randomized trial comparing the upright and supine positions for the second stage of labour. *British Journal of Obstetrics & Gynaecology, 104*(5), 567–571.

Eganhouse, D. J., & Burnside, S. M. (1992). Nursing assessment and responsibilities in monitoring the preterm pregnancy. *Journal of Obstetric, Gynecologic, and Neonatal Nursing, 21*(5), 355–363.

Elkington, K. W. (1991). At the water's edge: Where obstetrics and anesthesia meet. *Obstetrics and Gynecology, 77*(2), 304–308.

Enkin, M., Keirse, M., Neilson, J., Crowther, C., Duley, L., Hodnett, E., & Hofmeyer, J. (2000). *A guide to effective care in pregnancy and childbirth* (3rd ed.). Oxford, UK: Oxford University Press.

Eronen, M., Heikkila, P., & Teramo K. (2001). Congenital complete heart block in the fetus: Hemodynamic features, antenatal treatment, and outcome in six cases. *Pediatric Cardiology 22*(5), 385–392.

Feinstein, N. F., Sprague, A., & Trepanier, M. J. (2000). *Fetal heart rate auscultation.* Washington, D.C.: AWHONN.

Flamm, B. L. (1994). Electronic fetal monitoring in the United States. *Birth, 21*(2), 105–106.

Flynn, A. M., Kelly, J., Hollins, G., & Lynch, P. F. (1978). Ambulation in labor. *British Medical Journal, 2*(6137), 591–593.

Freeman, R. K., Garite, T. J., & Nageotte, M. P. (1991). *Fetal heart rate monitoring* (2nd ed.). Baltimore: Williams & Wilkins.

Friedman, E. A. (1978). *Labor: Clinical evaluation and management* (2nd ed.). Norwalk, CT: Appleton-Century-Crofts.

Garfield, R. (1987). Cellular and molecular bases for dystocia. *Clinical Obstetrics and Gynecology, 30*(1), 3–18.

Garite, T. J. (2002). Intrapartum fetal evaluation. In S. G. Gabbe, J. R. Niebyl, & J. L. Simpson (Eds.), *Obstetrics: Normal and problem pregnancies* (4th ed., pp. 395–429). New York: Churchill Livingstone.

Garite, T. J., Weeks, J., Peters-Phair, K., Pattillo, C., & Brewster, W. R. (2000). A randomized controlled trial of the effect of increased intravenous hydration on the course of labor in nulliparous women. *American Journal of Obstetrics and Gynecology, 183*(6), 1544–1548.

Grylack, L. J., Chu, S. S., & Scanlon, J. W. (1984). Use of intravenous fluids before cesarean section: Effects on perinatal glucose, insulin, and sodium homeostasis. *Obstetrics and Gynecology, 63*(5), 654–658.

Gupta, J. K., Brayshaw, E. M., & Lilford, R. J. (1989). An experiment of squatting birth. *European Journal of Obstetrics, Gynecology and Reproductive Biology, 30*(3), 217–220.

Hammacher, K. (1969). The clinical significance of cardiotocography. In P. Huntingford, K. Hüter, & E. Saling (Eds.), *Perinatal medicine: 1st European Congress, Berlin* (p. 81). Stuttgart, Germany: Thieme.

Hodnett, E. D. (2002). Caregiver support for women during childbirth (Cochrane Review). In: *The Cochrane Library,* Issue 4.

Hodnett, E. D., Lowe, N. K., Hannah, M. E., Willan, A. R., Stevens, B., Weston, J. A., Ohlsson, A., Gafni, A., Muir, H. A., Myhr, T. L., & Stremler, R. (2002). Effectiveness of nurses as providers of birth labor support in North American hospitals: A randomized controlled trial. *Journal of American Medical Association, 288*(11), 1373–1381.

Hofmeyr, G. J., & Kulier, R. (2002). Operative versus conservative management for "fetal distress" in labour (Cochrane Review). In *The Cochrane Library,* Issue 4.

Hohn, A., & Stanton, R. (2002). The cardiovascular system. In A. Fanaroff, & R. Martin (Eds.), *Neonatal-perinatal medicine: Diseases of the fetus and infant* (7th ed., pp. 883–940). St. Louis, MO: Mosby-Year Book.

Holland, R. L., & Smith, D. A. (2000). Care during the second stage of labor. In I. Chalmers, M. Erkin, & M. J. N. C. Keirse (Eds.), *A guide to effective care in pregnancy and childbirth* (pp. 1129–1144). Oxford, UK: Oxford University Press.

Huszar, G., & Roberts, J. M. (1982). Biochemistry and pharmacology of the myometrium and labor: Regulation at the cellular and molecular levels. *American Journal of Obstetrics and Gynecology, 142*(2), 225–237.

Iams, J. D., Newman, R. B., Thom, E. A., Goldenberg, R. L., Mueller-Heubach, E., Moawad, A., Sibai, B. M., Caritis, S. N., Miodovnik, M., Paul, R. H., Dombrowski, M. P., Thurnau, G., & McNeil, S. D. (2002). Frequency of uterine contractions and the risk of spontaneous preterm delivery. *New England Journal of Medicine, 346*(4), 250–252.

Ikuo, S., Akio, I., & Taro, T. (1992). Longitudinal measurement of fetal heart rate (FHR) monitoring in second trimester. *Early Human Development, 29*(1–3), 251–257.

King, T. L., & Simpson, K. R. (2001). Fetal assessment during labor. In K. R. Simpson & P. Creehan (Eds.), *Perinatal Nursing* (pp. 378–416). Philadelphia: Lippincott.

Klavin, M., Laver, A., & Boscola, M. (1977). *Clinical concepts of fetal heart rate monitoring.* Andover, MA: Hewlett-Packard Company.

Kopecky, E. A., Ryan, M. L., Barrett, J. F., Seaward, P. G., Ryan, G., Koren, G., & Amankwah, K. (2000). Fetal response to maternally administered morphine. *American Journal of Obstetricians and Gynecologists, 183*(2), 424–430.

Lederman, R. P., Lederman, E., Work, B. A. Jr., & McCann, D. S. (1978). The relationship of maternal anxiety, plasma catecholamines, and plasma cortisol to progress in labor. *American Journal of Obstetrics and Gynecology, 132*(5), 495–500.

Lotgering, F. K., Wallenburg, H. C., & Schouten, H. J. (1982). Interobserver and intraobserver variation in the assessment of antepartum cardiotocograms. *American Journal of Obstetricians and Gynecologists, 144*(6), 701–705.

Magann, E. F., Cleveland, R. S., Dockery, J. R., Chauhan, S. P., Martin, J. N., & Morrison, J. C. (1993). Acute tocolysis for fetal distress: Terbutaline versus magnesium sulphate. *Australian and New Zealand Journal of Obstetrics and Gynaecology, 33*(4), 362–364.

Martin, C. B. Jr. (1982). Physiology and clinical use of fetal heart rate variability. *Clinics in Perinatology, 9*(2), 339–352.

May, K., & Mahlmeister, L. (1994). *Comprehensive maternity nursing.* Philadelphia: Lippincott-Raven.

Mayberry, L. J., Hammer, R., Kelly, C., True-Driver, B., & De, A. (1999). Use of delayed pushing with epidural anesthesia: Findings from a randomized, controlled trial. *Journal of Perinatology, 19,* 26–30.

Mayberry, L. J., Wood, S. H., Strange, L. B., Lee, L., Heisler, D. R., & Nielson-Smith, K. (2000). *Second stage labor management: Promotion of evidence-*

based practice and a collaborative approach to patient care. Washington, D.C.: AWHONN.

Menihan, C. A., & Zottoli, E. K. (2001). *Electronic fetal monitoring: Concepts and applications.* Philadelphia: Lippincott.

Mercer, B. M., & Lewis, R. (1997). Preterm labor and preterm premature rupture of the membranes: Diagnosis and management. *Infectious Disease Clinics of North America, 11*(1), 177–201.

Moawad, A. H., Goldenberg, R. L., Mercer, B., Meis, P. J., Iams, J. D., Das, A., Caritis, S. N., Miodovnik, M., Menard, M. K., Thurnau, G. R., Dombrowski, M., & Roberts, J. M. (2002). The Preterm Prediction Study: The value of serum alkaline phosphatase, alpha-fetoprotein, plasma corticotrophin-releasing hormone, and other serum markers for the prediction of spontaneous preterm birth. *American Journal of Obstetricians and Gynecologists, 186*(5), 990–996.

Modanlou, H. D., & Freeman, R. K. (1982). Sinusoidal fetal heart rate pattern: Its definition and clinical significance. *American Journal of Obstetrics and Gynecology, 142*(8), 1033–1038.

Morrison, J. (1992). *Assessment and management of preterm labor.* Statement presented at the Armed Forces District Conference, Norfolk, VA.

Morton, K. E., Jackson, M. C., & Gillmer, M. D. (1985). A comparison of the effects of four intravenous solutions for the treatment of ketonuria during labour. *British Journal of Obstetrics and Gynaecology, 92*(5), 473–479.

Muller, J. S., Antunes, M., Behle, I., Teixeira, L., & Zielinsky, P. (2002). Acute effects of maternal smoking on fetal-placental-maternal system hemodynamics. *Arquivos Brasileiros De Cardiologia, 78*(2), 148–155.

Murray, M. (1997). *Antepartal and intrapartal fetal monitoring.* Albuquerque, NM: Learning Resources International.

Myers, R. E. (1975). Maternal psychological stress and fetal asphyxia: A study in the monkey. American *Journal of Obstetrics and Gynecology, 122*(1), 47–59.

Naef, R., Morrison, J. C., Washburne, J. F., McLaughlin, B. N., Perry, K. G., & Roberts, W. E. (1994). Assessment of fetal well-being using the nonstress test in the home setting. *Obstetrics and Gynecology, 84*(3), 424–426.

National Institute of Child Health and Human Development (NICHD) Research Planning Workshop, (1997). Electronic fetal heart rate monitoring: Research guidelines for interpretation. American *Journal of Obstetrics and Gynecology, 177*(6), 1385–1390, and *Journal of Obstetric, Gynecologic, and Neonatal Nursing, 26*(6), 635–640.

National Institutes of Health (NIH) (2000, August). *Antenatal corticosteroids revisited: Repeat courses.* Bethesda, MD: Author.

NIH. (2002, January). *Home Uterine Monitors Not Useful for Predicting Premature Birth.* Bethesda, MD: Author.

Newman, R., Campbell, B., & Stramm, S. (1990). Objective tocodynamometry identifies labor onset earlier than subjective maternal perception. *Obstetrics and Gynecology, 76,* 1089–1092.

Norwitz, E. R., Robinson, J. N., & Repke, J. T. (2002). Labor and delivery. In S. G. Gabbe, J. R. Niebyl, & J. L. Simpson (Eds.), *Obstetrics: Normal and problem pregnancies* (4th ed., pp. 353–394). New York: Churchill Livingstone.

O'Brien-Able, N. E., & Benedetti, T. J. (1992). Saltatory fetal heart rate patterns. *Journal of Perinatology, 12*(1), 13–17.

Omigbodun, A. O., Fajimi, J. L., & Adeleye, J. A. (1991). Effects of using either saline or glucose as a vehicle for infusion in labour. *East African Medical Journal, 68*(2), 88–92.

Oncken, C. A., Hardardottir, H., Hatsukami, D. K., Lupo, V. R., Rodis, J. F., & Smeltzer, J. S. (1997). Effects of transdermal nicotine or smoking on nicotine concentrations and maternal-fetal hemodynamics. *Obstetrics and Gynecology, 90*(4, Pt. 1), 569–574.

Oncken, C. A., Kranzler, H., O'Malley, P., Gendreau, P., & Campbell, W. A. (2002). The effect of cigarette smoking on fetal heart rate characteristics. *Obstetrics and Gynecology, 90*(5, Pt. 1), 751–755.

Oxorn, H. (1986). *Oxorn-Foote human labor and birth* (5th ed.). Norwalk, CT: Appleton-Century-Crofts.

Parer, J. T. (1999). Fetal heart rate. In R. K. Creasy, & R. Resnik (Eds.), *Maternal fetal medicine: Principles and practice* (4th ed., p. 270). Philadelphia: W.B. Saunders.

Parer, J. T. (1997). *Handbook of fetal heart rate monitoring* (2nd ed.). Philadelphia: W.B. Saunders.

Patkos, P., Boucher, M., Broussard, P. M., Phelan, J. P. & Platt, L. D. (1986). Factors influencing nonstress tests results in multiple gestation. *American Journal of Obstetricians and Gynecologists, 154*(5), 1107–1108.

Petrie, R. (1991). Intrapartum fetal evaluation. In S. Gabbe, J. Neibyl, & J. Simpson (Eds.), *Obstetrics: Normal and problem pregnancies* (2nd ed., p. 457). New York: Churchill Livingstone.

Pillai, M., & James, D. (1990). The development of fetal heart rate patterns during normal pregnancy, *Obstetrics and Gynecology, 76*(5, Pt. 1), 812–816.

Read, J. A., Miller, F. C., & Paul, R. H. (1981). Randomized trial of ambulation versus oxytocin for labor enhancement: A preliminary report. American *Journal of Obstetrics & Gynecology, 139*(6), 669–672.

Roberts, J. E., Mendez-Bauer, C., & Wodell, D. A. (1983). The effects of maternal position on uterine contractility and efficiency. *Birth, 10*(4), 243–249.

Roberts, J., & Woolley, D. (1996). A second look at the second stage of labor. *Journal of Obstetric, Gynecologic, and Neonatal Nursing, 25*(5), 415–423.

Rosen, M. G., & Dickinson, J. C. (1993). The paradox of electronic fetal monitoring: More data may not enable us to predict or prevent infant neurologic morbidity. *American Journal of Obstetrics and Gynecology, 168*(3, Pt. 1), 745–751.

Rotmensch, S., Liberati, M., Vishne, T. H., Celentano, C., Ben-Rafael, Z., & Bellati, U. (1999). The effects of betamethasone and dexamethasone on fetal heart rate patterns and biophysical activities: A prospective randomized trial. *Acta Obstetricia et Gynecologica Scandinavia, 78*(6), 493–500.

Rouse, D. J., Owen, J., & Hauth, J. C. (1999). Active phase labor arrest: Oxytocin augmentation for at least four hours. *Obstetrics and Gynecology, 93*(3), 323–328.

Sampselle, C. M., & Hines, S. (1999). Spontaneous pushing during birth: Relationship to perineal outcomes. *Journal of Nurse Midwifery, 44*(1), 36–39.

Schifrin, B. S., & Clement, D. (1990). Why fetal monitoring remains a good idea. *Contemporary OB/GYN, 35,* 70–86.

Schifrin, B. S., & Cohen, W. R. (1989). Labor's dysfunctional lexicon. *Obstetrics and Gynecology, 74*(1), 121–124.

Shermer, R. H., & Raines, D. A. (1997). Positioning during the second stage of labor: Moving back to basics. *Journal of Obstetric, Gynecologic, & Neonatal Nursing, 26*(6), 727–734.

Silverton, L. I. (1989). The thorny issue of intravenous fluids in normal labor. *Birth, 16*(1), 35.

Simkin, P. (1986). Stress, pain, and catecholamines in labor: Part 1. A review. *Birth, 13*(4), 227–233.

Simpson, K. R. (2002). *Cervical ripening and induction and augmentation of labor* (2nd ed.). Washington, D.C.: AWHONN.

Singhi, S. C., & Chookang, E. (1984). Maternal fluid overload during labour: Transplacental hypona-tremia and risk of transient neonatal tachypnea in term infants. *Archives of Disease in Childhood, 59*(12), 1155–1158.

Sleep, J., Roberts, J., & Chalmers, I. (2000). Care during the second stage of labor. In I. Chalmers, M. Erkin, & M. J. N. C. Keirse (Eds.), *A guide to effective care in pregnancy and childbirth* (pp. 1129–1144). Oxford, UK: Oxford University Press.

Society of Obstetricians, and Gynaecologists of Canada (SOGC). (2002). *Fetal health surveillance in labour* (SOGC Clinical Practice Guidelines No. 112). Ottawa, ON: Author

Stan, C., Boulvain, M., Hirsbrunner-Amagbaly, P., & Pfister, R. (2002). Hydration for treatment of preterm labour (Cochrane Review). In: *The Cochrane Library,* Issue 4.

Thacker, S. B., Stroup, D. F., & Peterson, H. B. (1998). Intrapartum electronic fetal monitoring: Data for clinical decisions. *Clinics of Obstetrics and Gynecology, 41*(2), 362–368.

Tucker, S. M. (2000). *Pocket guide to fetal monitoring and assessment.* St. Louis, MO: Mosby.

Turley, G. M. (2000). Essential forces and factors in labor. In S. Mattson and J. E. Smith (Eds.), *Core Curriculum for Maternal-Newborn Nursing* (2nd ed., pp. 204–240). Philadelphia: W.B. Saunders.

Wadhwa, P. D., Sandman, C. A., & Garite, T. J. (2001). The neurobiology of stress in human pregnancy: Implications for prematurity and development of the fetal central nervous system. *Progress in Brain Research, 133,* 131–142.

CHAPTER 7

Physiological Interventions for Fetal Heart Rate Patterns

Donna Adelsperger
Vickie J. Waymire

The goal of fetal monitoring is the ongoing assessment of fetal oxygenation. Both intrinsic and extrinsic influences affect the fetal oxygenation status. The clinician can best develop an understanding of the fetal physiologic response by thoroughly assessing the maternal medical and obstetric history, current risk factors and physical assessment findings, including fetal heart rate (FHR) characteristics and uterine activity. The selection of appropriate interventions to maximize fetal oxygenation is based on these assessments and other relevant clinical information.

When nonreassuring FHR characteristics are recognized, the inexperienced clinician may attempt one or more interventions in a random fashion. With a deeper understanding of fetal physiology, the clinician can focus on the problem and quickly choose appropriate interventions that support or maximize fetal oxygenation.

This chapter reviews concepts for the nursing process of collaborative diagnosis and interventions following assessment and interpretation of FHR characteristics (Figure 7-1). The Dynamic Physiologic Response Model (Figure 7-2) is used to conceptualize fetal status as the basis for interventions. Independent and collaborative interventions are discussed, with emphasis on fetal physiologic responses and the goal of supporting or improving fetal oxygenation.

☛ SYSTEMATIC INTERPRETATION OF THE FHR PATTERN

Appropriate interventions require an accurate interpretation of both the fetal heart and uterine activity characteristics. Attention should be given to the overall clinical picture and to the trends of the FHR pattern over time.

A systematic approach to interpretation encourages a more complete evaluation. Although the experienced clinician may perform many parts of the assessment simultaneously, a detailed and thorough evaluation of fetal heart characteristics and uterine activity should be performed when planning interventions. The method of monitoring used will determine which characteristics can be assessed.

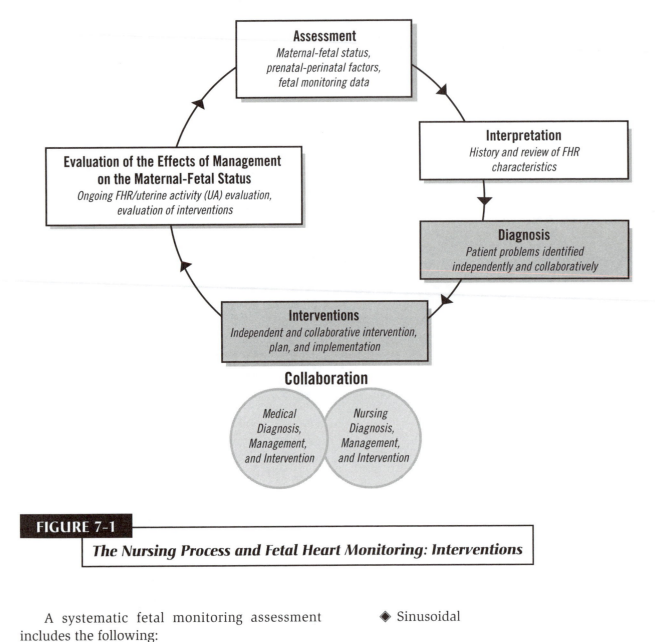

FIGURE 7-1

The Nursing Process and Fetal Heart Monitoring: Interventions

A systematic fetal monitoring assessment includes the following:

I. Uterine activity

◆ Frequency
◆ Duration
◆ Intensity
◆ Resting tone

II. Baseline FHR characteristics

◆ Baseline rate
◆ Rhythm
◆ Variability
  • Long-term variability (LTV)
  • Short-term variability (STV)

◆ Sinusoidal

III. Baseline changes

◆ Accelerations
◆ Periodic decelerations
  • Early
  • Variable
  • Late
  • Combined
◆ Nonperiodic decelerations
  • Variable
  • Prolonged

The terms *reassuring* and *nonreassuring* have been used to describe fetal monitoring patterns.

In some cases, the terms have been used to describe particular characteristics of a pattern. Generally, the terms are used more commonly to describe the overall fetal status.

A reassuring pattern reflects a fetus that demonstrates a favorable physiologic response during the perinatal period. "Reassuring" implies that the fetus may be assumed to have normal oxygen and acid-base status (ACOG, 1995). When the FHR pattern is reassuring, the probability that the fetus is well oxygenated is strong (Krebs, Petres, Dunn, & Smith, 1982; Parer, 1997; Paul, Suidan, Yeh, Schifrin, & Hon, 1975; Schifrin & Dame, 1972). The sensitivity of electronic fetal monitoring (EFM) is high, meaning that well-oxygenated fetuses are correctly identified. The clinician can be confident that the fetus is doing well in terms of oxygenation with a reassuring pattern.

A nonreassuring fetal heart pattern implies that the clinician is not reassured by the findings. A nonreassuring pattern reflects a fetus that demonstrates an unfavorable physiologic response. However, nonreassuring patterns are "nonspecific and cannot reliably predict whether a fetus will be well oxygenated, depressed or acidotic" (ACOG, 1995, p. 4). Not all fetuses with nonreassuring patterns

have neonatal depression or adverse outcomes. It is important to recognize that factors other than hypoxia such as fetal quiet sleep state, central nervous system (CNS) depressant drugs (e.g., narcotics, magnesium sulfate), anencephaly, defective cardiac conduction systems and congenital neurological abnormalities (e.g., acquired from infection) (Nijhuis, Crevels, & van Dongen, 1990; Phelan & Ahn, 1994; Schifrin, Hamilton-Rubinstein, & Shields, 1994) can result in nonreassuring patterns. Therefore, the specificity of EFM is said to be low.

Nonreassuring is a broad term that encompasses many pattern characteristics of varying significance. Because nonreassuring patterns can be associated with adverse neonatal outcomes related to hypoxia and because the clinician is unable to predict which fetuses may be affected, nonreassuring FHR patterns require careful evaluation and timely intervention.

The intent of intervention is to maximize the likelihood of favorable responses while addressing nonreassuring responses. The Dynamic Physiologic Response Model (Figure 7-2) provides a way of viewing patterns based on their characteristics. While the FHR patterns may change and may

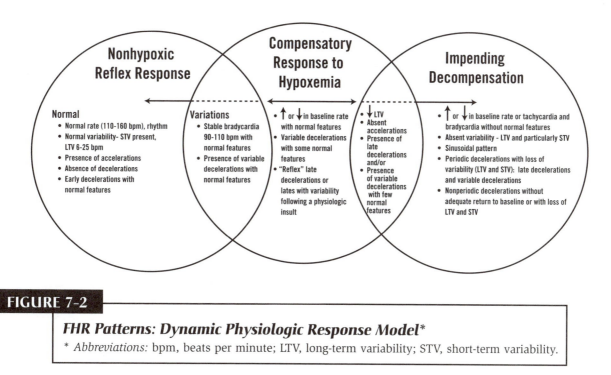

FIGURE 7-2

*FHR Patterns: Dynamic Physiologic Response Model**
* *Abbreviations:* bpm, beats per minute; LTV, long-term variability; STV, short-term variability.

become more reassuring after interventions, this model is not intended to imply a continuum that fetuses will go through in a particular order. What is notable in this model is that normal features—rate rhythm, variability, presence of accelerations and absence of decelerations—exist in the reassuring pattern. Early decelerations with normal features are not associated with hypoxemia. If a pattern becomes nonreassuring, there are often changes from the normal baseline rate (e.g., tachycardia, bradycardia), decelerations and decreased or absent variability. Other FHR patterns, such as some dysrhythmias, may not be categorized as either reassuring or nonreassuring.

☞ PHYSIOLOGIC-BASED INTERVENTIONS

The overarching goal of all interventions is the improvement of fetal oxygenation. The choice of a specific intervention is based on the understanding of the possible underlying physiologic mechanism affecting fetal oxygenation. It may be helpful to think of interventions as falling into four broad categories, or goals, as follows:

◆ Maximize placental blood flow

◆ Maximize umbilical circulation

◆ Maximize available oxygen

◆ Reduce uterine activity

These goals are applicable regardless of the mode of monitoring (auscultation and palpation or EFM). Additional detail regarding auscultation is included in Chapter 5. Specific actions or interventions may fall primarily into one category or overlap categories (see Table 7-1). The choice of intervention(s) will be based on the clinical assessments, pattern interpretation and underlying pathophysiologic factors. Interventions are neither random nor universal but are specifically chosen to maximize fetal oxygenation by addressing the underlying physiologic problem.

Nonreassuring FHR and uterine activity patterns can be related to maternal or fetal pathophysiology or both. Interventions are directed to promote fetal oxygenation by correcting the causative factor(s) if possible. Ideally, the pattern will improve and labor can continue. If a nonreassuring pattern does not improve, or worsens despite interventions, collaborative actions typically increase in number and intensity to promote intrauterine resuscitation. Operative interventions for a compromised fetus may not always be the most appropriate intervention. Yet, if all interventions are unsuccessful, operative delivery may be necessary. Interventions to maximize fetal perfusion and oxygenation should continue until reassuring status has been achieved or birth takes place.

☞ SELECTED INTERVENTIONS

The selection of specific interventions is individualized, based on observed maternal-fetal physiologic response. When acute nonreassuring patterns occur, fetal oxygenation can often be corrected if specific basic clinical interventions are performed in a timely fashion (Lindsay, 1999). Resolution of a nonreassuring pattern may result from one intervention, multiple interventions or other actions not included in the following discussion. The following discussion is intended to suggest possible actions and to guide thoughtful consideration of the many factors that may generate a specific pattern.

Interventions for Baseline Rate

Interventions for Tachycardia

◆ Assess maternal vital signs, specifically temperature and pulse

◆ Assess hydration (initiate or increase intravenous fluids if indicated)

◆ Initiate interventions to decrease maternal temperature if elevated

◆ Reduce anxiety, offer explanations, provide comfort measures and assist with breathing and relaxation techniques

◆ Assess variability and other fetal heart characteristics and consider the need for the following:

TABLE 7-1		
Four Physiologic Goals and Specific Interventions Associated with Maximizing Fetal Perfusion and Oxygenation*		
PHYSIOLOGIC GOAL	**POSSIBLE INTERVENTIONS**	**POSSIBLE PHYSIOLOGIC PROBLEM**
Maximize placental blood flow	Position laterally	Hypotension due to supine position
	Intravenous hydration	Hypotension due to hypovolemia
	Medication (ephedrine)	Hypotension due to vasodilation following epidural anesthesia, resulting in a decrease in maternal venous return and drop in maternal pressure
	Reduce pain/anxiety	Maternal blood shunted away from uterus due to maternal catecholamine production
Maximize umbilical circulation	Change maternal position	Umbilical cord compression due to position
	Lift fetal head off cord	Occult cord/cord prolapse
	Amioinfusion	Cord compression due to lack of cushion normally provided by amniotic fluid
Maximize available oxygen	Maternal position change (lateral)	Less than maximal maternal cardiac output due to position
	Give maternal oxygen	Decreased maternal-fetal oxygen gradient (effective transfer of oxygen may require maternal hyperoxia)
	Guide maternal breathing techniques	Hyperventilation causes hypocapnia, which leads to hypoventilation
		Decreased oxygen availability due to prolonged breath holding during pushing
	Correct underlying maternal disease	Maternal disease affecting oxygen available to fetus, such as diabetic ketoacidosis, pneumonia with hypoxemia, anemia, cardiopulmonary disease
Reduce uterine activity	Maternal position change (lateral)	Supine or standing positions increase uterine activity more than lateral position does
	Reduce/discontinue oxytocin or other uterotonic drugs	Excessive uterine stimulation
	Medication (tocolytics)	Excessive uterine activity

* These interventions may include both independent nursing action and collaborative actions. Examples of physiologic problems are paired with goals and actions.

- Change maternal position
- Administer oxygen (8–10 L/min given via a snug face mask)
- Decrease or discontinue oxytocin

◆ Assess possible drug use

◆ Assess for possible tachydysrhythmia

◆ If auscultating, intervene as needed and consider applying EFM to assess variability

When selecting interventions for tachycardia, the entire maternal-fetal "picture" is reviewed. Fetal heart and uterine activity characteristics are assessed, with attention to underlying physiologic factors associated with the development of fetal tachycardia. Each of the following situations illustrates such an assessment.

In a woman at low risk experiencing a normal pregnancy at term, mild tachycardia with average fetal heart variability and no accompanying periodic changes is not associated with fetal acidemia. The cause may be maternal fever. If maternal temperature is elevated, appropriate nursing, medical or collaborative management of the cause of the fever is indicated. Interventions should focus on eliminating the problem causing the fever. Position change may improve maternal circulation as well as perfusion to the placenta and improve blood flow through the umbilical cord. Hydration may prevent or alleviate the effects of dehydration. Antipyretics may also be used.

When the fetus is exhibiting tachycardia in response to maternal anxiety, pain or epinephrine stimulation, providing explanations, comfort measures and assistance with breathing and relaxation may be helpful. Tachycardia resulting from maternal medications, such as beta-sympathomimetics, may be expected and may not be entirely eliminated. Periodic assessment of maternal and fetal responses is warranted (e.g., pulse, FHR).

Tachycardia may also be noted transiently following an acute hypoxic event. This tachycardia is considered to be a physiologic response, which is secondary to adrenal stimulation causing a release of catecholamines (King & Parer, 2000). Tachycardia indicative of fetal acidemia is associated with variable or late decelerations and decreased variability. The focus of interventions will be on improving uteroplacental blood flow, umbilical cord blood flow and oxygenation, as well as on decreasing uterine activity. Collaborative care as well as further assessments and interventions are indicated.

When tachycardia is the result of a cardiac abnormality or dysrhythmia, medical management and collaborative care focus on the cause and effects of the tachycardia. Maternal positioning, oxygen administration and other actions may be warranted depending on the type and extent of the tachycardia. Fetal cardiac output depends on FHR and may be significantly decreased at rates over 200 bpm.

Interventions for Bradycardia

◆ Verify FHR versus maternal heart rate

◆ Assess fetal movement

◆ Perform fetal scalp stimulation

◆ Perform vaginal examination (if cord is prolapsed, elevate presenting part)

◆ Assess maternal vital signs, specifically blood pressure

◆ Assess hydration

◆ Depending on variability and other FHR assessment and uterine contraction pattern, consider the following actions:

- Maternal position change (right or left lateral or knee-chest)
- Discontinue oxytocin
- Instruct woman to modify or stop pushing
- Administer oxygen (8–10 L/min given via a snug face mask)

◆ If auscultating, intervene and consider applying EFM to assess variability

As with tachycardia, the fetal and maternal assessments may help the clinician identify the physiologic reason for bradycardia. There are both hypoxic and nonhypoxic causes of bradycardia. Technological artifact and maternal pulse should be ruled out before making an assessment of bradycardia.

Stable FHRs of greater than 80 bpm with the presence of variability and accelerations are not associated with acidemia and require only routine assessments and interventions (King & Parer, 2000). For example, fetal maturation may be associated with a normal, stable bradycardic rate such as this. Further assessment to verify fetal well-being may include review of gestational age, asking the mother about changes in the pattern of fetal movement, vaginal examination for rapid descent or prolapsed cord, fetal scalp stimulation or application of spiral electrode to assess STV.

End-stage bradycardia is an example of a pattern that can lead to hypoxia. This term refers to a prolonged bradycardic change from a previously normal rate. It frequently occurs from head compression, which causes vagal stimulation. The fetus tolerates this type of bradycardia as long as the baseline FHR is greater than 80 bpm and variability is present (Parer, 1997). Unresolved bradycardia may progress to fetal hypoxia due to decreased fetal cardiac output, decreased umbilical flow and decreased oxygen transport from the placenta (Parer, 1997). Bradycardia of less than 60 bpm or associated with decreased variability needs immediate attention and collaborative management.

Cardiac dysrhythmias may be the underlying cause of bradycardia. Complete heart block is an example of a nonhypoxic bradycardia. In the presence of a cardiac conduction defect, hypoxia is not usually the cause of bradycardia, especially in the absence of other nonreassuring FHR findings. Further evaluation and interventions as described in the previous section are warranted.

Interventions for Variability

Long-Term Variability (LTV)

Interventions for Average LTV

When LTV is average, the intervention may be only continued routine assessments and interventions, as the presence of LTV is a reassuring finding. Interventions will focus on maintaining the presence of variability and removing any additional stressors, such as cord compression, if present.

Interventions for Decreased LTV

◆ Observe for alternating periods of average variability and accelerations

◆ Change maternal position to left or right lateral

◆ Assess hydration (initiate or increase intravenous fluids)

◆ Perform scalp stimulation or use vibroacoustic stimulator

◆ Discontinue oxytocin (or other uterotonics) if indicated

◆ Provide reassurance and comfort measures to reduce anxiety

◆ Encourage the woman to change her breathing pattern

◆ Assess medication influence and possible use of illicit drugs, alcohol, tobacco

◆ Administer oxygen (8–10 L/min given via a snug face mask) if indicated

When periods of decreased variability occur prior to or following episodes of normal variability, the cause of decreased LTV may be an effect of sleep or medication. Continued assessments and routine care may be all that is warranted.

When the initial tracing shows decreased variability or decreased variability occurs for lengthy periods of time, assessment might include an evaluation of the woman's use of nicotine, illicit drugs, prescription medications, narcotics, or alcohol. Minimal variability is rarely associated with hypoxia in the intrapartum period in the absence of decelerations (King & Parer, 2000). Interventions may include fetal stimulation. Spontaneous or elicited accelerations are reassuring with persistently decreased variability. Other nonhypoxic causes of decreased variability are discussed along with STV later in this chapter.

If the LTV is decreasing with other FHR changes, such as variable or late decelerations, or is decreasing while other FHR changes are occurring and normal causes have been ruled out, a blood flow problem (uteroplacental or cord), an oxygenation problem or both may exist. Interventions will focus on increasing uteroplacental and umbilical blood flow, decreasing uterine activity if indicated, and improving oxygenation. Variability is a significant indicator of how well the fetus is tolerating a given stressor. Further actions, such as validating the monitoring data, changing to a spiral electrode for improved assessment of LTV and STV and assessing fetal response to stimulation and/or fetal scalp pH, may be indicated to further evaluate fetal status.

Interventions for Marked/Saltatory LTV

◆ Change maternal position (right or left lateral)

◆ Assess hydration

◆ Discontinue oxytocin (or other uterotonic drugs) if indicated

◆ Administer oxygen (8–10 L/min given via a snug face mask)

◆ Instruct woman to alter her breathing and pushing patterns

◆ Provide information and comfort techniques to reduce anxiety

◆ Administer tocolytics if indicated

A saltatory pattern may be seen during the intrapartum period. Contributing factors include increased fetal activity, fetal stimulation or a compensatory response to fetal hypoxemia (Parer, 1997). Evaluating the etiology and selecting the appropriate intervention(s) should take into consideration the entire clinical picture. The woman should be asked about her perception of fetal movement, and uterine activity should be assessed to rule out hyperstimulation or hypertonus. Interventions are initiated to promote uteroplacental and umbilical cord blood flow, to decrease uterine activity and to promote maternal cardiac and hemodynamic functioning (Menihan & Zottoli, 2001).

Short-Term Variability (STV)

Interventions for Present STV

When present, STV provides reassurance about the oxygen reserves available and the functioning of the medulla oblongata and autonomic nervous system, particularly the parasympathetic nervous system. Nonhypoxic causes of decreased FHR variability may include prematurity, fetal sleep (perhaps the most common cause), medication effects, fetal anomalies, tachycardia and dysrhythmia. When STV is present with other patterns, such as late or variable decelerations, it may indicate that oxygen reserves are still present, but interventions are warranted to remove or minimize the stressors. Examples of hypoxic causes of absent STV include cord compression or prolapse, maternal hypotension, uterine hyperstimulation, abruptio placentae, tachycardia and dysrhythmia (Menihan & Zottoli, 2001).

Interventions for Absent STV

◆ Change maternal position (left or right lateral)

◆ Assess hydration (initiate or increase intravenous fluids)

◆ Discontinue oxytocin (or other uterotonic drugs if indicated)

◆ Palpate uterus to ensure relaxation between uterine contractions

◆ Assess tracing for most recent acceleration(s)

◆ Administer oxygen (8–10 L/min given via a snug face mask)

◆ Assess maternal vital signs

◆ Perform scalp stimulation, vibroacoustic stimulation or scalp sampling

◆ Consider fetal pulse oximetry (if available)

◆ Assess for further nonreassuring signs (e.g., rising baseline FHR; late, variable or prolonged decelerations)

◆ Notify the primary health care provider

◆ Plan for delivery and care of neonate as needed

Absence of STV may represent the failure of fetal compensatory mechanisms to maintain cerebral oxygenation (Parer, 1997). Nursing interventions to support fetal oxygenation should be timely, with notification of the primary care provider. It is important to note that nonhypoxic causes of absent STV may not require all intervention listed above. However, the nursing interventions described for absent STV are usually appropriate until further evaluation is performed or etiology is determined.

Interventions for Undulating FHR Patterns

When an undulating pattern is observed, the etiology may range from a minor and temporary change related to narcotic analgesia or illicit drug use to a more serious and persistent change due to fetal anemia or fetal hypoxia as in isoimmunization. It is important to differentiate undulating patterns that are pseudosinusoidal from sinusoidal patterns.

Sinusoidal-appearing patterns that do not exist before analgesia administration frequently can be attributed to the analgesic. The sinusoidal-appearing pattern usually has periods of normal FHR baseline, baseline variability and other reassuring characteristics, such as FHR accelerations. The presence of STV is reassuring.

A true sinusoidal pattern may be associated with isoimmunization, fetal anemia or acute onset of significant hypoxia and is nonreassuring. Determination of Rh status and the possibility of isoimmunization should be pursued. Signs and symptoms of abruption, including pain, vaginal bleeding and an increase in uterine resting tonus, should be assessed, and risk factors associated with abruption, including abdominal trauma, rapid decompression of the uterus and cocaine use, also should be evaluated. If the woman's history indicates potential fetal–maternal hemorrhage, a sonographic examination may be performed to observe the fetus for ascites and/or hydrops.

The interventions begin with a reexamination of the patient's history, as well as a physical assessment. Supportive measures for a sinusoidal pattern include improving uterine blood flow and oxygenation.

Interventions for sinusoidal patterns are as follows:

◆ Position the woman laterally

◆ Administer oxygen (8–10 L/min given via a snug face mask)

◆ Provide intravenous hydration

◆ Notify the primary health care provider

In addition, depending on the etiology of the patterns, the following interventions may be considered:

◆ Kleihauer Betke test

◆ Expeditious delivery

◆ Intrauterine fetal blood transfusion via cordocentesis

Interventions for Fetal Dysrhythmias

The types of fetal heart irregularities that can be identified are outlined in Chapter 13. When an irregularity is detected, further assessment to determine etiology and severity is undertaken. An intermittent irregularity with normal heart rate, average STV and fetal reactivity often requires only observation and maintenance of uterine blood flow and oxygenation, as well as reporting the findings to the primary care provider.

The etiology and type of the dysrhythmia will determine the intervention. A persistent tachycardia (supraventricular tachycardia) with fixed R-wave to R-wave intervals or absence of STV may require further ultrasound diagnosis and pharmacologic therapy, such as digoxin.

Review of maternal history may indicate chronic disease, such as systemic lupus erythematosus, drug use or uncontrolled diabetes, as they may be associated with dysrhythmias. Treatments may include administration of antiarrhythmic drugs to the woman, use of steroids or other medications to decrease maternal antibodies or delivery. Additional treatment may be given to the newborn (Menihan & Zottoli, 2001).

Interventions for Variable Decelerations

◆ Change maternal position to determine best location for maintaining FHR (left or right lateral, knee-chest or upright)

◆ Perform vaginal examination to check for prolapsed cord or imminent delivery

◆ Elevate presenting part (if prolapse is present)

◆ Perform amnioinfusion as ordered

◆ Assess variable decelerations for shoulders

◆ Provide explanation and reduce anxiety

◆ Administer oxygen if variable decelerations are persistent, fetal baseline rate is increasing and variability is decreasing or if overshoots are present (8–10 L/min given via a snug face mask)

◆ Discontinue oxytocin (or other uterotonic drugs)

◆ Assess for accelerations

◆ Perform scalp stimulation or fetal scalp sampling or consider fetal pulse oximetry

◆ Consider need for for tocolytic agent

◆ Instruct woman to alter her pushing technique (if in second stage of labor)

◆ Notify the primary health care provider

◆ Plan for delivery and management of neonate

◆ When abrupt FHR decreases from baseline are heard with auscultation, intervene as above and consider applying EFM to assess variability and pattern characteristics

Variable decelerations in the presence of a stable baseline and average variability require no intervention other than position change in an attempt to stop the decelerations. Observation of an acceleratory phase before and after the deceleration provides additional reassurance. When baseline FHR increases and variability decreases, additional interventions as outlined above need to be considered. Although various criteria have been proposed to quantify the severity of variable decelerations, the most important factor to observe is the retention of variability (Parer, 1997).

The primary intervention to improve umbilical cord perfusion is maternal position change to decrease pressure on the umbilical cord and improve fetal and maternal blood flow. Maternal position changes are intended to change the position of the cord so that the variable deceleration pattern will either resolve or improve. It should be noted, however, that some maternal positions may increase compression of the umbilical cord and decrease fetal blood flow. Options available to correct umbilical cord compression include maternal position change to the left or right lateral recumbent position, hands and knees or high Fowler's position with lateral tilt. Positions causing supine hypotension resulting from decreased uteroplacental blood flow should be avoided. During the second stage of labor, open glottal pushing or pushing with every other contraction may be helpful to minimize the severity of the cord compression.

Overshoots associated with variable decelerations necessitate repositioning and observation of fetal heart variability. If variability decreases, application of a spiral electrode will provide information regarding fetal reserve. Additional interventions include oxygen administration, discontinuing oxytocin, assessment of hydration and color of amniotic fluid and notification of the primary care provider. As with all interventions, the nurse should reassure the patient and provide an explanation for the interventions.

Amnioinfusion

Amnioinfusion, the transcervical instillation of fluid into the amniotic cavity, is a simple, inexpensive procedure. The rationale for amnioinfusion is that expansion of amniotic fluid volume decreases the risk of umbilical cord compression and prolonged decelerations by providing a cushioning effect (Lindsay, 1999; Miyazaki & Nevarez, 1985; Nageotte, Bertucci, Towers, Lagrew, & Mondanlou, 1990; Strong, 1995). Amnioinfusion should be performed according to hospital policies and protocols. An intrauterine pressure catheter with a patent single- or double-lumen catheter is used to administer an infusant similar to normal fetal electrolyte concentration, such as normal saline or lactated Ringer's solution. Protocols for instillation of fluid vary, but most recommend an initial bolus up to 800 mL, followed by a maintenance infusion to replace fluid that is lost (ACOG, 1995). Some authorities recommend titration of the fluid bolus until decelerations are resolved, followed by an additional 250 mL (ACOG, 1995; Miyazaki & Nevarez, 1985).

Evaluating the effectiveness of amnioinfusion for significant variables may require at least 20–30 minutes (ACOG, 1995). If a tracing shows improvement with amnioinfusion, a reassuring fetal heart pattern is likely to continue. If the variable deceleration pattern does not improve despite an adequate bolus of infusant and replacement of lost fluid, or is accompanied by decreased variability, interventions should be continued and the physician or midwife should be notified. The amnioinfusion may be discontinued in some cases while other interventions are continued. The woman's response to the procedure should be evaluated, including uterine resting tone, contraction frequency and intensity and the amount of fluid output (Wallerstedt, Higgins, Kasnic, & Curet, 1994). Box 7-1 provides further discussion regarding amnioinfusion.

Interventions for Late Decelerations

◆ Change maternal position (left or right lateral)

◆ Discontinue oxytocin (or uterotonic agent)

◆ Assess hydration (initiate or increase intravenous fluids)

◆ Administer oxygen (8–10 L/min given via a snug face mask)

◆ Palpate uterus at rest to ensure relaxation

◆ Consider/request order for tocolytic drug

◆ Reduce anxiety, provide explanation, provide comfort measures and assist the woman with breathing and relaxation techniques

◆ Consider scalp stimulation or vibroacoustic stimulation

◆ Assist with scalp sampling or fetal pulse oximetry if available

◆ Notify primary health care provider/anesthesia provider

◆ Plan for delivery and neonatal care as needed

When acute nonreassuring fetal status is found, fetal oxygenation may be improved if clinical interventions are performed in a timely fashion. The interventions to improve placental perfusion include moving the patient to a lateral position to maximize uteroplacental blood flow and avoid supine hypotension and rapidly infusing intravenous fluids to maximize maternal fluid volume and improve oxygen saturation. Oxygen is more volume-dependent than diffusion-dependent. Therefore, a bolus of intravenous fluids may be an appropriate intervention unless contraindicated for medical reasons. Intravenous fluids with dextrose should not be used before delivery because dextrose may contribute to fetal hyperglycemia and rebound hypoglycemia. Ephedrine is effective in treating hypotension secondary to conduction anesthesia. It increases vascular tone, leading to restoration of normal blood pressure (Lindsay, 1999).

If uterine stimulation by oxytocin or another uterine stimulant is being provided to the woman, it should be discontinued in the presence of late decelerations, and the primary health care provider should be notified.

Administration of oxygen to the woman may maximize oxygenation to the fetus by increasing maternal oxygen content. Administration of oxygen is maintained when there is decreased or absent variability. If the pattern is corrected and variability is present, the oxygen may be discontinued and the fetal response assessed.

The most important components of placental exchange are the rates of blood flow on each side of the placenta as well as the area for exchange (Parer, 1997). Uterine tachysystole and hypertonus exacerbate the normal interruption of intervillous space perfusion and decrease maternal fetal oxygen exchange. Tocolysis is used to provide uterine relaxation and thereby increase uterine blood flow. Tocolytics have a rapid pharmacologic effect, increasing maternal cardiac output and heart rate and thus increasing uteroplacental blood flow and allowing some fetal recovery before delivery. In addition, tocolytics enhance the transfer of glucose to the fetus, which may offer protection against hypoxic CNS injury (Lindsay, 1999).

Intrapartum fetal oxygen saturation monitoring is an adjunct method of assessing fetal status during labor. It can help the practitioner

BOX 7-1. Amnioinfusion

RATIONALE FOR PROCEDURE

Amnioinfusion is a common procedure used during the intrapartum period to supplement an inadequate amount of amniotic fluid or to dilute thick, meconium-stained fluid (AAP & ACOG, 2002; Spong, 1997).

Increasing amniotic fluid volume has been reported to decrease the occurrence and severity of variable and prolonged fetal heart decelerations by providing "cushioning" for the umbilical cord (Hofmeyr, 2002a; Spong, 1997). Amnioinfusion also has been associated with a decreased need for operative interventions (Hofmeyr, 2002b; Pierce, Gaudier, & Sanchez-Ramos, 2000), and improved cord blood gasses (Pierce et al., 2000). Trials of transabdominal amnioinfusion, though small, suggest results similar to those of transcervical amnioinfusion (Hofmeyr, 2002a). No advantage has been demonstrated with prophylactic versus therapeutic amnioinfusion for oligohydramnios in labor when decelerations are not present (Hofmeyr, 2002b).

The use of amnioinfusion versus no amnioinfusion for moderate or thick meconium has been associated with reduced heavy meconium staining, variable decelerations, and cesarean sections, and may decrease meconium aspiration (Hofmeyr, 2000c). Studies have found that where perinatal surveillance was limited, amnioinfusion was associated with decreased meconium aspiration in newborns, neonatal hypoxic ischemic encephalopathy, and neonatal ventilation or intensive care admission (Hofmeyr, 2002c).

PROTOCOL AND PRINCIPAL ELEMENTS OF PROCEDURE

The hospital protocol should address the following issues:

- Contraindications to amnioinfusion (e.g., vaginal bleeding, uterine anomalies, active infection such as human immunodeficiency virus [HIV] or herpes, impending delivery or anomalous fetus)
- Who can perform the amnioinfusion
- Who can place the IUPC
- What type of fluid may be used (normal saline vs. Ringer's lactate)
- Which instillation method should be used (gravity flow and/or infusion pump)
- Which infusion techniques should be used (bolus, continuous or a combination of both)
- When and why the procedure should be altered (e.g., loss of large amount of fluid due to position change or coughing, increased uterine resting tone, reappearance of abnormal FHR or no uterine fluid return)

General guidelines for the procedure are as follows:

- The procedure requires rupture of membranes and placement of a single- or double-lumen intrauterine pressure catheter by a qualified provider according to facility protocol.
- Instill a bolus dose of up to 800 mL or per hospital protocol.
- Maintain infusion at a rate of 120–180 mL/h or per hospital protocol. (Many authorities recommend giving a bolus until the FHR improves, then adding 250 mL.)
- Warming of the solution is not necessary for full-term fetuses but may be appropriate for preterm or growth-restricted fetuses (ACOG, 1995; Wenstrom, Andrews, & Maher, 1995). If the amnioinfusion solution is warmed, acceptable temperatures are 93–96°F (34–37°C) (Nageotte et al., 1990; Schrimmer, Macri, & Paul, 1991; Strong, Hetzler, Sarno, & Paul, 1990).

BOX 7-1 (cont.)

A few anecdotal cases have reported that rapid infusion of cold fluid can cause bradycardia in a full-term fetus. Other studies have found no difference in outcomes when comparing the use of warmed versus room-temperature solutions (Glantz & Letteney, 1996; Strong, 1995). Blood warmers and fluid warmers specifically designed for fluid administration may be used if temperature settings are regulated. Warmers used for blankets and other fluids and microwave ovens should not be used since temperature settings may be inconsistent or dangerously high (Burrows, Gervasi, Kosty, Dierker, & Mann, 1995; Wallerstedt et al., 1994).

- Assess uterine resting tone and evaluate fluid output during amnioinfusion to avoid iatrogenic polyhydramnios (overdistention of the uterus). Overdistention is more likely to occur when the vertex obstructs flow. Releasing or withdrawing fluid may correct this situation.
- In addition to assessments appropriate for the stage of labor, additional assessments may include the following:
  - —Vital signs prior to placement, then assessment of maternal temperature every 2 hours and as required
  - —Fundal height and leakage of fluid (to prevent iatrogenic polyhydramnios)
  - —Amount, color and odor of fluid leaking from vagina
  - —Fetal response (resolution of decelerations, description of meconium)
- Observe resting tone of uterus carefully when evaluating uterine activity.
- Documentation should reflect purpose of the procedure, fetal and maternal response to procedure, uterine resting tone, fluid output and type, rate and volume of infusant.

The time required for an amnioinfusion to reach a therapeutic result or increase the amniotic fluid index is approximately 30 minutes (ACOG 1995; Snell, 1993).

decide whether it is safe for labor to continue or whether interventions are needed. A fetal oxygen saturation result of 30% or more is considered reassuring and usually means the fetus is adequately oxygenated and labor can continue (Garite et al., 2000). As is true of EFM, a single reading does not accurately reflect fetal condition, and the trend should be considered along with other clinical assessments (Yam, Chua, & Arulkumaran, 2000).

The correction of late decelerations implies that their etiology is a physiologic event that can be improved or corrected. However, when a late deceleration pattern persists despite corrective measures, other members of the health care team should be summoned. If the pattern persists, variability is decreased and/or the baseline becomes

tachycardic, preparations for an expedient delivery should be initiated.

Interventions for Early Decelerations

No interventions are recommended for early decelerations unless variability is absent or decreased. In such situations, the caregiver needs to be sure that the decelerations are early and not late decelerations. If variability is absent or decreased, the caregiver needs to assess fetal heart response to stimulation (through scalp, abdominal or vibroacoustic assessment), reevaluate the management plan and provide interventions described earlier in this chapter.

Interventions for Prolonged Decelerations

◆ Change maternal position (left or right lateral)

◆ Discontinue oxytocin (or other uterotonics)

◆ Assess hydration (initiate or increase intravenous fluids)

◆ Perform vaginal examination to check for cord prolapse or entrapment or fetal descent

◆ Evaluate presenting part (rule out breech presentation)

◆ Elevate presenting part

◆ Perform amnioinfusion as ordered

◆ Administer oxygen (8–10 L/min given via a snug face mask)

◆ Reduce anxiety, provide explanation and assist the woman with breathing and relaxation techniques

◆ Administer tocolytics as ordered

◆ Notify the primary health care provider and/or the anesthesia provider

◆ Plan for delivery and neonatal care

◆ If auscultating, intervene as stated and consider applying EFM to assess variability and pattern characteristics

The first intervention for the prolonged deceleration should be maternal position change. Assessing for identifiable causes may take place simultaneously with other interventions such as fluid bolus, oxygen administration or discontinuation of uterine stimulants (e.g., oxytocin or another uterotonic) to decrease of uterine contractions. Administration of a tocolytic, such as terbutaline, may be administered according to provider's order or hospital protocol. These actions may allow for intrauterine resuscitation.

When a tocolytic is administered to a patient whose fetus is demonstrating a prolonged deceleration, the rapid decrease in uterine activity may decrease umbilical cord compression or improve uteroplacental blood flow and, therefore, improve fetal oxygenation. Frequently, the FHR demonstrates an immediate improvement.

If the deceleration cannot be corrected, immediate delivery may be necessary. Persistent prolonged decelerations may be caused by irreversible umbilical cord accidents, significant placental abruption, decreased blood flow to the fetus that cannot be corrected or complications within the fetus itself.

Interventions for Combined Decelerations

Decelerations can occur in combination. For example, variable decelerations with an overshoot may be followed by a late deceleration. In combined deceleration patterns, the assessment of the pattern should be based on the most nonreassuring component of the pattern (Tucker, 2000). The interventions performed for one pattern frequently help to alleviate another.

Combined decelerations occur predominantly late in the first stage of labor and are often associated with abnormal uterine activity. Hyperstimulation of the uterus (sometimes associated with spontaneous labor but more often with infusion of oxytocin) may produce fetal bradycardia, prolonged or late decelerations or combined decelerations.

Interventions for Accelerations

Accelerations observed as a response to sympathetic stimulation are indicative of a well-oxygenated CNS, and no interventions are needed other than reassurance of the patient. Assessment of an accurate baseline rate is important when accelerations are present. The correct baseline may be perceived as decelerations if incorrectly interpreted (Freeman, Garite, & Nageotte, 1991). Regardless of whether accelerations are noted in the baseline or in association with a contraction, the fetus is demonstrating a reassuring response.

◻ SUMMARY

Decisions about interventions and use of further measures should be individualized in each patient situation on the basis of ongoing assessments. The nurse and other caregivers have the respon-

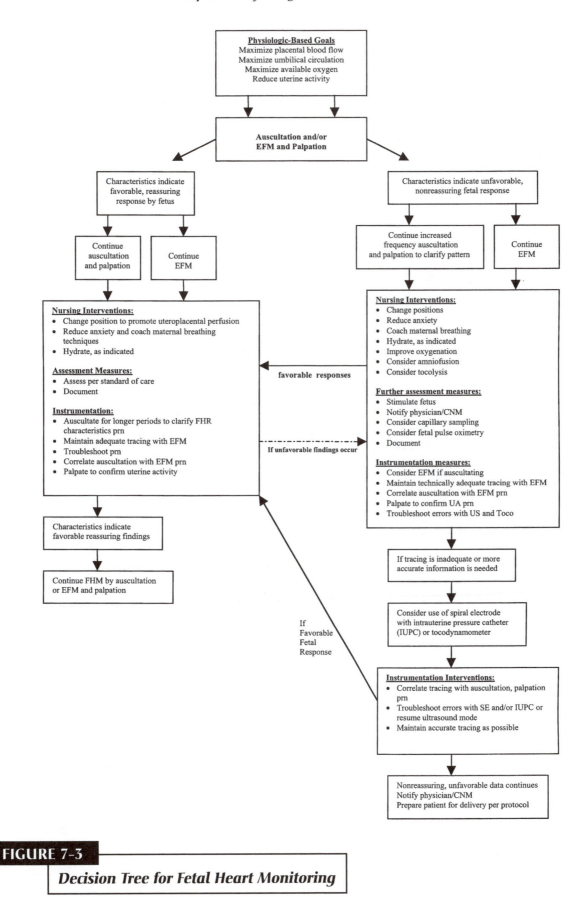

FIGURE 7-3

Decision Tree for Fetal Heart Monitoring

sibility to remain calm, provide clear directions to the patient as well as other members of the health care team, decrease patient anxiety and perform tasks confidently and competently. When explaining the situation to the patient, the caregiver should calmly, quickly and factually state any concerns about the fetus, along with the need to provide interventions that may improve fetal status. During the time interventions are in progress, concise instructions and an evaluation of events can be provided to the patient.

Figure 7-3 offers a decision-making tree that addresses the issues of intrapartum goals, physiologic interventions and the use of additional measures/actions, such as instrumentation. This decision-making tree provides a general process outline, which must be interpreted and modified, as appropriate, in light of the health care team's clinical assessment of the fetus.

☞ REFERENCES

American Academy of Pediatric, & American College of Obstetricians and Gynecologists (2002). *Guidelines for perinatal care*. Washington, D.C.: Author.

American College of Obstetricians and Gynecologists. (1995). *Fetal heart rate patterns: Monitoring, interpretation, and management* (ACOG Technical Bulletin No. 207). Washington, D.C.: Author.

Burrows, W. R., Gervasi, L., Kosty, D., Dierker, L. J., & Mann, L. I. (1995). Warming fluid for amnioinfusion during labor. *Journal of Reproductive Medicine, 40*(2), 123–126.

Freeman, R. K., Garite, T. J., & Nageotte, M. P. (1991). *Fetal heart monitoring* (2nd ed.). Baltimore: Williams & Wilkins.

Garite, T. J., Dildy, G. A., McNamara H., Nageotte, M. P., Boehm, F. H., Dellinger, E. H., et al. (2000). A multicenter controlled trial of fetal pulse oximetry in the intrapartum management of nonreassuring fetal heart rate patterns. *American Journal of Obstetrics and Gynecology, 183*(5), 1049–1058.

Glantz, J. C., & Letteney, D. L. (1996). Pumps and warmers during amnioinfusion: Is either necessary? *Obstetrics & Gynecology, 87*(1), 150–155.

Hofmeyr, G. J. (2002a). Amnioinfusion for umbilical cord compression in labor (Cochrane Review) In: *The Cochrane Library*, issue 2. Oxford: Update Software.

Hofmeyr, G. J. (2002b). Prophylactic versus therapeutic amnioinfusion for oligohydramnios in labour (Cochrane Review). In: *The Cochrane Library*, Issue 4. Oxford: Update Software.

Hofmeyr, G. J. (2002c). Amnioinfusion for meconium-stained liquor in labour (Cochrane Review). In: *The Cochrane Library*, Issue 4. Oxford: Update Software.

King, T., & Parer, J. (2000). The physiology of fetal heart rate patterns and perinatal asphyxia. *Journal of Perinatal and Neonatal Nursing, 14*(3), 19–39.

Krebs, H. B., Petres, R. E., Dunn, L. J., & Smith, P. J. (1982). Intrapartum fetal heart rate monitoring. VI. Prognostic significance of accelerations. *American Journal of Obstetrics & Gynecology, 142*(3), 297–305.

Lindsay, M. K. (1999). Intrauterine resuscitation of the compromised fetus. *Clinics in Perinatology, 26*(3), 569–584.

Macri, C. J., Schrimmer, D. B., Leung, A., Greenspan, J. S., & Paul, R. H. (1992). Prophylactic amnioinfusion improves outcome of pregnancy complicated by thick meconium and oligohydramnios. *American Journal of Obstetrics and Gynecology 167*(1), 117–121.

Menihan, C. A., & Zottoli, E. K. (2001). *Electronic fetal monitoring: Concepts and applications*. Philadelphia: Lippincott Williams & Wilkins.

Miyazaki, F. S., & Nevarez, F. (1985). Saline amnioinfusion for relief of repetitive variable decelerations: A prospective randomized study. *American Journal of Obstetrics and Gynecology, 153*(3), 301–306.

Moen, M. D., Besinger, R. E., Tomich, P. G., & Fisher, S. G. (1995). Effect of amnioinfusion on the incidence of postpartum endometritis in patients undergoing cesarean delivery. *Journal of Reproductive Medicine, 40*(5), 383–386.

Nageotte, M. P., Bertucci, L., Towers, C. J., Lagrew, D. C., & Mondanlau, H. (1990). Prophylactic amnioinfusion in pregnancies complicated by oligohydramnios or thick meconium: a prospective study [abstract]. In Proceedings of 9th Annual Meeting of the Society of Perinatal Obstetricians (p. 78).

Nijhuis, J. G., Crevels, A. J., & van Dongen, P. W. (1990). Fetal brain death: The definition of a fetal heart rate pattern and its clinical consequences. *Obstetrical and Gynecological Survey, 45*(4), 229–232.

Parer, J. T. (1997). *Handbook of fetal heart rate monitoring* (2nd ed.). Philadelphia: W.B. Saunders.

Paszkowski, T. (1994). Amnioinfusion: A review. *Journal of Reproductive Medicine, 39*(8), 588–594.

Paul, R. H., Suidan, A. K., Yeh, S., Schifrin, B. S., & Hon, E. H. (1975). Clinical fetal monitoring. VII. The evaluation and significance of intrapartum baseline FHR variability. *American Journal of Obstetrics and Gynecology, 123*(2), 206–210.

Phelan, J. P., & Ahn, M. O. (1994). Perinatal observations in forty-eight neurologically impaired term infants. *American Journal of Obstetrics and Gynecology, 171*(2), 424–431.

Pierce, J., Gaudier, F. L., & Sanchez-Ramos, L. (2000). Intrapartum amnioinfusion for meconium-stained fluid: Meta-analysis of prospective clinical trials. *Obstetrics and Gynecology, 95*(6, Pt. 2), 1051–1056.

Sadovsky, Y., Amon, E., Bade, M. E., & Petrie, R. H. (1989). Prophylactic amnioinfusion during labor complicated by meconium: A preliminary report. *American Journal of Obstetrics and Gynecology, 161*(3), 613–617.

Schifrin, B. S., & Dame, L. (1972). Fetal heart rate patterns: Prediction of Apgar score. *Journal of the American Medical Association, 219*(10), 1322–1325.

Schifrin, B. S., Hamilton-Rubinstein, T., & Shields, J. R. (1994). Fetal heart rate patterns and the timing of fetal injury. *Journal of Perinatology, 14*(3), 174–181.

Schrimmer, D. B., Macri, C. J., & Paul, R. H. (1991). Prophylactic amnioinfusion as a treatment for oligohydramnios in laboring patients: A prospective randomized trial. *American Journal of Obstetrics and Gynecology, 165*(4, Pt. 1), 972–975.

Snell, B. J. (1993) The use of amnioinfusion in nurse-midwifery practice. *Journal of Nurse-Midwifery, 38* (2 Suppl.), 62S–71S.

Spong, C. Y. (1997). Amnioinfusion: Indications and controversies. *Contemporary OB/GYN, 42*(8), 138–139, 143–149.

Strong, T. H. (1995). Amnioinfusion. *Journal of Reproductive Medicine, 40*(2), 108–114.

Strong T. H., Hetzler, G., Sarno, A. P., & Paul, R. H. (1990). Prophylactic intrapartum amnioinfusion: A randomized clinical trial. *American Journal of Obstetrics and Gynecology, 162*(6), 1370–1374.

Tucker, S. M. (2000). *Pocket guide to fetal monitoring and assessment* (4th ed.). St. Louis: Mosby.

Wallerstedt, C., Higgins, P., Kasnic, T., & Curet, L. B. (1994). Amnioinfusion: An update. *Journal of Obstetric, Gynecologic, and Neonatal Nursing, 23,* 573–578.

Wenstrom, K., Andrews, W. W., & Maher, J. E. (1995). Amnioinfusion survey: Prevalence, protocols, and complications. *Obstetrics and Gynecology, 86*(4, Pt 1), 572–576.

Yam, J., Chua, S., & Arulkumaran, S. (2000). Intrapartum fetal pulse oximetry. Part 2: Clinical application. *Obstetrics and Gynecology, 55*(3), 173–183.

CHAPTER 8

Assessment of Fetal Oxygenation and Acid-Base Status

Rebecca L. Cypher
Donna Adelsperger

Through the years, research has focused on the metabolic processes of fetal oxygenation and acid-base status in terms of detecting fetal hypoxia, identifying fetuses that are most likely to develop hypoxia and giving providers the means to intervene before the damage occurs (Garite & Porreco, 2001). Although electronic fetal monitoring (EFM) has not resulted in the elimination of fetal/neonatal morbidity and mortality, there is agreement among experts that fetal heart rate (FHR) accelerations usually indicate that a fetus is nonacidotic. Fetal heart auscultation also allows detection of the presence of accelerations associated with a nonacidotic fetus.

Although the primary focus of this text is fetal heart monitoring (EFM and intermittent auscultation), it is important to understand how normal glucose metabolism as well as uteroplacental physiologic factors affect intrapartum acid-base assessment and fetal oxygenation. Additional tools are used as adjuncts to EFM and intermittent auscultation to provide indirect and direct information about the acid-base status of the fetus and newborn, and these are briefly reviewed in this chapter. General guidelines for the use of selected indirect and direct tools to assess fetal oxygenation are provided. Hospital guidelines and protocols should be consulted and followed when implementing the procedures described in this chapter.

FETAL ACID-BASE BALANCE: KEY CONCEPTS

Fetal acid-base balance is determined by many factors, including the acid-base balance of the mother prior to the onset of labor. Once labor begins, the arteries supplying blood flow to the uterus are constricted, resulting in a decrease in the flow and exchange of oxygen and carbon dioxide to and from the fetus during uterine contractions. The fetus with an adequate oxygen reserve will adapt to this normal decrease in oxygen exchange when there are adequate rest periods between contractions. If the fetus does not have adequate oxygen reserves, there may be a progressive accumulation of carbon dioxide (hypercapnia) that could lead to respiratory acidemia and decreased oxygen (hypoxemia), which could also result in metabolic acidemia or a combination of both types of acidemia (Greene, 1999). The following section describes how the fetus meets its normal metabolic needs, as well as physiologic and pathophysiologic factors that may affect the fetal acid-base balance.

Normal Fetal Glucose Metabolism

The fetus meets its metabolic needs through the oxidation of glucose to water and carbon dioxide in the presence of oxygen (Greene, 1999). In normal cellular glucose metabolism, energy is released during glycolysis (splitting) of the glucose molecules and during the oxidation of the end products of glycolysis. During an early anaerobic phase of carbohydrate metabolism, glucose is initially converted to pyruvic acid through a series of chemical reactions. Eventually, through the Krebs cycles, chemical reactions within the cell mitochondria result in carbon dioxide and hydrogen atom formation. Subsequently, oxidation of the hydrogen atom occurs. Adenosine triphosphate, which is energy for use by the cells, is formed during these processes, with the largest amount formed during oxidation of the hydrogen atoms (Guyton & Hall, 1997).

During anaerobic metabolism, when oxygen is not available for the oxidation of the hydrogen atoms, cellular oxidation of the hydrogen cannot take place. Small amounts of energy may be released through the initial breakdown of glucose into pyruvic acid. With extended periods of decreased oxygen, the end products of chemical reactions build up. The build up of hydrogen and pyruvic acid leads to lactic acid formation through chemical reactions. In the absence of oxygen, lactic acid cannot be broken down and it accumulates, resulting in metabolic acidemia. With the addition of oxygen (at the cellular level), lactic acid is then converted, resulting in formation of carbon dioxide, which enters the umbilical arteries and is transported into the maternal circulation for excretion through the maternal system. The process of reversing metabolic acidosis with adequate oxygenation can take 20–30 minutes or

longer, depending on the degree of acidosis. Therefore, fetuses with progressive metabolic acidosis in utero may exhibit decreased variability, possible loss of variability, neurological compromise and intrauterine death.

When umbilical cord compression or occlusion occurs, carbon dioxide produced by lactic acid conversion cannot be removed from the fetal circulation, which results in a build up of carbon dioxide. The excess carbon dioxide is hydrolyzed, and carbonic acid is formed, potentially resulting in respiratory acidosis. However, respiratory acidosis is easily reversed, as the carbon dioxide is quickly diffused into the maternal circulation for excretion through the maternal system.

Physiologic and Pathophysiologic Factors Affecting Intrapartum Acid-Base Assessment

The placenta is the fetal organ for respiration. When the placenta is functioning to the fullest capacity, this organ will provide sufficient oxygen for fetal growth and development under conditions of aerobic metabolism. Fetal acid-base status depends on maternal regulation and transplacental transfer of gases. The normoxic fetus has a pH level slightly lower than the maternal pH level and is affected by the acid-base balance of the mother. During labor, uterine arteries are constricted decreasing blood flow to the fetus and carbon dioxide away from the fetus. Normally the fetus can adapt to the decrease in oxygen. If fetal oxygen reserves are depleted there may be a progressive accumulation of carbon dioxide (hypercapnia) that may result in respiratory acidemia and lack of oxygen (hypoxemia) that could result in metabolic acidemia (Greene, 1999). Two classes of acids are produced when the fetus exhibits normal metabolism: volatile acids (e.g., carbonic acid) and nonvolatile acids (e.g., lactic acid), also known as fixed acids (Thorp & Rushing, 1999).

The end result of aerobic metabolism in the fetus is carbonic acid, which is formed by the hydration of carbon dioxide during oxidative metabolism. It is found in very low concentrations in the plasma. During pregnancy, increased respiratory effort by the pregnant woman increases the amount of carbon dioxide the fetus must dispose of through the placenta. Carbon dioxide diffuses across the placenta very rapidly as long as there is adequate intervillous and umbilical blood flow (Menihan & Zottoli, 2001).

Acidemia, whether respiratory, metabolic or mixed, is an abnormal increase in the hydrogen ion concentration in the blood due to an accumulation of an acid or a loss in the base. Accumulated carbonic acids (weak acids) combine with hydrogen ions and then break down into carbon dioxide and water, which are quickly excreted across the placenta if blood flow is restored in a reasonable time. This principle applies to the adult as well as the fetus.

The fetus can develop respiratory acidemia in several scenarios, including prolonged second stage of labor, an acute onset of decreased umbilical cord perfusion or uteroplacental perfusion. If these problems are not corrected, respiratory acidemia may occur. For example, repeated umbilical cord compression may occur during a labor complicated by oligohydramnios. With adequate cord release, a healthy fetus will be able to resuscitate itself in utero. Depending on the duration of the temporary insult, the fetus will excrete carbon dioxide across the placenta if allowed sufficient time. Otherwise, the fetus will develop respiratory acidemia.

Metabolic acidemia in the fetus results from a restricted placental transfer of oxygen and an accumulation of nonvolatile acids (lactic acid) that form as a result of anaerobic metabolism (glycolysis). This is secondary to inadequate levels of oxygen (hypoxemia). Buffers in the blood permit the maintenance of the pH at a relatively constant level. Plasma bicarbonate and hemoglobin are the two most important buffers in the blood (Gilstrap, 1999).

The fetal renal system is unable to excrete the nonvolatile acids due to the immaturity of the active transport systems. These acids must cross the placenta into the maternal circulation for excretion by the maternal kidneys, but this diffusion is much slower than carbon dioxide diffusion. It may require hours rather than seconds, even if sufficient oxygen is restored. When these acids accumulate, fetal metabolic acidemia occurs (Thorp & Rushing, 1999).

During labor, a mild maternal metabolic acidemia may develop due to muscle activity, catecholamine release or relative starvation. A mixture of both respiratory and metabolic acidemia also may occur. When the supply of oxygen and the removal of carbon dioxide and fixed acids by the placenta are in balance, the fetus will maintain a normal acid-base balance within a narrow range. If these processes are interrupted, the fetus may develop acidemia (Thorp & Rushing, 1999).

🖢 FETAL OXYGENATION AND ACID-BASE ASSESSMENT

As previously stated, care providers sometimes need to employ additional methods to further assess fetal oxygenation and acid-base status. Fetal well-being can be evaluated when EFM or intermittent auscultation is used with other adjunct methods of evaluation, including indirect and direct approaches (Garite, 2002b; SOGC, 1995, 2002, Tucker, 2000). Direct methods are those in which actual blood sampling occurs; indirect methods are those in which acid-base levels are implied on the basis of a less direct measure or the fetal response or both.

Indirect Methods of Acid-Base Assessment

Indirect methods for evaluation of acid-base values include fetal movement counting, fetal scalp stimulation and vibroacoustic stimulation (VAS). Some of these tools can be used to further evaluate fetal status by attempting to elicit or evaluate a reactive fetal heart response—an acceleration of 15 beats per minute (bpm) in amplitude for a duration of 15 seconds. This fetal response is predictive of a nonacidotic fetus, generally with a pH of 7.20 or more and a normoxic central nervous system. While reactivity is associated with fetal well-being, the absence of an acceleration does not serve as a diagnosis for acidemia or predict fetal compromise. Fetal pulse oximetry has been used in the presence of nonreassuring FHR patterns as a further assessment of fetal acid-base levels, although its use has not yet been recommended as a general standard of care (ACOG, 2001; SOGC, 2002). Decisions to use additional direct assessments of acid-base status are based on various factors, including the maternal-fetal history, labor progress, current maternal status and individual institutional guidelines.

Fetal Movement

The maternal perception of fetal movement is the oldest, simplest and least expensive method of monitoring fetal well-being (Gegor, Paine & Johnson, 1991). The pregnant woman senses about 70–80% of gross fetal movement (Druzin, Gabbe & Reed, 2002). In general, the presence of fetal movement is a reassuring sign of fetal well-being associated with an intact fetal central nervous system.

Numerous techniques for monitoring fetal movements have been described. Unfortunately, there are no universal counting criteria or set values for evaluating fetal movement. Examples of counting methods include counting three fetal movements over 60 minutes and noting the amount of time to count 10 fetal movements (Gegor et al., 1991; Pearson & Weaver, 1976; Rayburn, Zuspan, Motley & Donaldson, 1980; Sadovsky, Yaffe & Polishuk, 1974). Regardless of the method used, research has demonstrated that when fetal activity is chronically reduced, fetal hypoxemia may be suspected. Researchers are currently establishing norms for fetal movement based on observations of fetuses at different gestational ages and are attempting to determine characteristic changes associated with hypoxia (Lindsay, 1999). See Chapter 12 for additional information on fetal movement assessment and other antepartum tests for fetal well-being.

Fetal Scalp Stimulation

Another indirect method used to evaluate fetal status is fetal scalp stimulation (Box 8-1). This method is accomplished by applying firm digital pressure on the fetal scalp during a vaginal examination to elicit a reactive response. A well-oxygenated fetus will respond with an acceleration of 15-bpm in amplitude or more for a duration of

15 seconds or more, which usually reflects a pH of 7.0 or greater (see Figure 8-1). Clark, Gimovsky and Miller (1984) demonstrated that induced accelerations reflect a fetus with an intact central nervous system. These researchers also demonstrated that when an acceleration is elicited, either induced or spontaneous, the fetus is not acidotic. As stated earlier, the absence of an acceleration does not diagnose acidemia or predict fetal compromise. Further observation and assessment measures may be indicated.

Vibroacoustic Stimulation (VAS)

Vibroacoustic stimulation (VAS) is an indirect method used to further assess the acid-base status of the fetus when fetal accelerations do not occur spontaneously. VAS evaluates the FHR response to acoustic stimulation.

The acoustic environment of the fetus is composed of continuous cardiovascular, respiratory, and intestinal sounds of the pregnant woman. Vibrations on the external surface of the mother's abdomen can also induce sounds within the uterus. Sounds penetrate the tissues and fluid surrounding the fetal head and stimulate the inner ear through a bone conduction route. The fetus hears low-frequency sounds below 300 Hz. In fact, the fetus can likely detect vowels and rhythmic patterns of music (Gerhardt & Abrams, 2000).

Vibroacoustic stimulators or artificial larynxes are hand-held or attached by a connector to the fetal monitor. The stimulation, which is atraumatic to the fetus, can produce a change in fetal state (usually from quiet to active sleep) and elicit an acceleration. Yao et al. (1990) reported that movements occurred more frequently after VAS set at 103 dB and 109 dB. If the artificial larynx is set at 103 dB it will usually be sufficient to elicit accelerations (Yao et al., 1990). The static and dynamic forces of the vibrator and the distance from the fetal head are also factors in the transmission of the sound (Gerhardt & Abrams, 2000).

Vibroacoustic stimulation is easy to perform and inexpensive. It is also noninvasive and may decrease testing time for the nonstress test (NST) and the incidence of nonreactive NSTs (AAP & ACOG, 2002; ACOG, 1999; Marden, McDuffie,

BOX 8-1

Fetal Scalp Stimulation

Fetal scalp stimulation is used to elicit an acceleration when the auscultated FHR characteristics or EFM pattern interpretation is inconclusive or nonreassuring. After the fetal scalp is digitally stimulated, the EFM tracing is observed or the FHR is auscultated for an acceleration that peaks 15 bpm or greater above the baseline FHR and lasts 15 seconds or more.

GENERAL GUIDELINES:

- Explain the procedure to the patient.
- Place the patient in a lateral position.
- Perform a vaginal examination.
- Apply gentle digital pressure on the fetal scalp. Avoid stimulation during a deceleration because the sympathetic nerves are already compromised and thus may alter the response or decrease a reactive response.
- Document the procedure and response per institutional policy.

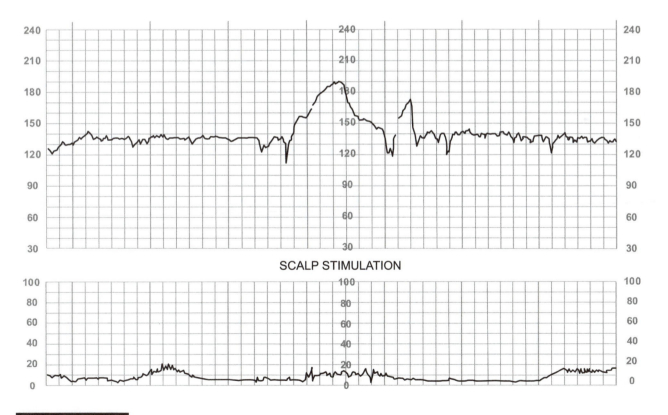

SCALP STIMULATION

FIGURE 8-1

Fetal Scalp Stimulation Elicits FHR Acceleration
Note: The FHR accelerates from a baseline of 135–140 bpm up to 190 bpm.

Allen & Abitz, 1997; Saracoglou, Gol, Sabin, Turkkani & Oztopeu, 1999; Smith, Phelan, Platt, Broussard & Paul, 1986; Tan & Smyth, 2001). Use of VAS has also reduced false-positive rates for NSTs (Marden et al., 1997; Saracoglu et al., 1999). Fetuses that respond to VAS with an acceleration on an NST or a startle response on a biophysical profile have very low rates of death within 1 week of the test (Smith-Levitin, Petrikovsky & Schneider, 1997). Box 8-2 describes the performance and interpretation of VAS and related safety concerns.

While professional interpretation of its use during labor and its role in the intrapartum setting have been debated, VAS has been used as an alternative to fetal scalp sampling. In 1994, Smith found VAS to be as reliable as fetal scalp sampling for determining acidemia during the first stage of labor. Of those fetuses that responded to VAS with an acceleration exceeding 15 bpm for a 15-second duration, none were found to have an acidotic pH. Likewise, of the fetuses that did not respond to VAS, 53% had a scalp pH of less than 7.20.

Occasionally, a fetus will respond to VAS with prolonged tachycardia or bradycardia, particularly when oligohydramnios is present (Miller, Rabello & Paul, 1996). Some medications have been associated with altered responses to VAS. These include beta-adrenergic blocking agents and magnesium sulfate, which have been associated with decreased reactivity and a blunted response (Sherer & Bentolili, 1998). The effect of intrauterine growth restriction on fetal response to VAS has also been studied. It has been noted that FHR accelerations are shorter in duration and body movements fewer in these fetuses when compared with normal-size fetuses (Porter & Clark, 1999). In fetuses between 26 and 32 weeks of gestation that are small for gestational age, researchers reported a limited response, suggestive of delayed functional maturation of fetal sensory receptors (Gagnon, Hunse & Foreman, 1989).

Fetal Pulse Oximetry

The use of EFM provides indirect measures of fetal oxygenation, making it sensitive but not specific for detecting compromised fetal well-being. In May 2000, the Food and Drug Administration (FDA) approved an additional method of assessing fetal oxygen status during labor. Fetal oxygen saturation ($FSpO_2$) monitoring is the first major technological advance in fetal assessment since EFM was introduced four decades ago. Such monitoring can be used as an adjunct to EFM in the presence of a nonreassuring FHR pattern. The adoption of fetal pulse oximetry in clinical practice as a standard of care has not yet been endorsed by the American College of Obstetricians and Gynecologists (ACOG, 2001) or the Society of Obstetricians and Gynaecologists of Canada (SOGC, 2002). Additional research is recommended regarding efficacy and cost evaluation (ACOG, 2001).

Oximetry was developed in the United States and Great Britain during World War II when military aircraft did not have pressurized cabins. This technology allowed for the measurement of hemoglobin oxygen saturation in blood or tissue on the basis of the Lambert-Beer relationship (Dildy, Clark & Loucks, 1996). Pulse oximeters were developed for medical use in the late 1970s and are found in most operating rooms and critical care units (Garite & Porreco, 2001).

The theory behind pulse oximetry is that oxyhemoglobin (hemoglobin with oxygen) and deoxyhemoglobin (hemoglobin without oxygen) will absorb light. Oxyhemoglobin weakly absorbs red light and strongly absorbs infrared light. Conversely, deoxyhemoglobin strongly absorbs red light and weakly absorbs infrared light. During pulse oximetry, red and infrared light are alternately emitted into the tissue through a sensor. The oximeter calculates the ratio of oxygen-saturated and unsaturated hemoglobin by measuring the absorption of each color. The fraction is displayed as a percentage, known as arterial oxygen saturation, via the pulse oximeter (Garite & Porreco, 2001; Mallinckrodt, Inc., 2000b; Simpson & Porter, 2001).

Pulse oximetry involves the application of a sensor to a finger, toe, ear or the bridge of the nose. The patient is monitored via a transmission type of sensor in which the optical components are positioned across from each other so the light passes through the tissue. The absorption of light is measured as it shines across the tissue's vascular beds (Simpson, 1998; Simpson & Porter, 2001;

BOX 8-2

VAS

Vibroacoustic stimulation is an indirect method of assessing the acid-base status of the fetus when fetal accelerations do not occur spontaneously. The goal is to elicit accelerations of 15 bpm or greater above the baseline FHR for a duration of 15 seconds or more. A hand-held, commercially distributed vibroacoustic stimulator or a battery-powered artificial larynx or both are used to deliver auditory and vibratory stimulus to the fetus. Vibroacoustic stimulation may be used as an adjunct to reduce false-positive rates for NSTs (Marden et al., 1997; Saracoglu et al., 1999) and biophysical profiles (Garite, 2002a: Smith-Levitin et al., 1997).

GENERAL GUIDELINES:

Procedure

- Explain the procedure to the patient.
- Evaluate the FHR baseline prior to stimulation.
- Place the vibroacoustic stimulator on the woman's abdomen in the area of the fetal head. The distance of the stimulator does not seem to affect the results, although intrauterine sound levels decrease if the distance is increased (Eller et al., 1992).
- Although the intensity of the stimulus may vary, it is usually between 80 and 110 decibels. The duration of the stimulus should be at least 3 seconds, yet no greater than 5 seconds.
- If the fetus does not respond to the initial VAS, a second stimulation may be applied 3–10 minutes later. If no response is achieved after the second VAS, further evaluation may be required (e.g., contraction stress test, oxytocin challenge test or biophysical profile).
- Documentation should include a description of the tracing prior to VAS, the type of stimulus used, duration and position of stimulus applied and the response to the stimulus by the fetus (per institutional policy and procedures).

Interpretation

Interpretation will depend on individual institutional guidelines. Sample guidelines are as follows:

- Reactive: Accelerations of 15 bpm above the FHR baseline for more than 15 seconds' duration in a 20-minute period
- Nonreactive: No acceleration in the allotted time
- Equivocal:
  —One acceleration meeting the stated criteria
  —Accelerations not meeting the stated criteria
  —Uninterpretable/unreadable fetal tracing

Evaluate the baseline FHR prior to performing VAS since a tachycardic FHR may result from the stimulation and may last as long as 1 hour. If this should occur, observe the tachycardic rate for normal baseline characteristics. Continue observation of the fetus until the FHR returns to the range before stimulation. Some investigators have suggested the magnitude and duration of FHR accelerations correspond to the state of fetal health (Polzin, Blakemore, Petrie & Amon, 1988).

(Box continues)

BOX 8-2 (cont.)

VAS

The effect of gestational age on VAS results is being explored. The incidence of reactive NSTs with the use of VAS may increase as much as 89–100% in fetuses 26 weeks of gestation or more (Smith, 1995). After 30 weeks of gestation, there is significant and prolonged increase in baseline fetal heart rate lasting up to 1 hour (Gagnon, Benzaquen & Hunse, 1992).

The fetal response to VAS may be diminished or absent with the rupture of membranes and may decrease as labor progresses (Sleutel, 1989). There have been concerns about VAS resulting in prolonged FHR decelerations in pregnancies complicated by oligohydramnios. Sarno, Ahn, Phelan & Paul (1990) found that amniotic fluid was not related to the occurrence of prolonged decelerations.

Safety

Smith (1994) found that while prolonged exposures to sound levels of greater than 110 decibels could result in injury, it was unlikely to be harmful with a brief, nonrepetitive stimulus. Arulkumaran and associates (1991) found no evidence of hearing loss in infants that received VAS in utero.

Tucker, 2000). This type of adult sensor could not be applied to the fetus. Modifying the technology for fetal application involved addressing challenges specific to fetal physiology, including difficulty detecting arterial pulsations from fetal blood vessels, which are smaller than those of adult and pediatric patients; a lower normal fetal oxygen saturation level than that of adults and children; and changes in light wavelength in the fetus (Dildy, Clark and Loucks, 1996).

The intrauterine environment also presented unique challenges. Thick, particulate meconium and vernix can occlude the reflectance sensor, which would interfere with light transmission and signal acquisition. The sensor can be displaced with fetal movement. The technology needed to be adapted to the fetus using a sensor specifically developed for the fetus and computer software that incorporated lower oxygen saturation values, smaller arterial pulsations and application to the fetus in utero (Mallinckrodt, 2000c).

A reflectance device then was developed that could display oxygen saturation of the fetus via the fetal temple, cheek or forehead and accounted for the physiological factors that support the fetus in an oxygen-poor environment (Mallinckrodt, 2000b). In utero, the fetus is supported by a number of characteristics: a higher affinity for oxygen, a higher hemoglobin value, a preferred streaming of oxygenated blood from the right atrium to the left atrium via the foramen ovale and up the aorta to the brain and upper body, more capillaries per unit of tissue than an adult and a higher cardiac output and heart rate (Porter, 2000).

The fetal sensor is different from conventional pulse oximetry in that it is a reflectance sensor instead of a transmission sensor. In the traditional transmission sensor, the light emitting electrodes (LEDs) and photodetector are positioned opposite each other to determine light absorption across the vascular beds. In the reflectance sensor used with fetal pulse oximetry, the LEDs and photodetectors are positioned adjacent to one another on the same skin surface.

The Critical Threshold

Use of fetal pulse oximetry requires a thorough understanding of the concept of the *critical threshold:* the point below which hypoxia would likely cause metabolic acidosis or above which there would be almost no risk for acidosis (Garite & Porreco, 2001). Persistent fetal hypoxia may lead to acidosis, neurological injury, tissue and organ damage and, ultimately, death (Dildy, Clark and Loucks, 1996). However, because the fetus often becomes hypoxemic for short periods of time and may revert to a normal acid-base balance without becoming acidotic, it was necessary to establish a critical threshold. The goal of intrapartum monitoring is to intervene early enough to avoid these complications whenever possible.

After years of animal and human studies, values for normal and abnormal fetal oxygen saturation measured by pulse oximetry were identified and validated. The methodology for establishing a critical threshold was established by researchers at Mallinckrodt, Inc. (Swedlow, 2000). The methodology for research included the following: retrospective search of the literature for evidence demonstrating the existence of a critical threshold for fetal oxygen saturation, prospective animal research demonstrating existence of a threshold using a standard obstetric model, retrospective examination of the distribution of fetal oxygen saturation values in the human fetus during normal-outcome labor and the definition of the threshold at or below the fifth percentile and prospective study for the presence of an acceptable predictive agreement between fetal oxygen saturation and fetal scalp pH (Swedlow, 2000).

Based on the current research, normal oxygen saturation for the fetus in labor is 30–65% saturation (Dildy, Thorp, Yeast & Clark, 1996; Nijland, Jongsma, Nijhuis, van den Berg & Oeseburg, 1995; Richardson, Carmichael, Homan & Patrick, 1992). The fetus is presumed to be adequately oxygenated at this value. Metabolic acidosis does not develop until the saturation level falls below 30% for at least 10–15 minutes (Seelbach-Göbel, Heupel, Kühnert & Butterwegge, 1999). Thus, the critical threshold was established at 30%. This value was also validated in a randomized, controlled trial conducted concurrently in nine medical centers across the United States (Garite et al., 2002b).

Interpretation and Clinical Management

The use of EFM or auscultation may provide data indicating potential hypoxemia (Garite & Porreco, 2001). However, patterns or fetal heart characteristics heard with auscultation are sometimes confusing or nonreassuring. The fetal pulse oximeter can be used as an adjunct to EFM in these situations.

Fetal pulse oximetry is an adjunct and does not replace the intrauterine resuscitation techniques currently used to improve fetal oxygenation. Therefore, techniques to improve fetal oxygenation need to be implemented when confusing FHR patterns and characteristics occur. Such interventions include maternal position changes, oxygen administration, administration of intravenous fluids, a decrease or elimination of uterine activity and amnioinfusion or tocolytic medications if indicated (Kühnert et al., 1998). If these techniques do not lead to reassuring data about the fetus or the FHR tracing is uninterpretable, fetal pulse oximetry may be indicated as an additional assessment. If the FHR continues to be nonreassuring but the fetal oxygen saturation reading is ≥30% between contractions, the fetus is assumed to be adequately oxygenated. If the fetal oxygen saturation remains below 30% despite intrauterine resuscitation measures, consideration should be given to expediting delivery (Kühnert et al., 1998).

A uniform system for classifying reassuring, nonreassuring and ominous FHR patterns was established for the multi-center randomized controlled clinical trial of fetal pulse oximetry (Garite et al., 2000). In February 2003, the classifications for nonreassuring and ominous FHR patterns were revised. (Swedlow & Bolling, personal communication, February 3, 2003). Based on these revisions, at least one of the criteria for nonreassuring patterns outlined in Box 8-3 should be present when deciding to initiate fetal pulse oximetry. If an ominous pattern is present, fetal pulse oximetry should not be used. Additional criteria and contraindications are found in Box 8-4.

Sensor Insertion/Placement and Position

Early fetal pulse oximetry devices were attached with suction cups, glue or clips directly attached to the fetal scalp (Dildy, Clark and Loucks, 1996). Eventually, these evolved into the fetal pulse oximetry system in use today. The actual fetal sensor contains the LEDs, the photodetectors and contact electrodes. This sensor is attached to a sensor

BOX 8-3

(NOTE: These FHR pattern classifications are provided to guide decision making about the use of fetal pulse oximetry but do not replace the definitions of FHR patterns presented in Chapter Six of this textbook.)

FHR Class	FHR Pattern
I	**REASSURING** Any FHR pattern that does not meet criteria for Class II or III. Typically, a Class I trace is characterized by a baseline between 110 and 160 bpm, with longterm variability between 5 and 25 bpm, and either no decelerations or only early decelerations.

II	**NONREASSURING**
	Any one of the following for more than 15 minutes:
	• Persistent late decelerations (> 50% of contractions)
	• Sinusoidal pattern[a]
	• Variable decelerations with one or more of the following:
	   —A relative drop of ≥ 70 bpm or an absolute drop to ≤ 70 bpm for more than 60 seconds[b]
	   —Persistent slow return to baseline
	   —Long term variability < 5 bpm[c]
	   —Tachycardia > 160 bpm
	• Recurrent prolonged decelerations (2 or more < 70 bpm for more than 90 seconds)
	Any one of the following for more than 60 minutes
	• Tachycardia > 160 bpm with longterm variability < 5 bpm[c]
	• Persistent decreased variability (≤ 5 bpm for more than 60 minutes)[c]

III	**OMINOUS** • Prolonged deceleration to < 70 bpm for more than 7 minutes[d] • Markedly decreased or absent variability with persistent late decelerations • Markedly decreased or absent variability with severe variable decelerations

a. Sinusoidal pattern is defined as regular oscillations about the baseline, 5–15 bpm in magnitude, with 2 to 5 cycles per minute on an otherwise normal baseline with absent short-term variability.
b. Variable decelerations are to be timed from the beginning of the deceleration to the end of the deceleration (i.e., more than 60 seconds in duration).
c. Decreased variability not otherwise explained by the clinical situation (e.g., narcotic administration).
d. It is not necessary to wait for more than 7 minutes of prolonged deceleration before initiating intervention (e.g., evaluation of the cause, non-surgical intervention, and preparation for delivery), even with reassuring $FSpO_2$.

Source: D. Swedlow and M. Bolling, personal communication February 3, 2003. Re: changes in the management protocol for use of fetal pulse oximetry. Reprinted with permission of Nellcor Puritan Bennett, Inc., Pleasanton, California.

cable. On the back of the sensor cable is a removable stylet that assists with placement. The cable is attached to the fetal pulse oximetry module that interfaces with the EFM. A permanent record of fetal oxygen saturation levels can then be recorded on the FHR strip (Mallinckrodt, Inc., 2000a).

Placement of the sensor is similar to the technique used with the intrauterine pressure catheter (see Figure 8-2). Fetal lie should be determined by Leopold's maneuvers. A vaginal examination should be done to determine fetal head position by palpating the sagittal suture and one or both

BOX 8-4

Fetal Pulse Oximetry

The fetal pulse oximetry system is an adjunct to fetal heart rate monitoring that allows the provider to better assess fetal status in the presence of a nonreassuring FHR pattern. It measures fetal oxygenation during labor, enabling the provider to determine if the fetus is adequately oxygenated.

CRITERIA FOR USE

- Singleton fetus
- 36 weeks of gestation or more
- Vertex presentation
- Ruptured membranes
- Cervix 2 cm dilated or more
- Fetal station of –2 or below
- Nonreassuring FHR pattern as identified in Box 8-3

CONTRAINDICATIONS

- Documented or suspected placenta previa
- Ominous FHR pattern requiring immediate intervention
- Need for immediate delivery (unrelated to FHR pattern), such as active uterine bleeding
- Infectious diseases such as human immunodeficiency virus (HIV), active genital herpes, hepatitis B or hepatitis E seropositivity or other infection precluding internal monitoring

WARNINGS

- Do not use with an electrosurgical unit.
- Do not use in presence of flammable anesthetics.
- The sensor can be left in place during maternal defibrillation, but data may be inaccurate.
- Do not use to monitor patients during water births, whirlpools, showers or in any situation in which patient is immersed in water.
- Do not leave fetal oxygen sensor in place during vacuum extraction, forceps delivery or cesarean delivery.
- Do not attempt to rupture membranes with sensor.

CLINICAL USE

- Providers should have demonstrated expertise in determining fetal presentation and head position, as well as proficiency in placing fetal scalp electrodes and intrauterine pressure catheters.
- Remove sensor from package. Each fetal oxygen sensor is supplied as a sterile, single-use, disposable device. Do not attempt to clean, reprocess, resterilize or reuse the sensor, as this may result in malfunction, infection or false data.
- Do not attempt to insert sensor if the cervix is dilated less than 2 cm or if amniotic membranes are not ruptured.

(Box continues)

BOX 8-4 (cont.)

Fetal Pulse Oximetry

- Introduce the sensor through the examining fingers once presentation, cervical dilation and station have been determined. It may be easier to insert the sensor posteriorly at either the 5-o'clock or 7-o'clock position.
- Guide the sensor along the fingers until the sensor meets the midpoint of the sagittal suture.
- Insert the sensor approximately perpendicular to the sagittal suture but pointed slightly toward the anterior fontanel, allowing alignment to the fetal cheek or temple.
- Insert deeply enough into the uterus so that the sensor is past the fetal hairline.
- During a contraction, stop insertion and resume placement once the contraction stops.
- If the FHR slows during vaginal examination or sensor insertion, stop the procedure. Do not proceed with sensor placement, as this can cause a reflex bradycardia stimulus. Wait for the FHR to return to the previous range before proceeding.
- Do not force sensor placement if there is resistance; guide the sensor to a more satisfactory site and continue.
- If there is no resistance, continue to insert the sensor until the 15 cm tactile ridge is felt at the midpoint of the presenting part. This means the tactile ridge is crossing the tip of the examining fingers.
- Slowly advance the sensor another 3–4 cm to ensure optimal placement.
- Sensor cable marks should be approximately 25–27 cm at the introitus if the fetus is at –2 station.
- Use the monitor display, audible fetal pulse tones and feedback from the indicator to evaluate whether optimal placement has been reached. Suboptimal sensor placement, excessive vernix, fetal hair or motion artifact (due to uterine contractions or maternal position changes) may result in no fetal oxygen saturation values being displayed or erroneous values.
- When the sensor lifted indicator is extinguished, remove the stylet with opposite hand, while continuing to hold the sensor in position with gloved fingers.
- Do not attempt to reinsert a stylet into the sensor cable chamber once it has been completely removed during sensor placement. This may result in fetal or maternal injury. Sensor adjustments can be accomplished without the stylet.

Adapted from *Clinical Use Guide*, by Mallinckrodt, Inc., Copyright © 2000 by. Mallinckrodt, Inc. Reprinted with permission.

---

fontanels (Mallinckrodt, Inc., 2000a).

The optimal placement for the sensor is the cheek or temple of the fetal head. A fulcrum tip helps hold the sensor against the fetal face between uterine contractions. The fulcrum is a smooth and flexible lever arm that holds the sensor against the fetal skin. The sensor takes up any remaining space between the fetal head and the adjacent uterine wall, which helps to ensure con-tinuous contact between the sensor and the skin so that an accurate saturation measurement is obtained (Mallinckrodt, Inc., 2000c). At present, the technology does not always allow for registration of the signal because of interference throughout the labor course (Menihan & Zottoli, 2001). The sensor usually descends with the fetus, although adjustments may need to be made (Simpson, 1998).

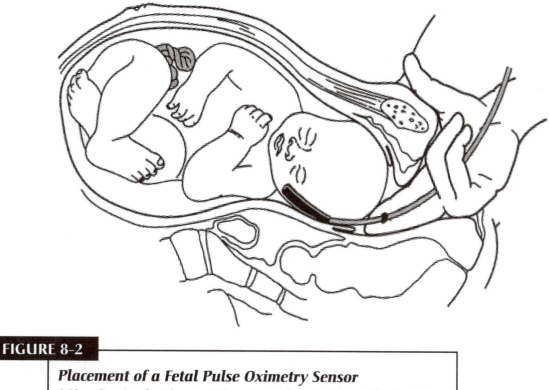

FIGURE 8-2

Placement of a Fetal Pulse Oximetry Sensor

* *Note:* Reprinted with permission. Copyright © 2000 by Mallinckrodt, Inc.

The Role of the Nurse

According to Simpson and Porter (2001), the nurse involved with fetal oxygen saturation monitoring will be challenged with a variety of responsibilities. They include identification of the patient with a nonreassuring tracing, via exclusion and inclusion criteria, who may require fetal oxygen saturation monitoring; sensor insertion; data interpretation; medical record documentation and communication with the provider responsible for the patient. These roles should be outlined in the individual labor and delivery unit's policies and procedures.

Once monitoring has been initiated, the fetal oxygen saturation values are recorded on the uterine activity channel of the EFM tracing. The nurse is responsible for documenting these data on the labor flow sheet or the form identified by the institution's guidelines. The data are recorded as a range of 5% (e.g., $FSpO_2 = 35\text{–}40\%$).

Currently, there are no guidelines from the American College of Obstetricians and Gynecolo-gists about the frequency of assessment or documentation of these data during labor. Because the use of this monitoring implies a higher risk status for the fetus, fetal assessment should occur every 15 minutes during the active phase of labor and every 5 minutes during the second stage of labor. More frequent assessment may be warranted, especially when the fetal oxygen saturation values are below 30% between contractions for more than 10 minutes. Documentation should include the ranges of the fetal oxygen saturation values, the intrauterine resuscitation techniques used and notification of the provider, if necessary.

Direct Methods of Acid-Base Assessment

Research has shown the most accurate assessment of fetal acid-base status is achieved when EFM and intermittent auscultation are used in conjunction with a variety of direct measurement tools (Tucker, 2000), such as fetal scalp sampling (Enkin et al., 2000). These tools may help identify the earliest stages of hypoxia during the intrapartum period, as well as provide information about acid-base status of the newborn after delivery.

When the fetal status is unclear following auscultation or EFM or when fetal heart and uterine activity patterns are confusing, direct measurement tools, such as scalp blood sampling and umbilical cord blood sampling, may be helpful. Umbilical cord sampling may be considered at delivery to provide retrospective information as well as information that may be useful for newborn stabilization (Sonek & Nicolaides, 1994). Other examples of direct assessment include sampling obtained via in utero methods (e.g., cordocentesis or percutaneous umbilical blood sampling [PUBS]), but these methods are less commonly used.

Fetal Scalp Sampling

When the auscultated FHR characteristics or EFM pattern interpretation is inconclusive and the fetus has not responded to stimuli, further assessment may be indicated. In many cases of nonreassuring FHR pattern, neither hypoxia nor acidosis occurs. Alternative methods of assessing acid-base status, such as fetal scalp sampling, may prevent unnecessary intervention (Low, Victory & Derrick, 1999). Although the steps for fetal scalp sampling are simple, sampling involves ruptured membranes and requires appropriate care and experience. Box 8-5 describes fetal scalp sampling technique.

Although there may be some variation of preference by institution and practitioner, the following indications are often used by those who employ fetal scalp sampling. These include cases of persistent nonreassuring FHR patterns implying fetal or maternal compromise or cases in which acidemia cannot be ruled out. In these cases, maternal intervention or expedient delivery may be indicated (ACOG, 1995).

Nonreassuring FHR Patterns

Fetal heart rate patterns and characteristics that may be indications for fetal scalp sampling include the following:

◆ Unexplained, decreased or minimal long-term variability/absent short-term variability without periodic or nonperiodic changes

◆ Undulating or sinusoidal pattern of unknown origin

◆ Late decelerations with absent or decreasing short-term variability and long-term variability

◆ Abnormal or unusual FHR patterns/characteristics

Contraindications

The principle relative contraindications for this procedure are listed below. Limiting factors may include availability of equipment and practitioners experienced in fetal scalp sampling. The risks and benefits of this procedure are controversial, and relative contraindications should be considered.

◆ Fetal coagulopathy, whether determined or suspected (e.g., hemophilia, thrombocytopenia)

◆ Active maternal genital infections (e.g., herpes, group B streptococcus)

◆ Suspected or documented HIV or hepatitis

◆ Chorioamnionitis

Factors Affecting Sampling and Interpretation of Results

There are factors to be considered during the sampling process that may or may not be controlled by the skill of the practitioner obtaining the sample. Some factors that may affect sampling and interpretation of results include the following:

◆ Fetal presentation, position and station; maternal cervical dilation and effacement

◆ Maternal positioning

◆ Accuracy of sampling and measurement (e.g., presence of hair, caput, air contamination from slow blood flow, difficulty in equipment calibration or function, presence of cephalhematoma, fontanels and/or meconium)

◆ Time lapse for filling the capillary tube

◆ Machine calibration

BOX 8-5

Technique of Fetal Scalp Sampling

The procedure for fetal scalp sampling is described in manuals, textbooks and by manufacturers of sampling kits. Although the steps are simple, the sampling technique requires experience and should be conducted only by a trained, qualified professional. Sampling requires that the patient have ruptured membranes, cervical dilation of at least 3–5 cm, and a vertex fetus at −1 station.

The equipment needed includes a cone-shaped endoscope with a light source, blade and blade holder, sponges and holder, preheparinized capillary tube, ethyl chloride and silicone grease. The micro (small) sample of blood is analyzed by a blood gas machine for pH level.

GENERAL GUIDELINES:

- Explain the procedure to the patient.
- Place the patient in a lateral position with top leg on raised side rail or held by assistant or in lithotomy position with a wedge under the hip.
- Place the endoscope in the vagina and visualize the fetal scalp.
- Provide a light source.
- Clean the fetal scalp with swabs.
- Spray scalp with ethyl chloride to induce hyperemia (as per hospital protocol).
- Place silicone on area of skin to be punctured to contain blood droplet.
- Perform a single or x-shaped puncture, being careful to avoid sutures, fontanels and areas of caput.
- Collect free-flowing blood in the preheparinized capillary tube.
- Mix blood using magnet and metal device in the capillary tube.
- Collect two samples and then apply pressure to the area sampled using a sponge or swab until bleeding stops (at least through two uterine contractions).
- Analyze specimen per hospital protocol.
- Document the time of the procedure, the fetal response and the results in the medical record (per institutional policies and procedures).

◆ Maternal acid-base balance, especially among obstetric patients with complications who may need to be sampled simultaneously for comparative evaluation with the fetus

◆ Relationship of the time of the sample to FHR characteristics and patterns, uterine contraction pattern activity at the time of sampling, and clinical circumstances

◆ Fetal trauma related to the procedure (e.g., hemorrhage, abscess)

◆ Laboratory results report pH value, but do not measure base deficit or base excess

◆ Contamination of the sample

◆ Cooperation of the patient

◆ Blood clotting in capillary tube before sample reaches the laboratory

Important Considerations in Fetal Scalp Sampling

The need for fetal scalp sampling has been dramatically reduced by the use of other noninvasive tests, such as fetal scalp stimulation and VAS (Ecker & Parer, 1999). If fetal scalp sampling is used, several factors must be considered. Regardless of the pH value used as the delineation between nonacidemia and acidemia, it is important to view the value as a trend. The clinician should evaluate whether the pH is rising or falling. This perspective may be the most useful in evaluating both the tracing and the results of the scalp sampling in the clinical setting (International Federation of Gynecology and Obstetrics, 1995). Furthermore, pH is a less satisfactory measure of acidemia than a combination of pH and base deficit because of variations of acidemia that may be present at the time of blood sampling (SOGC, 1995, 2002).

Umbilical Cord Blood Sampling

During the past decade, umbilical cord blood analysis has been recognized as a reliable indication of fetal oxygenation and acid-base condition at birth (Thorp & Rushing, 1999). Box 8-6 describes the process of neonatal cord blood sampling. Fetal cord blood gases for both the term and preterm infant supply specific information on the intrauterine environment at the time just preceding collection of the sample. A finding of normal umbilical blood gas measurements precludes the presence of acidemia at or immediately before delivery (Gregg & Weiner, 1993) and is a more objective measure than the Apgar score. Cord blood gas measurements provide an objective assessment of neonatal status (Dickinson, Erikson, Meyer & Parisi, 1992). Wide ranges of nor-

---

BOX 8-6

Neonatal Umbilical Cord Blood Gases

Blood gas analysis of the umbilical cord blood collected at delivery provides an objective means of assessing fetal oxygenation and acid-base status at birth (Thorp & Rushing, 1999). Obtaining cord blood samples will document the presence and type of acidemia, as well as provide information for resuscitation efforts and neonatal care.

GENERAL GUIDELINES:

- Obtain two or three preheparinized syringes with a short, small-gauge needle.
- Prepare labels with the name of the patient, medical record number and sample site.
- Obtain a 10–30-mL double-clamped cord segment after the original cord clamping. Double clamping should be performed immediately after delivery, because even brief delays of 20–30 seconds can affect the blood gas values.
- Obtain a blood sample from the umbilical artery first, because it is often more difficult to sample and the umbilical vein may help support the umbilical artery.
- Carefully expel any excess air from each syringe, then cap each syringe.
- Label the specimen(s). Send specimen(s) to the laboratory immediately. In some cases, the specimen(s) is set aside until a decision about blood gas analysis is made. If set aside, the specimen may be placed on ice. However, specimens remain relatively stable in a double-clamped segment of umbilical cord or in syringes for up to 1 hour at room temperature (Thorp & Rushing, 1999).
- Document that the umbilical cord blood samples were collected and sent to the laboratory for analysis; document the results when available.

TABLE 8-1

*Normal Ranges of Umbilical Cord Arterial Blood Gas Values**

ARTERIAL MEASURE[a]	NORMAL MEAN VALUE RANGE[b]	RANGE (± 2 SD)
pH	7.20–7.29	7.02–7.43
pCO_2 (mmHg)	49.2–56.3	21.5–78.3
Bicarbonate (mEq/L)	22.0–24.1	14.8–29.2
Base deficit (mEq/L)	2.7–8.3	−2.0–16.3
pO_2 (mmHg)	15.1–23.7	2.0–37.8

Adapted from information in Thorp & Rushing, 1999.

* *Abbreviations:* pCO_2, partial pressure of carbon dioxide; pO_2, partial pressure of oxygen; SD, standard deviations.

[a] Venous values reflect maternal acid-base status and are generally higher than arterial values that reflect fetal acid-base status. Venous values may be normal despite arterial values reflecting fetal acidemia.

[b] These figures represent the range of normal mean values reported in a review of studies of umbilical arterial cord blood gases (Thorp & Rushing, 1999).

mal umbilical cord blood values have been suggested in the research literature (Thorpe & Rushing, 1999) (see Table 8-1).

Umbilical cord blood gas analysis can be used to assist with neonatal management. It is possible to obtain a double-clamped section of cord at all deliveries and delay analysis until a neonatal indication is identified. The cord blood can then be analyzed if needed (SOGC, 1995, 2002).

Indications and Contraindications

Umbilical cord blood sampling may be helpful in clarifying fetal acid-base status and may also assist planning the clinical management of selected newborns (Thorp & Rushing, 1999). Indications for umbilical cord blood sampling may include the following:

◆ Nonreassuring FHR characteristics or tracing

◆ Thick meconium

◆ Low Apgar scores

◆ Preterm birth

◆ Use of forceps or vacuum extraction

◆ Emergency cesarean delivery

◆ Delivery of high-risk patients

◆ Newborn depression (Thorp & Rushing, 1999)

There are no known contraindications for the use of umbilical cord blood sampling.

Factors Affecting Sampling and Interpretation of Results

Factors that may affect umbilical cord blood sampling and interpretation include the following:

◆ Differences in methodology, such as duration of procedure or air bubbles in a sample

◆ Differences in heparin concentration use, such as the following:

   • Spurious metabolic acidemia resulting from use of too much heparin or too concentrated a solution (Thorp & Rushing, 1999)

   • Bicarbonate and partial pressure of carbon dioxide (pCO_2) values show an inverse relationship with the volume of heparin (Duerbeck, Chaffin & Seeds, 1992)

◆ Sampling of venous and not arterial blood

TABLE 8-2

Significance of Deviation from Normal Values

TYPE OF ACIDOSIS	PH	PCO$_2$	HCO$_3$	BASE DEFICIT
Respiratory	Decreased	Increased	Normal	Normal
Metabolic	Decreased	Normal	Decreased	Increased
Mixed	Decreased	Increased	Decreased	Increased

If a low 1-minute Apgar score accompanies a low pH value, the pCO$_2$, partial pressure of oxygen (pO$_2$) and base deficit values will assist in determining whether the insult is acute or chronic and represents respiratory, metabolic or mixed acidemia (Table 8-2) (Fields, Entman & Boehm, 1983). The terms *fetal asphyxia* or *birth asphyxia* frequently are used inappropriately or incorrectly. These terms should not be used unless a diagnosis is made (see Table 8-3). Furthermore, the term *asphyxia* should only be used to describe a neonate with all of the conditions (AAP & ACOG, 2002) identified in Table 8-3. For example, non-reassuring FHR patterns or low 1-minute Apgar scores alone cannot predict long-term neurologic injury or cerebral palsy (AAP & ACOG, 2002).

Interpretation of Umbilical Cord Blood Acid–Base Values

Interpretation of the results of cord blood gas analysis requires basic understanding of both respiratory and metabolic acidosis and the clinical implications of each. As previously discussed, respiratory acidosis occurs when an elevated pCO$_2$ level is present (i.e., the value is greater than two standard deviations above the mean). Normally, carbon dioxide diffuses rapidly across the placenta. The rate of carbon dioxide diffusion is related to the rate of blood flow on both sides of the placenta. Respiratory acidosis can develop rapidly, but also can be corrected rapidly.

Metabolic acidosis takes longer to develop and longer to resolve; it is present when levels of lactic acid and other acids become elevated. These acids are the end product of anaerobic metabolism. Elevation of the acids causes the fetal system of buffers to drop. The term *base deficit* refers to a below-normal amount of buffers available in the plasma; the term *base excess* indicates an above-normal amount of buffer available. Metabolic acidosis is more serious than respiratory acidosis because it reflects a more prolonged hypoxic insult (Wallman, 1997).

A fetus may experience respiratory and metabolic acidosis simultaneously. If this occurs, it is referred to as *mixed acidosis* (Menihan & Zottoli, 2001). Values above 7.25 for scalp pH are considered normal, while values between 7.20 and 7.25 are borderline. Values below 7.20 for scalp pH represent acidemia.

For umbilical cord blood, the normal mean arterial blood pH values ranged from 7.20 to 7.29 in a review of studies that monitored umbilical cord arterial blood gas values, with a full range of normal pH values (± two standard deviations) from 7.02 to 7.43 (Thorp & Rushing, 1999). While historically, cord blood pH values below 7.20 have been considered to be pathologic or clinically significant it has now been well established that this number is not appropriate (Goldaber and Gilstrap, 1993). Values between 7.10 and 7.19 have been reported as lower ranges of normal values (Sykes et al., 1982; Gilstrap, Leveno, Burris, Williams & Little, 1989). Blood pH values below 7.00 have been associated with adverse neonatal outcomes and more clearly represent a threshold for significant fetal acidemia (Gilstrap et al., 1989).

TABLE 8-3

Factors Consistent with a Diagnosis of Intrapartum Asphyxial Brain Damage

FHR pattern with absent FHR variability at birth which will be noted with decelerations (usually severe variables, lates, or bradycardia)

Umbilical artery pH < 7.0 (more convincing if < 6.8)

Umbilical artery base excess < –15mEq/L (more convincing if < –20)

Apgar score < 3 at 5 min (more convincing if still < 3 at 10 min)

Neurologic signs in newborn (more convincing if seizures)

Multiorgan damage in newborn (renal, heart, etc.)

Note: From *Handbook of Fetal Heart Rate Monitoring* (2nd ed., p. 205), by J. T. Parer. Copyright © 1997 W. B. Saunders. Reprinted with permission.

TABLE 8-4

*Single-Digit Value Guideline for Initial Assessment of Normal and Abnormal Umbilical Cord Blood Acid-Base Values**

	NORMAL VALUES	METABOLIC ACIDEMIA	RESPIRATORY ACIDEMIA
pH	> 7.10	< 7.10	< 7.10
pO_2 (mmHg)	> 20	< 20	Variable
pCO_2 (mmHg)	< 60	< 60	> 60
Bicarbonate (mEq/L)	> 22	< 22	> 22
Base deficit (mEq/L)	< 10	> 10	< 10
Base excess (mEq/L)	> –10	< –10	> –10

* The values presented are suggested as a guide for evaluating acid-base status. All umbilical cord blood values should be evaluated in relation to the specific clinical findings and situation for a given patient. Note that greater absolute values of base deficit or excess are associated with acidemia.

Although normal blood values are often described in ranges, it may be helpful to identify a specific number to use as a frame of reference when evaluating cord blood values (see Table 8-4). All umbilical cord blood values should be evaluated in relationship to the specific clinical findings and situation for any given patient. In addition to pH levels, the pO_2, pCO_2, bicarbonate and base deficit or excess values are often considered.

Decreased pH reflects higher acid level and, therefore, acidemia. Plasma bicarbonate is one buffer used to raise pH levels. In metabolic acidosis, an excess of hydrogen ions is released. As a result, bicarbonate—a base—is depleted (Cohen & Schifrin, 1983; Gimovsky & Caritis, 1982). The decrease in base is reflected as an increased base deficit or decreased base excess. The base deficit or excess is not measured directly, but is calculated from the pH, pCO_2 and bicarbonate blood values.

Base deficit measures the amount of base buffers below normal levels. A large, positive base deficit indicates that base buffers have been used to buffer acids, that sufficient base reserves are not present and that metabolic acidosis is present. Base excess measures the amount of base buffers above normal levels. Therefore, a large, negative base excess also indicates that base buffers have been used to buffer acids, that sufficient base reserves are not present and that metabolic acidosis is present. The use of base deficit vs. base excess often depends on the laboratory. Regardless of what specific values are used, it is important to assess the trends of serial pH values obtained from scalp and cord blood values when assessing the situation for recovery.

⌨ SUMMARY

Electronic fetal monitoring and fetal auscultation continue to be the commonly used methods for assessing fetal well-being, but, clearly, additional assessment strategies are needed. Technical advances in acid-base monitoring have markedly improved medical care in such fields as anesthesiology, critical care and newborn intensive care (Dildy, Thorp, Yeast and Clark, 1996). These technical advances are slowly paving the way to more accurate assessment of fetal oxygenation. The fetus is an extraordinary and complex being that has a remarkable built-in system for responding to periods of hypoxemia. Unfortunately, this system may be challenged enough to cause the fetus to compensate during these periods of oxygen deprivation, resulting in a nonreassuring tracing on EFM or nonreassuring characteristics found with fetal auscultation. Health care providers are challenged to understand the circumstances that affect fetal oxygenation, select the appropriate method of acid-base assessment, and intervene in a timely manner to maximize fetal oxygenation.

REFERENCES

American Academy of Pediatrics & American College of Obstetricians and Gynecologists. (2002). *Guidelines for Perinatal Care* (5th ed.). Washington, D.C.: Author.

American College of Obstetricians and Gynecologists. (1994). *Inappropriate use of the terms fetal distress and birth asphyxia* (Committee Opinion No. 197). Washington, D.C.: Author.

American College of Obstetricians and Gynecologists. (1995). *Fetal heart rate patterns: Monitoring, interpretation, and management* (Technical Bulletin No. 207). Washington, D.C.: Author.

American College of Obstetricians and Gynecologists. (1999). *Antepartum fetal surveillance* (Practice Bulletin No. 9). Washington, D.C.: Author.

American College of Obstetricians and Gynecologists. (2001). *Fetal pulse oximetry* (Committee Opinion No. 258). Washington, D.C.: Author.

Arulkumaran, S., Skurr, B., Tong, H., Kek, L. P., & Ratnam, S. S. (1991). No evidence of hearing loss due to fetal acoustic stimulation test. *Obstetrics & Gynecology, 78*(2), 283–285.

Clark, S. L., Gimovsky, M. L., & Miller, F. C. (1984). The scalp stimulation test: A clinical alternative to fetal scalp sampling. *American Journal Obstetrics and Gynecology, 148*(3), 274–277.

Cohen, W. R., & Schifrin, B. S. (1989). Clinical management of fetal hypoxemia. In W. R. Cohen, Acker, W. R. & E. A. Friedman (Eds.), *Management of Labor* (pp. 283–316). Baltimore, MD: University Park Press.

Dickinson, J. E., Erikson, N. L., Meyer, B. A. & Parisi, V. M. (1992). The effect of preterm birth on umbilical cord blood gases. *Obstetrics and Gynecology, 79*(4), 575–578.

Dildy, G. A., Clark, S. L., & Loucks, C. A. (1996). Intrapartum fetal pulse oximetry: Past, present, and future. *American Journal of Obstetrics and Gynecology, 175*(1), 1–9.

Dildy, G. A., Thorp, J. A., Yeast, J. D., & Clark, S. L. (1996). The relationship between oxygen saturation and pH in umbilical blood: Implications for intrapartum fetal oxygen saturation monitoring. *American Journal of Obstetrics and Gynecology, 175*(3), 682–687.

Druzin, M. L., Gabbe, S. G., & Reed, K. L. (2002). Antepartum fetal evaluation. In S. G. Gabbe, J. R. Niebyl, & J. L. Simpson (Eds.), *Obstetrics: Normal and Problem Pregnancies* (4th ed.) (pp. 313–349). New York: Churchill Livingstone.

Duerbeck, N. B., Chaffin, D. G., & Seeds, J. W. (1992). A practical approach to umbilical artery pH and blood gas determinations. *Obstetrics and Gynecology, 79*(6), 959–962.

Ecker, J. L., & Parer, J. T. (1999). Obstetric evaluation

of fetal acid-base balance. *Critical Reviews in Clinical Laboratory Sciences, 36*(5), 407–451

Eller, D. P., Robinson, L. J., & Newman, R. B. (1992). Position of the vibroacoustic stimulator does not affect fetal response. *American Journal of Obstetrics and Gynecology, 167,* 1137–1139.

Enkin, M., Keirse, M., Neilson, J., Crowther, C., Duley, L., Hodnett, E., & Hofmeyer, J. (2000). *A guide to effective care in pregnancy and childbirth* (3rd ed.). Oxford, UK: Oxford University Press.

Fee, S. C., Malee, K., Deddisch, R., et al (1990). Severe acidosis and subsequent neurologic status. *American Journal of Obstetrics and Gynecology, 162:*802.

Fields, L. M., Entman, S. S., & Boehm, F. H. (1983). Correlation of the one minute Apgar score and the pH value of umbilical arterial blood. *Southern Medical Journal, 76*(12), 1477–1479.

Gagnon, R., Hunse, C., & Foreman, J. (1989). Human fetal behavioral states after vibratory stimulation. *American Journal of Obstetrics and Gynecology, 161*(6 Pt 1), 1470–1476.

Garite, T. J., (2002a). Antepartum fetal evaluation. In S. G. Gabbe, J. R. Niebyl, & J. L. Simpson (Eds.), *Obstetrics: Normal and Problem Pregnancies* (4th ed.) (pp. 327–330). New York: Churchill Livingstone.

Garite, T. J. (2002b). Intrapartum fetal evaluation. In S. G. Gabbe, J. R. Niebyl, & J. L. Simpson (Eds.), *Obstetrics: Normal and Problem Pregnancies* (4th ed.) (pp. 395–429). New York: Churchill Livingstone.

Garite, T. .J., Dildy, G. A., McNamara, H., Nageotte, M. P., Boehm, F. H., Dellinger, E. H., Knuppel, R. A., Porreco, R. P., Miller, H. S., Sunderji, S., Varner, M. W., & Swedlow, D. B. (2000). A multicenter controlled trial of fetal pulse oximetry in the intrapartum management of nonreassuring fetal heart rate patterns. *American Journal of Obstetrics and Gynecology, 183*(5), 1049–1058.

Garite, T. J., & Porreco, R. P. (2001). Evaluating fetal hypoxia with pulse oximetry. *Contemporary OB/GYN, 46*(7), 12–26.

Gegor, C. L., Paine, L. L., & Johnson, T. R. (1991). Antepartum fetal assessment: A nurse-midwifery perspective. *Journal of Nurse-Midwifery, 36*(3), 153–167.

Gerhardt, K. J., & Abrams, R. M., (2000). Fetal exposures to sound and vibroacoustic stimulation. *Journal of Perinatology, 20*(8 Pt 2), S21–30.

Gilstrap, L. C. (1999). Fetal acid-base balance. In Creasy, R. K., & Resnik, R. (Eds.), *Maternal-Fetal Medicine* (4th ed) (pp. 331–340). Philadelphia: W.B. Saunders.

Gilstrap, L. C., Leveno, K. J., Burris, J., Williams, M. L., & Little, B. B. (1989). Diagnosis of birth asphyxia on the basis of fetal pH, Apgar score, and newborn cerebral dysfunction. *American Journal of Obstetrics and Gynecology, 161*(3), 825–830.

Gimovsky, M. L., & Caritis, S. N. (1982). Diagnosis and management of the hypoxic fetal heart rate patterns. *Clinics in Perinatology, 9*(2), 313–324.

Goodwin, T. M., Milner-Masterson, L., & Paul, R. H. (1994). Elimination of fetal scalp sampling on a large clinical service. *Obstetrics and Gynecology, 83*(6), 971–974.

Greene, K. R. (1999). Scalp blood gas analysis. *Obstetrics and Gynecology Clinics of North America, 26*(4), 641–656.

Gregg, A. R., & Weiner, C. P. (1993). "Normal" umbilical arterial and venous acid-base and blood gas values. *Clinical Obstetrics and Gynecology, 36*(1), 24–32.

Guyton, A. C., & Hall, J. E. (1997). *Human physiology and mechanisms of disease* (6th ed.). Philadelphia: W.B. Saunders.

International Federation of Gynecology and Obstetrics (IFGO) Study Group on the Assessment of New Technology. (1995). Intrapartum Surveillance: Recommendations on current practice and overview of new developments. *International Journal of Gynecology and Obstetrics, 49*(2), 213–231.

Kühnert, M., Seelbach-Göbel, B., Di Renzo, G. C., Howarth, E., Butterwegge, M., & Murphy, J. M. (1998). Guidelines for the use of fetal pulse oximetry during labor and delivery. *Prenatal and Neonatal Medicine, 3*(4), 432–433.

Lindsay, M. K. (1999). Intrauterine resuscitation of the compromised fetus. *Clinics in Perinatology, 26*(3), 569–584.

Low, J. A., Victory, R., & Derrick, E. J. (1999). Predictive value of electronic fetal monitoring for intrapartum fetal asphyxia with metabolic acidosis. *Obstetrics and Gynecology, 93*(2), 285–291.

Mallinckrodt, Inc. Healthy Mother and Baby Division. (2000a). *Oxifirst fetal oxygen saturation monitoring system: The technology.* Pleasanton, CA: Author.

Mallinckrodt, Inc. Healthy Mother and Baby Division. (2000b). *Introduction to Oxifirst fetal oxygen saturation monitoring.* Pleasanton, CA: Author

Mallinckrodt, Inc. Healthy Mother and Baby Division (2000c). *Questions and answers for medical professionals.* Pleasanton, CA: Author.

Marden, D., McDuffie, R. S., Allen, R., & Abitz, D. (1997). A randomized controlled trial of a new fetal acoustic stimulation test for fetal well-being. *American Journal of Obstetrics and Gynecology, 176*(6), 1386–1388.

Menihan, C. A., & Zottoli, E. K. (2001). *Electronic fetal monitoring: Concepts and applications.* Philadelphia: Lippincott.

Miller, D. A., Rabello, Y. A., & Paul, R. H. (1996). The modified biophysical profile: Antepartum testing in the 1990s. *American Journal of Obstetrics and Gynecology, 174*(3), 812–817.

Nijland, R., Jongsma, H. W., Nijhuis, J. G., van den Berg, P. P, & Oeseburg, B. (1995). Arterial oxygen saturation in relation to metabolic acidosis in fetal lambs. *American Journal of Obstetrics and Gynecology, 172*(3), 810–819.

Parer, J. T. (1997). *Handbook of Fetal Heart Rate Monitoring* (2nd ed.). Philadelphia: W.B. Saunders.

Pearson, J. F., & Weaver, J. B. (1976). Fetal activity and wellbeing. *British Medical Journal, 1*(6021), 1305–1307.

Polzin, G. B., Blakemore, K. J., Petrie, R. H., & Amon, E. (1988). Fetal vibro-acoustic stimulation: Magnitude and duration of fetal heart rate accelerations as a marker of fetal health. *Obstetrics and Gynecology, 72*(4), 621–626.

Porter, M. L. (2000). Fetal pulse oximetry: An adjunct to electronic fetal heart rate monitoring. *Journal of Obstetric, Gynecologic, and Neonatal Nursing, 29*(5), 537–548.

Porter, T. F., & Clark, S. L. (1999). Vibroacoustic and scalp stimulation. *Obstetrics and Gynecology Clinics of North America, 26*(4), 657–669.

Rayburn, W., Zuspan, F., Motley, M. E., & Donaldson, M. (1980). An alternative to antepartum fetal heart rate testing. *American Journal of Obstetrics and Gynecology, 138*(2), 223–226.

Richardson, B. S., Carmichael, L., Homan, J., & Patrick, J. (1992). Electrocortical activity, electrocular activity, and breathing movements in fetal sheep with prolonged and graded hypoxemia. *American Journal of Obstetrics and Gynecology, 167*(2), 553–558.

Sadovsky, E., Yaffe, H., & Polishuk, W. (1974). Fetal movement monitoring in normal and pathological pregnancy. *International Journal of Gynecology and Obstetrics, 12*, 75.

Saling, E. (1996). Fetal pulse oximetry during labor: Issues and recommendations for clinical use. *Journal of Perinatal Medicine, 24*(2), 467–478.

Sarinoglu, F., Gol, K., Sabin, I., Turkkani, B., & Oztopeu, C. (1999). The predictive value of fetal acoustic stimulation. *Journal of Perinatology, 19*(2), 103–105.

Sarno, A. P., Ahn, M. O., Phelan, J. P. et al. (1990). Fetal acoustic stimulation in the early intrapartum period as a predictor of subsequent fetal condition. *American Journal of Obstetrics & Gynecology, 162*: 762–767

Seelbach-Göbel, B., Heupel, M., Kühnert, M., & Butterwegge, M. (1999). The prediction of fetal acidosis by means of intrapartum fetal pulse oximetry. *American Journal of Obstetrics and Gynecology, 180*(1 Pt 1), 73–81.

Sherer, D. M.and Bentolili, E. (1998). Blunted fetal response to vibroacoustic stimulation following chronic exposure to propanolol. *American Journal of Perinatology, 15*: 495-498.

Simpson, K. R. (1998). Intrapartum fetal oxygen saturation monitoring. *Lifelines, 2*(6), 20–24.

Simpson, K. R., & Porter, M. L. (2001). Fetal oxygen saturation monitoring: Using this new technology for fetal assessment during labor. *Lifelines, 5*(2), 26–33.

Sleutel, M. (1989). An overview of vibroacoustic stimulation. *Journal of Obstetric, Gynecologic, and Neonatal Nursing, 18*(6), 447–452.

Smith, C. V. (1994). Vibroacoustic stimulation for risk assessment. *Clinics in Perinatology, 21*(4), 797–808.

Smith, C. V. (1995). Vibroacoustic stimulation. *Clinical Obstetrics and Gynecology, 38*(1), 68–77.

Smith, C. V., Nguyen, H. N., Phelan, J. P., & Paul, R. H. (1986). Intrapartum assessment of fetal well-being: A comparison of fetal acoustic stimulation with acid-base determinations. *American Journal of Obstetrics and Gynecology, 155*(4), 726–728.

Smith, C. V., Phelan, J. P., Platt, L. D., Broussard, P., & Paul R. H. (1986). Fetal acoustic stimulation testing: A randomized clinical comparison with the nonstress test. *American Journal of Obstetrics and Gynecology, 155*(1), 131–134.

Smith-Levitin, M., Petrikovsky, B., & Schneider, E. P. (1997). Practical guidelines for antepartum fetal surveillance. *American Family Physician, 56*(8), 1981–1988.

Society of Obstetricians and Gynaecologists of Canada (SOGC). (1995). SOGC Policy Statement: Fetal health surveillance in labour. *Journal of SOGC, 17*(9), 865–901.

Society of Obstetricians, and Gynaecologists of Canada. (2002). Fetal health surveillance in labour (SOGC Clinical Practice Guidelines No. 112). Ottawa, Ontario, Canada: Author

Sonek, J., & Nicolaides, K. (1994). The role of cordocentesis in the diagnosis of fetal well-being. *Clinics in Perinatology, 21*(4), 743–764.

Swedlow, D. B. (2000). *Review of evidence for a fetal SPO₂ critical threshold of 30 percent* (Reference Note No. 2). Pleasanton, CA: Mallinckrodt.

Swedlow, D., & Bolling, M. (personal communication February 3, 2003). Letter to clinicians regarding changes in the management protocol for use of fetal pulse oximetry. Retrieved June 11, 2003 from www.fda.gov/cdrh/psn/show16-Nellcor.html.

Sykes, G. S., Molloy, P. M., Johnson, P., Gu, W., Ashworth, F., Stirrat, G. M., & Turnbull, A. C. (1982). Do Apgar scores indicate asphyxia? *Lancet, 1*(8270), 494–496.

Tan, K. H., & Smyth, R. (2001). Fetal vibroacoustic stimulation for facilitation of tests of fetal wellbeing (Cochrane Review). In *The Cochrane Library* (Issue 2). Oxford: Update Software.

Thorp, J. A., & Rushing, R. S. (1999). Umbilical cord blood gas analysis. *Obstetrics and Gynecology Clinics of North America, 26*(4), 695–709.

Tucker, S. M. (2000). *Pocket guide to fetal monitoring and assessment.* St Louis: Mosby.

Wallman, C. M. (1997). Interpretation of fetal cord blood gases. *Neonatal Network 16*(1), 72–75.

Yao, Q. W., Jakobsson, J., Nyman, M., Rabaeus, H., Till, O., & Westgren, M. (1990). Fetal response to different intensity levels of vibroacoustic stimulation. *Obstetrics and Gynecology, 75*(2), 206–209.

Yeoman, E. R., Hauth, J. C., Gilstrap, L. C., & Strickland, D. M. (1985). Umbilical cord pH, PCO2, and bicarbonate following uncomplicated term vaginal deliveries. *American Journal of Obstetrics and Gynecology, 151*(6), 798–800.

SECTION FIVE

Application of Fetal Heart Monitoring Data

CHAPTER 9

Communication of Fetal Heart Monitoring Information

Kathleen Rice Simpson
G. Eric Knox

☞ PURPOSE AND SIGNIFICANCE

Communication is an integral component of nursing care. The quality of communication can have a significant influence on quality of care and outcomes for mothers and babies. Communication that is open, direct, accurate, and concise will increase the likelihood that information about patient status is known by all those who need to know it and that it is acted on in a clinically timely manner. Common communication channels include those from the nurse to the laboring woman and her family or support persons, from the nurse to the primary health care provider, and from the nurse to other nurses. Although most of the communication between the nurse and the patient is verbal, it is important to consider that nonverbal cues from the nurse may influence how the woman interprets the message. Communication from the nurse to the primary health care provider and from the nurse to other nurses is both verbal and written. Verbal communication between providers may not always be face to face. For example, communication about ongoing maternal-fetal status during labor can occur while the nurse is at the bedside and the physician or certified nurse midwife (CNM) is in the office or at home. Medical record documentation serves to communicate the previous and ongoing patient condition and care to the nurse, CNM, physician, and other members of the health care team. This chapter covers communications about fetal status, including discussions between professional colleagues and discussions with the woman and her family and support person(s). Strategies to promote respectful collaborative communication among colleagues are included. Trends and issues related to medical record documentation are discussed with examples that can be used or adapted according to individual institutional protocols. Finally, perspectives on risk management, conflict resolution, and the chain of command as they relate to fetal assessment are presented as suggestions to promote safe care for mothers and babies and to decrease liability exposure.

☞ COMMUNICATION AMONG PROFESSIONAL COLLEAGUES

Perinatal services in each institution are performed by teams of professional colleagues. Teamwork is a key factor to success in achieving excellence in clinical practice. In any situation requiring a real time combination of multiple skills, experiences, and judgment, teams—not individuals—create superior performance (Risser et al., 1999). Ideally, a perinatal team consists of health care professionals working collectively and in nonhierarchical fashion toward a mutually agreed upon and common goal: the best possible outcomes for mothers and babies (Simpson & Knox, 2001). Each member contributes and is valued for his or her talents, education, experience, background, and perspective. Individual member contributions are evaluated by merit without regard for the member's status in a traditional health care hierarchy. For example, the input of a staff nurse has as much value as that of an attending physician, and the input from a resident physician is considered just as important as that of an advanced-practice nurse (Sherwood, Thomas, Bennett, & Lewis, 2002). The hallmark of successful teamwork is effective communication.

Achieving an environment where perinatal teamwork is a reality can be a challenge because universal and institution-specific barriers may exist. Those barriers are complex and involve many interrelated factors (see Box 9-1). Although some of those factors can be changed or overcome, others represent challenges embedded in the structure of our current health care system (Simpson & Knox, 2001). Each of those factors has an influence on how well physicians, CNMs and nurses communicate.

Although teamwork is a key component of safe and effective perinatal care, nurses, CNMs, and physicians are responsible and accountable for their individual actions and contributions to the team. Professionals are responsible members of the health care team who have a body of knowledge and skills that contain an ethos of good practice. That ethos includes practice that is based on valid, current science; appropriate use of technology; a fiduciary relationship to the patient and family; and responsible behavior in relation to other health care providers to uphold patient safety standards (Benner, et al., 2002). Health care professionals are responsible for accurate and timely assessments, clinical interventions, follow-up, and documentation of all critical events in the medical record. The model of communication (see Figure 9-1) presented is part of the nursing process and includes key concepts and important content that

---

BOX 9-1

Current Factors That Impede Teamwork in Perinatal Care

- Historical roles of women in society
- Traditional roles of physicians and nurses
- Institutional territory and politics
- Licensure and professional accountability
- Type and quantity of education
- Different styles of learning and information exchange
- Socialization of each group
- Methods and amounts of compensation
- Power of social and professional position
- Unresolved conflict, setting the stage for the expectation of future discord

Note: From "Perinatal Teamwork: Turning Rhetoric into Reality," by K. R. Simpson and G. E. Knox, 2001, in K. R. Simpson and P. A. Creehan (Eds.), *AWHONN's Perinatal Nursing* (pp. 378–416). Philadelphia: Lippincott. Copyright: AWHONN.

should be shared between colleagues to promote effective communication.

Nurse to Primary Health Care Provider Communication

Nurse to primary health care provider (e.g., physician, CNM) communication includes: information about maternal-fetal assessments and needs, and in relation to FHM, the interpretation of fetal heart data; changes in maternal or fetal status; interventions provided and the maternal-fetal response(s); and specific requests for primary care provider orders or actions. As previously stated, communication should be direct, clear, concise, timely, and respectful. Communication among members of the health care team that is mutually respectful and direct can lead to a plan of care developed through the wisdom and experience of the knowledgeable professionals involved in patient care.

Interaction and communication between physicians and nurses commonly occurs in a hierarchical model (based on tradition and training). Based on the current research literature, physician-nurse communication patterns and the effects of

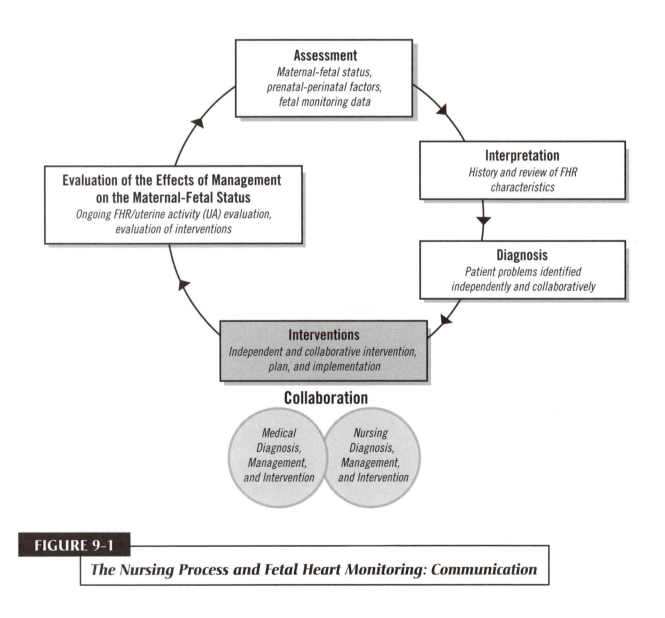

FIGURE 9-1

The Nursing Process and Fetal Heart Monitoring: Communication

those patterns have been examined whereas nurse and other care providers (e.g., nurse midwife) communication have not been studied. Therefore, the following discussion refers to nurse-physician communication. In a hierarchical model physicians give orders and nurses may be expected to follow those orders without question (Keenan, Cooke & Hillis, 1998; Sleutel, 2000). Communication of this nature about fetal status does not always create optimal patient care and has the potential to increase the risk of preventable adverse outcomes. Examples of situations where a traditional hierarchical model may create barriers to clear communication include (a) situations of rapidly changing fetal status, where the nurse at the bedside has more information than the physician or CNM at home or in the office; (b) teaching situations in which the nurse has more experience than the student or resident physician; and (c) situations where the nurse has learned important information from the woman or family that the family has chosen not to communicate with the physician. In circumstances such as those, experienced nurses may initiate strategies designed to overcome provider discomfort with nurses' critical thinking skills or clinical suggestions concerning how their patients should be cared for; thus violating the expected hierarchal model of communication (Simpson & Knox, 2001).

Instead of mutual direct communication leading to a plan of care developed through the wisdom and experience of knowledgeable professionals, nurses may revert to the so-called doctor-nurse game to achieve what they believe is in the patient's best interest (Stein, Watts, & Howell, 1990). Although this technique was first described in the literature over 30 years ago (Stein, 1967), it was used for many years before Dr. Stein's classic article was published and persists today. Tips on how to interact effectively with members of the health care team are often given by experienced nurses to new graduates as part of socialization to the role of the professional registered nurse (Willis & Parish, 1997). One technique often taught is how to encourage the physician to think a plan of action was their idea rather than that of the nurse. Using this communication technique may avoid open disagreement and/or conflict and allow the

nurse to give recommendations and the physician to request recommendations without appearing to do so (Peter, 2000). However, indirect, inefficient, and inaccurate communication can occur and may lead to preventable adverse outcomes in multiple ways such as: a) when nurses have difficulty finding the right "story" to convey the emergent nature of an evolving clinical situation (Knaus, Draper & Wagner, 1986); b) when the assessment is not complete because of a clinical fact known to the physician but not the nurse; or c) when the assessment is correct but the description is misunderstood by the physician. Dysfunctional communication using less direct and respectful techniques can impede patient care.

By contrast, one hallmark of team behavior is clear language agreed to and understood by all members (Simpson & Knox, 2001). Clear language is particularly important when communication does not occur face to face. Telephone communication with the physician or CNM should be direct and to the point. For example:

◆ "Based on my initial assessment, this patient is having variable decelerations and has meconium-stained fluid. May I have an order for an amnioinfusion, and can you please come in to see this patient as soon as possible?"

◆ "I am having difficulty obtaining a continuous tracing of the fetal heart rate. May I have an order to place a fetal spiral electrode? I'll call you back and let you know how the baby is doing after I have a period of fetal heart rate tracing with the spiral electrode."

◆ "I am uncomfortable with your order to start oxytocin because of the nonreassuring fetal heart rate pattern. I am going to wait until you are able to come in and see this patient and we can review the tracing together. When can I expect to see you?"

◆ "You ordered intermittent auscultation of the fetal heart rate, but what I am hearing during auscultation suggests decelerations. I'm calling to let you know that I am going to use continuous monitoring, at least for a while, until I have a reassuring fetal heart rate tracing. I'll call you back after I assess the patient and review the tracing to let you know what is happening with the baby."

◆ "Fetal status is deteriorating quickly, and I need you here now."

In a classic study of how the quality of interactions between nurses and physicians in an intensive care setting affects patient outcomes, Knaus, et al. (1986) demonstrated that the most powerful determinant of severity-adjusted patient death rates was how well nurses and physicians worked together in planning and subsequently delivering patient care. They concluded that a high degree of involvement and interaction between nurses and physicians directly influences patient outcomes. Other researchers found that for each severity level of medical condition studied, patients were at greater risk of dying or being readmitted when nurses and resident physicians failed to communicate and effectively work together (Baggs, Ryan, & Phelps, 1992). These findings were supported by a more recent study (Baggs, et al., 1999). In summary, knowledgeable, clear, direct and respectful communication is an important key to promoting patient safety.

Nurse to Nurse Communication

Communication of fetal assessment data from the nurse to other nurses varies with institutional practice models and staffing patterns. In units where primary nursing care is routine or where there is likely to be one nurse for each laboring women, communication from nurse to nurse may be limited to change-of-shift reporting. In reality, most labor and delivery units have a 1:2 (or greater) nurse-to-patient ratio. If a woman's condition changes so that she temporarily needs one-to-one care such as during epidural placement, a persistent nonreassuring fetal heart rate (FHR) pattern, second stage labor pushing, or birth—a significant amount of data about maternal-fetal status will need to be communicated accurately and concisely to the relief nurse who will be covering the other nurse's patient. Verbal report should be accompanied by complete and timely medical record documentation. Some practice models involve team nursing, where several

nurses care for a team of patients. It is important in this model to identify which nurse has primary responsibility for the patient and to keep all members of the team informed about ongoing maternal-fetal status. Sometimes an acute event necessitates one nurse's covering another nurse's patient without the benefit of a comprehensive verbal report. When medical record documentation is up-to-date, a review of the electronic fetal monitoring (EFM) tracing and labor flow record should be adequate for the nurse to assume care and ensure patient safety.

Communication between nurses during change of shift or change of responsibility for patient care should be comprehensive. For example, a report from nurse to nurse about a woman in labor should include the following:

◆ Key maternal-fetal admission data

◆ Current assessment including how the mother and fetus have tolerated labor

◆ Interventions or procedures that have been done

◆ Progress of labor

◆ Maternal vital signs

◆ Characteristics of the FHR and uterine activity

◆ Current and previous dosages of pharmacological agents that were used to ripen the cervix or induce or augment labor, if applicable

◆ Pain status, including current and previous pain relief and comfort measures that have been used

◆ The woman's desires for labor and birth

◆ Pertinent psychosocial issues

The nurses should review the medical record together, whenever possible, before the nurse who is giving the report leaves the unit. Doing so will ensure that all data are covered and give the nurse who is leaving an opportunity to answer questions and address concerns that the relief or oncoming nurse may have. Ideally, a report between nurses is followed by a visit to the patient's room, where the reporting nurse introduces the relief nurse to the patient and support persons in attendance.

🖙 STRATEGIES FOR SUCCESSFUL COMMUNICATION AMONG PROFESSIONAL COLLEAGUES

Selection and Use of a Common Language for Fetal Assessment in All Professional Communication and Medical Record Documentation

Each institution should have policies related to FHR pattern interpretation and medical record documentation, ideally developed by an interdisciplinary team. This mutually agreed upon language can then be routinely used by all providers to enhance both interdisciplinary communication and patient safety (Simpson & Knox, 2000). The potential for miscommunication between care providers, especially during telephone conversations about fetal status, are decreased when everyone is speaking the same language about EFM data. Thus, timely intervention for nonreassuring FHR patterns is more likely. Several FHR nomenclatures have been published in the literature, including those described in this text and taught in the Association of Women's Health, Obstetric and Neonatal Nurses (AWHONN) *Fetal Heart-Monitoring Principles and Practices* courses, as well as those described in the American College of Obstetricians and Gynecologists (ACOG) Technical Bulletin *Fetal Heart Rate Patterns: Monitoring, Interpretation, and Management* (1995); the Society of Obstetricians and Gynaecologists of Canada (SOGC) Policy Statement *Fetal Health Surveillance in Labour* (2002); and the results of the National Institute of Child Health and Human Development (NICHD) Research Planning Workshop (1997). None of those nomenclatures has been shown to be more reliable or valid than another. The key issue is to jointly select one set of definitions and consistently use it in all types of communication.

Joint Nurse-CNM-Physician Education about Fetal Assessment

Nurses, CNMs, and physicians jointly assess and mange maternal fetal status during labor. There-fore, interdisciplinary continuing education programs provide one way to promote effective communication among providers (Simpson & Knox, 2001). These interdisciplinary educational programs about electronic fetal monitoring can potentially:

◆ Decrease the frequency of clinical disagreement among physicians, CNMs and nurses regarding the description and interpretation of FHR patterns

◆ Increase the opportunity for interaction and role modeling professional communication techniques, and

◆ Promote collaborative problem-solving in the clinical setting.

EFM-tracing reviews work well as a form of interdisciplinary education because the presentation and discussion are associated with specific clinical cases and graphic display of FHR patterns. A group process can be used to review expected responses, appropriate interpretations, and related interventions. Team discussions can lead to an increased knowledge of EFM principles for everyone involved. Developing case studies containing clinical ambiguity can be an ideal way to clarify ongoing clinical issues where interpretation and expectations of provider groups may differ (Simpson, 2001). An interdisciplinary team in each institution can identify clinical situations that have or can result in varying opinions about management. For example, physicians may expect a series of nursing interventions for a specific FHR pattern that are not the routine of nurses on the unit. In another example, there may be clinical disagreement about what to do when uterine hyperstimulation is the result of oxytocin administration, but the FHR remains reassuring. Opinions may vary among nurses and primary care providers about when and under what circumstances oxytocin dosages should be increased or decreased and thus, be a source of frustration. An open and proactive discussion of physiologic principles related to oxytocin administration and rationale for a course of action can result in consensus regarding policies and enhanced communication among providers.

In summary, educational collaboration among nurses, CNMs, and physicians who are jointly responsible for FHR pattern interpretation and clinical interventions can enhance collaboration in everyday clinical interactions and thus promotes patient safety.

COMMUNICATION WITH PREGNANT WOMEN AND THEIR FAMILIES OR SUPPORT PERSONS

Preparation for applying the monitoring equipment should include an explanation of EFM and time for answering the woman and her support person(s)' questions. The nurse should explain the heart rate sounds and what the data on the tracing mean in lay terms. In addition, the nurse should discuss what might happen if the FHR pattern becomes nonreassuring so the woman and her family can be prepared if intrauterine resuscitation techniques are initiated quickly. In one study, the higher women rated the amount and quality of information about EFM provided by the nurse during initial monitor application, the more positively women viewed their overall EFM experience during labor (Simpson, 1991). In addition, women who felt that they were adequately informed about routine interventions during nonreassuring FHR patterns were less likely to be overly concerned when such patterns occurred.

Ideally, the most low-tech and least-invasive methods of fetal assessment are used for women in labor (AWHONN, 2000a). Intermittent auscultation of the FHR at prescribed frequencies during labor has been shown to be as efficacious as continuous EFM (AAP & ACOG, 2002) and so is recommended as the preferred method by some professional associations for low-risk women (SOGC, 2002). Women may know prior to labor that some form of EFM or auscultation may be used. Ideally, the primary health care provider should discuss common methods of fetal assessment during labor with the woman during the prenatal period so that potential concerns or objections may be reviewed prior to admission for childbirth.

MEDICAL RECORD DOCUMENTATION

Overview

Documentation has become one of the most time-consuming of nursing activities. Nurses often are concerned that medical record documentation forces them to focus on "paperwork" rather than patient care. Cumbersome documentation systems that require duplicate and triplicate entries of the same data can contribute to this real problem. There can be ramifications for inaccuracies and omissions in medical record documentation. Documentation deficiencies may result in decreased communication among team members, denied reimbursement by insurance carriers for care rendered, lost information for statistical or outcome data for quality purposes, and in the case of litigation, increased liability exposure for institutions and health care providers (Simpson & Chez, 2001). The ongoing challenge is to create a streamlined system for documentation that is cost-effective, easy to use, time efficient for the nurse, and sufficiently comprehensive for current or subsequent review.

The medical record should provide a factual and objective account of care provided, including direct and indirect communication with other members of the health care team. Only clinically relevant information should be documented. There should be guidelines in each institution about how to document initiation and steps of notification in the chain of command see Figure 9-2 for an example of a chain of command. Facility guidelines may include chain-of-command documentation in the medical record or on quality improvement or variance reports. It is important to be knowledgeable about and adhere to individual institutional policies about chain-of-command documentation.

Decreasing Liability Exposure Related to Documentation

The medical record is often the single most important document available in the defense of an allegation of negligent care (Berry, 1999). The time

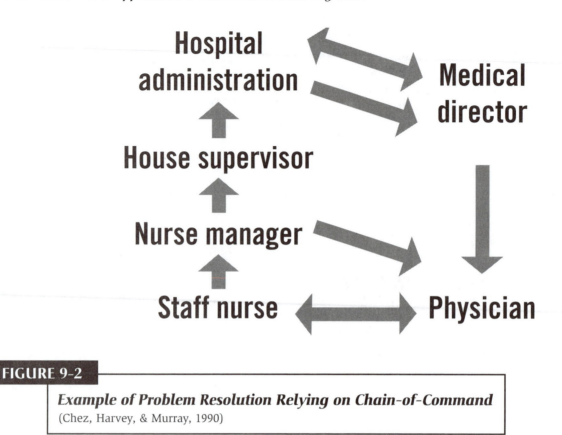

FIGURE 9-2

Example of Problem Resolution Relying on Chain-of-Command
(Chez, Harvey, & Murray, 1990)

from event to formal legal inquiry may involve several years and the nurse may have limited independent recall without documentation in the medical record. Therefore, frequently, in issues of litigation, the nurse relies on written nurses notes or data entered into an electronic medical record at the time of patient contact. A complete and legible medical record is an asset when defending against allegations of improper care (Berry, 1999; Rommal, 1996). Because lack of documentation can result in a presumed lack of care, omissions are challenging to defend. According to risk-claims data from a professional liability insurance carrier, documentation ranks second only to patient monitoring and assessment in the area of nursing-related risk exposure, accounting for 20.7% of all exposures (Berry, 1999).

Litigation can follow clinical events that result in adverse outcomes, regardless of whether the adverse outcome was preventable or nonpreventable. Documentation including the events preced-

ing, during, and following an emergent clinical situation should reflect all care provided. During emergent situations medical record documentation may occur retrospectively. The first priority during an emergency is to provide immediate patient care. Post-event documentation should focus on reconstructing a summary of all of the assessments, actions and communication that transpired as accurately and timely as possible. For example, in the case of a nonreassuring FHR of acute onset resulting in an emergent cesarean birth, summary documentation should include but may not be limited to the following:

◆ Time the nonreassuring fetal heart rate was recognized

◆ Nursing actions initiated for maternal and/or fetal resuscitation

◆ Continued FHM assessment to evaluate the fetal response to interventions

◆ Communication with team members and their responses

◆ Time the woman was taken to the surgical suite and time of the incision

◆ Chronologies of interventions performed (including by which personnel) for newborn resuscitation, if necessary, and

◆ A narrative note reflecting discussion between health care providers and the woman and her family.

During emergent intrapartum situations, some nurses feel that documentation directly on the fetal monitoring tracing can assist them in constructing notes after patient stabilization. If this approach is used, it is important to ensure that the content and times included in the narrative notes written later coincide with the fetal monitoring tracing annotations (including the time, if present on the fetal monitoring tracing). Retrospective charting is better than no documentation. However, late entries can be areas of focus in litigation if they are written days after the event. Give careful attention to ensuring that charting occurs as soon after the event as possible and that the data entered are accurate and objective. Do not alter the medical record to include data that are not accurate even if asked to do so.

While notations directly on the FHR tracing can be useful during emergent situations, the practice of duplicate documentation of routine care on both the FHR tracing and the medical record is no longer recommended (Chez, 1997; AWHONN, 1998; Simpson & Chez, 2001). Previously, perinatal nurses believed that there should be enough documentation on the FHR tracing so that the tracing could "stand alone" for subsequent review. However, hand writing on the tracing about routine care not only can decrease the amount of nursing time spent on patient care activities, but this practice also can lead to errors in documentation and can contribute to delays in transcription to the medical record (Chez, 1997). If the FHR tracings are electronically archived, hand-written notes on the tracing do not become part of the permanent medical record. As more institutions adopt electronic information systems with the

ability to enter data that can be noted electronically on both the FHR tracing and labor record, this issue may be minimized or eliminated.

It is appropriate for nurses and health care providers to document FHR patterns by name in the medical record. In 1986, ACOG and AWHONN (then known as NAACOG, the Nurses Association of the American College of Obstetricians and Gynecologists) issued a joint publication about electronic fetal monitoring that included recommendations for identification, documentation and communication of FHR patterns (*Joint ACOG/ NAACOG Statement on Electronic Fetal Monitoring*, 1986). According to this joint statement, fetal monitoring patterns have been given descriptive names (e.g., accelerations and early, late, and variable decelerations) and nurses should use these terms in written medical record documentation and in verbal communication about fetal status among providers. Since at least 1986, perinatal nurses have been encouraged to identify FHR patterns by the appropriate name in the medical record and it remains appropriate to do so (AAP & ACOG, 2002). In the past, nurses were often taught to provide extensive detail about all FHR decelerations (e.g., deceleration down to the 60s lasting for 70 seconds with a slow return to baseline or decelerations occurring after each contraction down to the 100s lasting for 40 seconds) in the medical record so that they would be able to reconstruct the FHR pattern from their notes. Describing FHR patterns in the narrative notes was previously taught for two reasons: 1) fear that the paper EFM tracing could be lost and these descriptions would be crucial if the case involved a future lawsuit and 2) "diagnosing" was not considered to be within the scope of nursing practice, thus descriptions of the patterns rather than identifying the FHR pattern by name was preferable. Detailed narrative descriptions of FHR patterns may only be necessary when there is uncertainty about how to name a pattern with mixed characteristics.

Routine detailed description of deceleration patterns is time consuming, may be unnecessary and in some situations may increase liability exposure. For example, if the nurse has documented descriptive details of decelerations in the narrative notes and a subsequent adverse outcome occurs followed by litigation, experts may disagree about the details of each FHR deceleration. Repeated expert testimony that decelerations lasted 60 seconds rather than 55 seconds and/or reached a low point of 100 bpm rather than 105 bpm may be challenging to defend when presented to a jury. There is typically little clinical significance between 100 bpm and 105 bpm, and/or a 5 second difference in the duration of the FHR deceleration, however these perceived differences in documentation can create the impression that the nurse was inaccurate in his or her interpretation of the clinical situation, when, in reality, there was no relationship between the FHR documentation and the condition of the infant (Simpson & Knox, 2000).

Electronic Information Systems

Over the past few years, many perinatal units have begun using electronic information systems. Electronic documentation systems capabilities may vary widely. Whatever information system is chosen should ideally streamline the overall documentation process, promote and improve communication among providers, and decrease time entering data. Some institutions use electronic information systems for central fetal monitoring surveillance and EFM tracing and medical record documentation and storage, while others use the fetal surveillance and archiving functions while continuing with traditional paper medical records. Each of these functions of an electronic information system has benefits and limitations. Before deciding to purchase and fully implement any electronic information system, perinatal nursing and medical leaders in consultation with direct health care providers should mutually decide (based on unit design, volume of patients, complexity of service) the goals to be accomplished, and a carefully review potential benefits and limitations. Potential benefits include the ability to view EFM tracings and other portions of the medical record from multiple areas on and off the unit; for example, in some cases, the tracings and medical record can be reviewed by providers at home, in their office or on personal data assistant handheld devices, ease of data entry,

clarity of medical record documentation, electronic storage (paperless) and retrieval, and cost savings over time. Potential limitations include an over reliance on technology, the risk of diminishing bedside care, substituting the central monitoring computer screens as the primary method of assessment of women and their fetuses in labor, time and expense needed to educate all users about the capabilities, operation, and maintenance of sophisticated documentation systems. In addition, there may be a potential loss of information if data are not entered and archived correctly or if electronic system downtime and malfunction occur. Other potential limitations include ongoing costs related to system upgrades as well as the need for a systems manager to coordinate all systems activities.

Currently, research data is sparse about the reliability and validity of maternal-fetal assessment data from computer screens. There have been few studies comparing interpretation of evolving fetal status via electronic computer screens versus interpretation based on the paper tracing. Learned proficiency in one method of acquiring, processing and interpreting data does not guarantee the ability to accurately interpret the same data when presented in a different format. Until further research has been published about reliability and validity of interpretation of maternal-fetal data solely based on visualization of the computer screen, consideration should be given to continuing the practice of printing of the paper tracing directly from the fetal monitor while care is being provided. As research studies are conducted and results analyzed, professional organizations such as AWHONN and ACOG will have evidence upon which to base recommendations for clinical practice.

In addition to the previous considerations, facilities may need backup systems for EFM tracing storage to insure later retrieval if necessary. The ink on the paper monitoring tracings has the potential to fade over time. Microfilming the tracings prior to storage or discarding them can prevent loss of data. Data disks in an archiving system are at risk for corruption like any other computerized storage system. Since many states have statutes of limitations for litigation related to labor and birth that extend to 21 years after the event, it is important to consider whether current data and their storage systems will be able to be accessed by information systems 21 years in the future.

If paper tracings are routinely discarded after microfilming, consider saving the paper tracings associated with a selected set of clinical indicators that reflect complex or challenging case scenarios for education and peer review. Facilities should have a mechanism in place to ensure safe storage of EFM tracings.

Flow Sheets and Narrative Notes

A written or electronic flow sheet at the point of care as the primary source of comprehensive data about maternal-fetal status, nursing interventions, and the events of labor and birth can facilitate timely and accurate medical record data entry (Simpson & Chez, 2001). Well-designed flow sheets are useful tools to prompt notations and practice consistent with unit guidelines, especially in the labor and birth setting (See Figure 9-3 for a sample labor flow sheet.) Routine assessments and interventions can easily be documented in the flow sheet format. See Figures 9-4, 9-5, 9-6, 9-7, 9-8, 9-9 and 9-10 for examples of documentation based on common clinical situations with EFM tracings. Examples of flow sheet documentation using nomenclature taught in the AWHONN *Fetal Heart Monitoring Principles and Practices* workshop and proposed by NICHD are provided in these figures. Figure 9-11 is an example of documentation based on intermittent auscultation and palpation. Abbreviations can be useful to the speed documentation process. If abbreviations are used, there should be a "key to abbreviations" on the labor flow record and the abbreviations should be consistent with the documentation policy of the institution. See Box 9-2 for a list of common abbreviations used for documentation of maternal-fetal assessment data.

Narrative notes should be used to document other than routine care or events that are not included on the flow sheet. Narrative notes may also be used to document:

◆ Nurse-physician communication

◆ Ongoing interventions for a nonreassuring FHR that does not resolve with the usual intrauterine resuscitation techniques

◆ Changes in maternal status

◆ Patient concerns or requests, and

◆ Details of emergent situations and the outcome.

Avoid forms with preprinted times and limited space for notations. These types of forms may contribute to inaccurate or inadequate documentation. Vital signs and other maternal/fetal assessments and/or emergencies do not always occur at predetermined 15-minute intervals. There are times when more documentation is required than can fit into limited pre-set boxes.

Fetal Heart Rate and Uterine Activity Assessment and Documentation

The frequency of FHR and uterine activity assessment and documentation are guided by professional organizations, institutional guidelines, and take into consideration the particular clinical circumstances (ACOG, 1995; AWHONN, 2000; SOGC, 1995, 2002). Guidelines for ongoing labor assessments are described in the Clinical Position Statement *Fetal Assessment* (AWHONN, 2000), *Guidelines for Perinatal Care* (AAP & ACOG, 2002), and the Technical Bulletin *Fetal Heart Rate Patterns: Monitoring, Interpretation, and Management* (ACOG, 1995). The *Comprehensive Accreditation Manual for Hospitals* (Joint Commission on Accreditation of Health Care Organizations [JCAHO], 2003), perinatal nursing textbooks, and some state board of health publications are other resources that provide guidelines for initial and ongoing nursing assessments of women in labor. Based on these guidelines, each perinatal center develops protocols related to maternal/fetal assessment. See Box 9-3 for suggested guidelines for maternal and fetal assessment and documentation during a normal, uncomplicated labor and Figure 9-3 for a sample medical record form for documentation during labor.

Labor Flow Record

Patient Name_____   Physician/CNM_____

Date/Time				Key
Fetal Assessment				**Monitor Mode**
Monitor Mode				Ext = External Ultrasound or Toco
Baseline FHR				FSE = Fetal Spiral Electrode
Baseline Variability				IUPC = Intrauterine Pressure Catheter
FHR Pattern				**Variability**
FSp0$_2$				STV = Absent (∅) or Present (+)
Uterine Activity				LTV
Monitor Mode				Min = Minimal/Decreased (≤ 5 bpm)
Frequency of Contractions				Ave = Average/WNL (6 to 25 bpm)
Duration of Contractions				Mark = Marked/Saltatory (> 25 bpm)
Intensity of Contractions				**FHR Pattern**
Uterine Resting Tone				A = Acceleration
Oxytocin (mU/min)				E = Early Deceleration
Cervical Status				L = Late Deceleration
Vaginal Exam by				V = Variable Deceleration
Dilation (cm)				P = Prolonged Deceleration
Effacement (%)				**Frequency of Contractions (Minutes)**
Station				∅ = None
Assessments/Interventions				Irreg = Irregular
Maternal Position				**Intensity of Contractions**
Activity				M = Mild
Oxygen per Face Mask (Amount)				Mod =Moderate
Pain Assessment				Str = Strong
Nurse Initials				By IUPC = mmHg
				Maternal Position
				LL = Left Lateral
				RL = Right Lateral
				SF = Semi-Fowlers
				Pain Assessment
				0 = None
				3 = Mild
				5 = Tolerable
				7 = Moderate
				10 = Severe

FIGURE 9-3

Sample Labor Flow Record

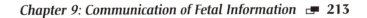
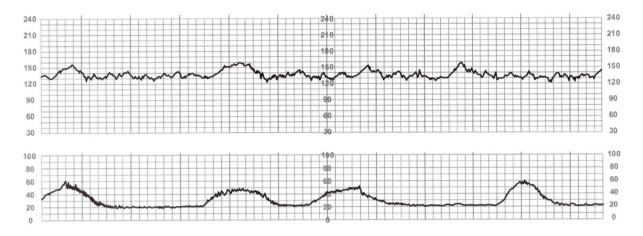

Labor Flow Record				
Patient Name_____		Physician/CNM_____		

Date/Time 12/22/2002	12:15			**Key**
Fetal Assessment				**Monitor Mode** Ext = External Ultrasound or Toco
Monitor Mode	Ext			FSE = Fetal Spiral Electrode
Baseline FHR	130-140			IUPC = Intrauterine Pressure Catheter
Baseline Variability	LTV Ave			**Variability**
FHR Pattern	A			STV = Absent (∅) or Present (+)
FSp0₂				LTV Min = Minimal/Decreased (≤ 5 bpm)
Uterine Activity				Ave = Average/WNL (6 to 25 bpm)
Monitor Mode	Ext			Mark = Marked/Saltatory (> 25 bpm)
Frequency of Contractions	Q 2-4			**FHR Pattern**
Duration of Contractions	80 sec			A = Acceleration
Intensity of Contractions	Mod/Palp			E = Early Deceleration
Uterine Resting Tone	Soft/Palp			L = Late Deceleration
Oxytocin (mU/min)	9			V = Variable Deceleration
Cervical Status				P = Prolonged Deceleration
Vaginal Exam by	KRS			**Frequency of Contractions (Minutes)**
Dilation (cm)	4			∅ = None
Effacement (%)	80			Irreg = Irregular
Station	-2			**Intensity of Contractions**
Assessments/Interventions				M = Mild
Maternal Position	LL			Mod =Moderate
Activity	Bedrest			Str = Strong
Oxygen per Face Mask (Amount)				By IUPC = mmHg
Pain Assessment	5			**Maternal Position** LL = Left Lateral
Nurse Initials	KRS			RL = Right Lateral
				SF = Semi-Fowlers
				Pain Assessment 0 = None
				3 = Mild
				5 = Tolerable
				7 = Moderate
				10 = Severe

FIGURE 9-4

Sample Documentation Using EFM: Reassuring Tracing, External Monitoring (AWHONN terminology)

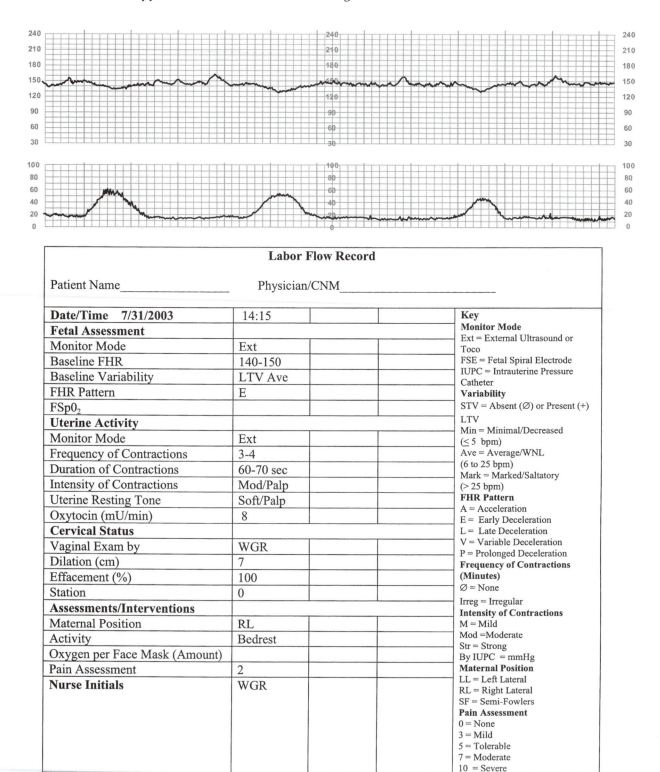

Labor Flow Record

Patient Name_____   Physician/CNM_____

Date/Time 7/31/2003	14:15			Key
Fetal Assessment				**Monitor Mode** Ext = External Ultrasound or Toco
Monitor Mode	Ext			
Baseline FHR	140-150			FSE = Fetal Spiral Electrode
Baseline Variability	LTV Ave			IUPC = Intrauterine Pressure Catheter
FHR Pattern	E			**Variability**
FSp0₂				STV = Absent (∅) or Present (+)
Uterine Activity				LTV
Monitor Mode	Ext			Min = Minimal/Decreased (≤ 5 bpm)
Frequency of Contractions	3-4			Ave = Average/WNL (6 to 25 bpm)
Duration of Contractions	60-70 sec			Mark = Marked/Saltatory (> 25 bpm)
Intensity of Contractions	Mod/Palp			**FHR Pattern**
Uterine Resting Tone	Soft/Palp			A = Acceleration
Oxytocin (mU/min)	8			E = Early Deceleration L = Late Deceleration
Cervical Status				V = Variable Deceleration
Vaginal Exam by	WGR			P = Prolonged Deceleration
Dilation (cm)	7			**Frequency of Contractions (Minutes)**
Effacement (%)	100			∅ = None
Station	0			Irreg = Irregular
Assessments/Interventions				**Intensity of Contractions** M = Mild
Maternal Position	RL			Mod =Moderate
Activity	Bedrest			Str = Strong
Oxygen per Face Mask (Amount)				By IUPC = mmHg
Pain Assessment	2			**Maternal Position** LL = Left Lateral
Nurse Initials	WGR			RL = Right Lateral SF = Semi-Fowlers
				Pain Assessment 0 = None 3 = Mild 5 = Tolerable 7 = Moderate 10 = Severe

---

FIGURE 9-5

Sample Documentation Using EFM: Early Decelerations, External Monitoring (AWHONN terminology)

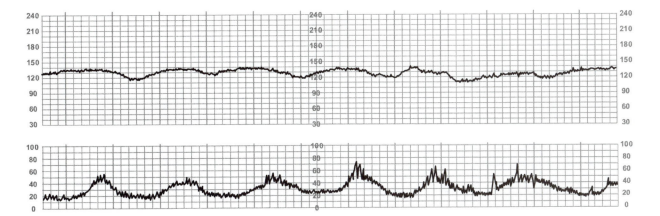

Labor Flow Record				
Patient Name_____		Physician/CNM_____		

				Key
Date/Time 8/28/2003	18:30			**Monitor Mode**
Fetal Assessment				Ext = External Ultrasound or Toco
Monitor Mode	FSE			FSE = Fetal Spiral Electrode
Baseline FHR	125-130			IUPC = Intrauterine Pressure Catheter
Baseline Variability	Min			**Variability**
FHR Pattern	L			Ab = Absent (none)
FSp0₂				Min = Minimal ($\leq$ 5 bpm)
Uterine Activity				Mod = Moderate (6 to 25 bpm)
Monitor Mode	Ext			Mark = Marked (> 25 bpm)
Frequency of Contractions	1 to 2			**FHR Pattern**
Duration of Contractions	60 sec			A = Acceleration
Intensity of Contractions	M/Palp			E = Early Deceleration
Uterine Resting Tone	Soft/Palp			L = Late Deceleration
Oxytocin (mU/min)	Off			V = Variable Deceleration
Cervical Status				P = Prolonged Deceleration
Vaginal Exam by	DJK			**Frequency of Contractions (Minutes)**
Dilation (cm)	3			$\varnothing$ = None
Effacement (%)	50%			Irreg = Irregular
Station	-2			**Intensity of Contractions**
Assessments/Interventions				M = Mild
Maternal Position	LL			Mod =Moderate
Activity	Bedrest			Str = Strong
Oxygen per Face Mask (Amount)	10			By IUPC = mmHg
Pain Assessment	3			**Maternal Position**
Nurse Initials	DJK			LL = Left Lateral
				RL = Right Lateral
				SF = Semi-Fowlers
				Pain Assessment
				0 = None
				3 = Mild
				5 = Tolerable
				7 = Moderate
				10 = Severe

Narrative Notes:

Hyperstimulation for last 10 minutes. Uterine resting tone soft. Late decelerations noted. Oxytocin remains off. O₂ at 10L per face mask. Turned to L Side. Dr. Smith notified of hyperstimulation, fetal status and interventions. She will be here within 20 minutes to see pt.

FIGURE 9-6

Sample Documentation Using EFM: Late Decelerations, FSE and External Monitoring (NICHD terminology)

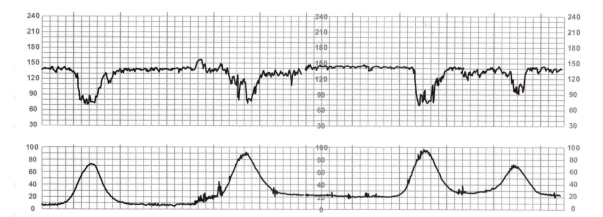

Labor Flow Record				Key

Patient Name_____   Physician/CNM_____

Date/Time 9/24/02	05:30			**Key**
Fetal Assessment				**Monitor Mode**
Monitor Mode	FSE			Ext = External Ultrasound or Toco
Baseline FHR	130-140			FSE = Fetal Spiral Electrode
Baseline Variability	STV +			IUPC = Intrauterine Pressure Catheter
	LTV Ave			**Variability**
FHR Pattern	V			STV = Absent (∅) or Present (+)
FSp0₂				LTV
Uterine Activity				Min = Minimal/Decreased (≤ 5 bpm)
Monitor Mode	IUPC			Ave = Average/WNL (6 to 25 bpm)
Frequency of Contractions	2-4			Mark = Marked/Saltatory (> 25 bpm)
Duration of Contractions	50-60 sec			**FHR Pattern**
Intensity of Contractions	70-90			A = Acceleration
Uterine Resting Tone	8-28			E = Early Deceleration
Oxytocin (mU/min)				L = Late Deceleration
Cervical Status				V = Variable Deceleration
Vaginal Exam by	DTS			P = Prolonged Deceleration
Dilation (cm)	9			**Frequency of Contractions (Minutes)**
Effacement (%)	100			∅ = None
Station	+2			Irreg = Irregular
Assessments/Interventions				**Intensity of Contractions**
Maternal Position	RL			M = Mild
Activity	Bedrest			Mod = Moderate
Oxygen per Face Mask (Amount)				Str = Strong
Pain Assessment	1			By IUPC = mmHg
Nurse Initials	DTS			**Maternal Position**
				LL = Left Lateral
				RL = Right Lateral
				SF = Semi-Fowlers
				Pain Assessment
				0 = None
				3 = Mild
				5 = Tolerable
				7 = Moderate
				10 = Severe

Narrative Notes:
Variable decelerations noted. VE now 9 cms. Turned to R side. Dr Jones notified of fetal status and rapid labor progress. On his way to hospital.

FIGURE 9-7

Sample Documentation Using EFM: Variable Decelerations, FSE and IUPC (AWHONN terminology)

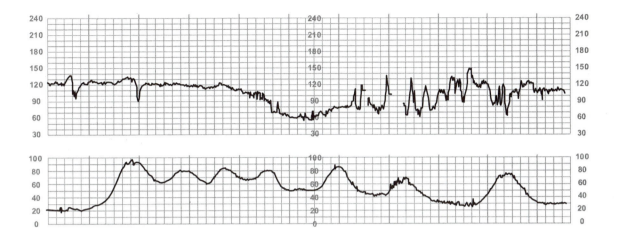

Labor Flow Record				
Patient Name_____	Physician/CNM_____			
Date/Time 5/1/2003	16:40			**Key** **Monitor Mode**
Fetal Assessment				Ext = External Ultrasound or Toco
Monitor Mode	FSE			FSE = Fetal Spiral Electrode
Baseline FHR	120-125			IUPC = Intrauterine Pressure Catheter
Baseline Variability	Min			**Variability**
FHR Pattern	P			Ab = Absent (none)
FSpO₂				Min = Minimal (≤ 5 bpm) Mod = Moderate (6 to 25 bpm)
Uterine Activity				Mark = Marked (> 25 bpm)
Monitor Mode	IUPC			**FHR Pattern** A = Acceleration
Frequency of Contractions	Hyperstim			E = Early Deceleration
Duration of Contractions	70			L = Late Deceleration
Intensity of Contractions	70-90			V = Variable Deceleration P = Prolonged Deceleration
Uterine Resting Tone	20-30			**Frequency of Contractions** **(Minutes)**
Oxytocin (mU/min)	Off			∅ = None
Cervical Status				Irreg = Irregular
Vaginal Exam by	ECS			**Intensity of Contractions**
Dilation (cm)	3-4			M = Mild Mod =Moderate
Effacement (%)	100			Str = Strong
Station	-1			By IUPC = mmHg
Assessments/Interventions				**Maternal Position**
Maternal Position	RL			LL = Left Lateral RL = Right Lateral
Activity	Bedrest			SF = Semi-Fowlers
Oxygen per Face Mask (Amount)				**Pain Assessment**
Pain Assessment	3			0 = None 3 = Mild
Nurse Initials	ECS			5 = Tolerable 7 = Moderate 10 = Severe

Narrative Notes:

Hyperstimulation with prolonged deceleration noted. Oxytocin discontinued. Turned to R side.
IV fluid bolus given. VE 3-4 cm. Dr. Brown notified.

FIGURE 9-8

Sample Documentation Using EFM: Prolonged Decelerations, FSE and IUPC (NICHD terminology)

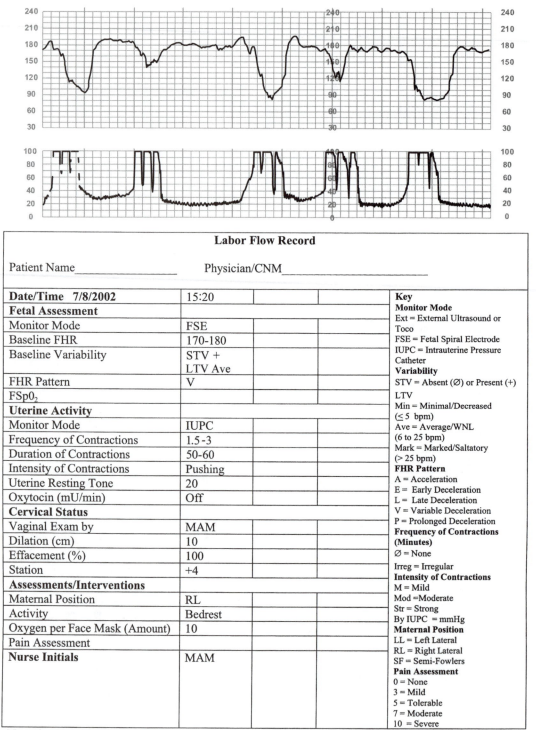

Labor Flow Record

Patient Name_____   Physician/CNM_____

Date/Time 7/8/2002	15:20			Key
Fetal Assessment				**Monitor Mode**
Monitor Mode	FSE			Ext = External Ultrasound or Toco
Baseline FHR	170-180			FSE = Fetal Spiral Electrode
Baseline Variability	STV + LTV Ave			IUPC = Intrauterine Pressure Catheter
FHR Pattern	V			**Variability** STV = Absent (∅) or Present (+)
FSp0₂				LTV
Uterine Activity				Min = Minimal/Decreased (≤ 5 bpm)
Monitor Mode	IUPC			Ave = Average/WNL (6 to 25 bpm)
Frequency of Contractions	1.5-3			Mark = Marked/Saltatory (> 25 bpm)
Duration of Contractions	50-60			**FHR Pattern**
Intensity of Contractions	Pushing			A = Acceleration
Uterine Resting Tone	20			E = Early Deceleration
Oxytocin (mU/min)	Off			L = Late Deceleration
Cervical Status				V = Variable Deceleration
Vaginal Exam by	MAM			P = Prolonged Deceleration **Frequency of Contractions**
Dilation (cm)	10			**(Minutes)**
Effacement (%)	100			∅ = None
Station	+4			Irreg = Irregular **Intensity of Contractions**
Assessments/Interventions				M = Mild
Maternal Position	RL			Mod =Moderate
Activity	Bedrest			Str = Strong By IUPC = mmHg
Oxygen per Face Mask (Amount)	10			**Maternal Position**
Pain Assessment				LL = Left Lateral RL = Right Lateral
Nurse Initials	MAM			SF = Semi-Fowlers **Pain Assessment** 0 = None 3 = Mild 5 = Tolerable 7 = Moderate 10 = Severe

Narrative Notes:

Maternal temp 100.4, Dr. at bedside coaching to push with contractions. On R side. Oxytocin remains off.

FIGURE 9-9

Sample Documentation Using EFM: Second Stage of Labor, Decelerations, FSE and IUPC (AWHONN terminology)

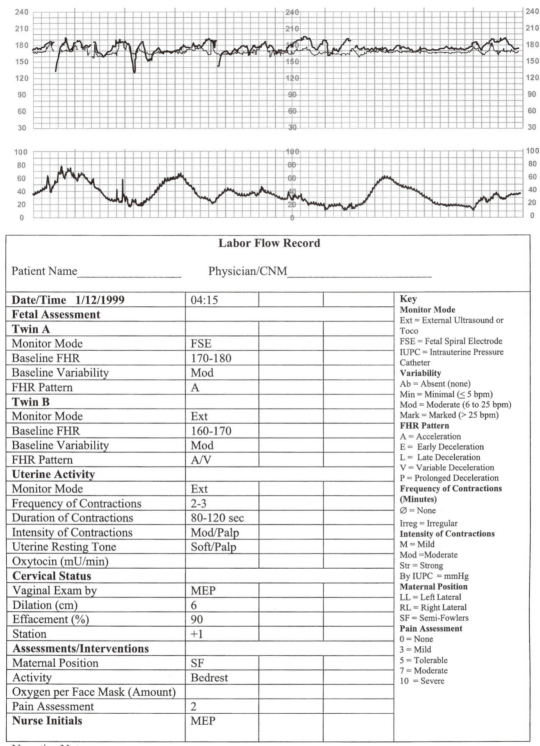

Labor Flow Record

Patient Name_____   Physician/CNM_____

Date/Time 1/12/1999	04:15			Key
Fetal Assessment				**Monitor Mode**
Twin A				Ext = External Ultrasound or Toco
Monitor Mode	FSE			FSE = Fetal Spiral Electrode
Baseline FHR	170-180			IUPC = Intrauterine Pressure Catheter
Baseline Variability	Mod			**Variability**
FHR Pattern	A			Ab = Absent (none)
Twin B				Min = Minimal (≤ 5 bpm)
Monitor Mode	Ext			Mod = Moderate (6 to 25 bpm)
Baseline FHR	160-170			Mark = Marked (> 25 bpm)
Baseline Variability	Mod			**FHR Pattern**
FHR Pattern	A/V			A = Acceleration
Uterine Activity				E = Early Deceleration
Monitor Mode	Ext			L = Late Deceleration
Frequency of Contractions	2-3			V = Variable Deceleration
Duration of Contractions	80-120 sec			P = Prolonged Deceleration
Intensity of Contractions	Mod/Palp			**Frequency of Contractions (Minutes)**
Uterine Resting Tone	Soft/Palp			Ø = None
Oxytocin (mU/min)				Irreg = Irregular
Cervical Status				**Intensity of Contractions**
Vaginal Exam by	MEP			M = Mild
Dilation (cm)	6			Mod =Moderate
Effacement (%)	90			Str = Strong
Station	+1			By IUPC = mmHg
Assessments/Interventions				**Maternal Position**
Maternal Position	SF			LL = Left Lateral
Activity	Bedrest			RL = Right Lateral
Oxygen per Face Mask (Amount)				SF = Semi-Fowlers
Pain Assessment	2			**Pain Assessment**
Nurse Initials	MEP			0 = None
				3 = Mild
				5 = Tolerable
				7 = Moderate
				10 = Severe

Narrative Notes:
FHR reassuring both twins. Comfortable with epidural. Sitting up watching TV. Dr. Jackson here to see patient.

FIGURE 9-10

Sample Documentation Using EFM: Twins (NICHD terminology)

Labor Flow Record

Patient Name_____   Physician/CNM_____

Date/Time 2/28/2003	08:00			Key
Fetal Assessment				**Monitor Mode** Ext = External Ultrasound or Toco
Monitor Mode	Auscultation			
Baseline FHR	140s/Regular			FSE = Fetal Spiral Electrode IUPC = Intrauterine Pressure Catheter
Baseline Variability				
FHR Pattern	A to 160s			**Variability** STV = Absent (∅) or Present (+)
Uterine Activity				LTV
Monitor Mode	Palpation			Min = Minimal/Decreased (≤ 5 bpm)
Frequency of Contractions	3-4			
Duration of Contractions	60-70 sec			Ave = Average/WNL (6 to 25 bpm)
Intensity of Contractions	Mod/Palp			Mark = Marked/ Saltatory (> 25 bpm)
Uterine Resting Tone	Soft/Palp			
Oxytocin (mU/min)				**FHR Pattern** A = Acceleration
Cervical Status				E = Early Deceleration
Vaginal Exam by	SAF			L = Late Deceleration V = Variable Deceleration
Dilation (cm)	3			P = Prolonged Deceleration
Effacement (%)	80			**Frequency of Contractions (Minutes)**
Station	-1			∅ = None
Assessments/Interventions				Irreg = Irregular
Maternal Position	LL			**Intensity of Contractions** M = Mild
Activity	Birthing Ball			Mod =Moderate
Oxygen per Face Mask (Amount)				Str = Strong
Pain Assessment	3			By IUPC = mmHg
Nurse Initials	SAF			**Maternal Position** LL = Left Lateral RL = Right Lateral SF = Semi-Fowlers
				Pain Assessment 0 = None 3 = Mild 5 = Tolerable 7 = Moderate 10 = Severe

Narrative Notes: Contracting q 3-4 minutes X 60 to 70 seconds. Moderate by palpation. Resting tone soft. FHR 140 bpm by intermittent auscultation, regular rhythm. Accelerations up to 160 bpm. Tolerating contractions well with coaching. Using the birthing ball.

FIGURE 9-11

Sample Documentation of Intermittent Auscultation and Palpation (AWHONN terminology)

BOX 9-2

Common Abbreviations Used in Medical Record Documentation During Labor

Abbreviation	Term
AFI	Amniotic fluid index
AFV	Amniotic fluid volume
bpm	Beats per minute
ED	Early deceleration
EFM	Electronic fetal monitoring
FHR	Fetal heart rate
FSE	Fetal spiral electrode
IA	Intermittent auscultation
IUPC	Intrauterine pressure catheter
LD	Late deceleration
LTV	Long-term variability
MVU	Montevideo units
PD	Prolonged deceleration
STV	Short-term variability
TOCO	Tocodynamometer
UC	Uterine contractions
US	Ultrasound
VAS	Vibroacoustic stimulation
VD	Variable deceleration
VE	Vaginal examination

Documentation reflects the systematic assessment of the FHR and uterine activity. Systematic assessment and documentation of the FHR via auscultation includes FHR baseline rate, rhythm, accelerations, and decreases from the baseline rate. Systematic assessment and documentation of the FHR via EFM includes determination of the baseline rate, variability, and presence or absence of accelerations and/or decelerations (see Table 9-1). If decelerations are noted with EFM, further assessment is required to determine the type and duration. Systematic assessments of uterine activity including frequency, duration, intensity, and resting tonus are documented according to the method of uterine activity monitoring being used (see Table 9-2). For example, intensity refers to the strength of the contraction and is described as mild, moderate, or strong by palpation, or millimeters of mercury (mmHg) of intraamniotic pressure with an intrauterine pressure catheter (IUPC). The external tocodynamometer method provides information about frequency and duration; however, resting tone and intensity must be determined by palpation. Contraction frequency, duration, intensity, and uterine resting tone can be evaluated by both palpation and an IUPC.

During the active phase of the first stage of labor, the FHR should be assessed at 30 minute intervals, preferably just after a contraction, and during the second stage of the labor the FHR should be assessed at 15 minute intervals, unless fetal risk status or response to labor indicates the need for more frequent assessment (AAP & ACOG, 2002; AWHONN, 2000). If risk factors are present

BOX 9-3

Suggestions for Maternal-Fetal Assessment and Documentation

ASSESSMENT AND DOCUMENTATION FOR ANY HOSPITAL ADMISSION OF PREGNANT WOMEN

Pregnant women may come to the hospital's labor and birth unit not only for obstetric care, but also for treatment of any sign or symptom of illness. Pregnant women presenting to a hospital for care, taking into consideration gestational age, should be assessed for the following:

- maternal vital signs
- fetal heart rate (FHR), and
- uterine contractions.

The responsible obstetric care provider should be informed promptly if any of the following findings are present: vaginal bleeding, acute abdominal pain, temperature of 100.4°F or higher, preterm labor, preterm premature rupture of membranes, hypertension and a nonreassuring FHR (AAP & ACOG, 2002).

ASSESSMENT AND DOCUMENTATION DURING THE ADMISSION FOR LABOR PROCESS

Any patient who is suspected to be in labor or who has rupture of the membranes or vaginal bleeding should be evaluated promptly in an obstetric service area.

When a pregnant woman is evaluated for labor the following factors should be assessed and recorded in the patient's medical record:

- maternal vital signs,
- frequency and duration of uterine contractions,
- documentation of fetal well-being,
- urinary protein and glucose concentration,
- cervical dilatation and effacement, unless contraindicated (e.g., placenta previa),
- fetal presentation and station of the presenting part,
- status of the membranes,
- date and time of the woman's arrival and notification of the provider, and
- estimation of fetal weight and assessment of maternal pelvis (AAP & ACOG, 2002).

If the patient is in prodromal or early labor and she has no complications, admission to the labor and delivery area may be deferred after initial evaluation and documentation of fetal well-being.

If the woman has had prenatal care and a recent examination has confirmed the normal progress of pregnancy, her admission evaluation may be limited to an interval history and physical examination directed at the presenting complaint. Previously identified risk factors should be recorded in the prenatal record. If no new risk factors are found, attention may be focused on the following historical factors:

- time of onset and frequency of contractions,
- status of the membranes,
- presence or absence of bleeding,
- fetal movement,

BOX 9-3 (cont.)

Suggestions for Maternal-Fetal Assessment and Documentation

- history of allergies, time,
- content and amount of most recent food or fluid ingestion, and
- use of any medication (AAP & ACOG, 2002).

ASSEMENT AND DOCUMENTATION DURING LABOR AND BIRTH

Maternal Vital Signs

Maternal vital signs should be assessed and recorded at regular intervals, at least every 4 hours. This frequency may be increased, particularly as active labor progresses according to clinical signs and symptoms (AAP & ACOG, 2002).

Fetal Heart Rate

The method of FHR monitoring for fetal surveillance during labor may vary, depending on the risk assessment at admission, the preferences of the patient and obstetric staff, and department policy.

If no risk factors are present at the time of the patient's admission, a standard approach to fetal surveillance is to determine and record the auscultated FHR just after a contraction at least every 30 minutes in the active phase of the first stage of labor and at least every 15 minutes in the second stage of labor (AAP & ACOG, 2002; AWHONN, 2000a).

In Canada, the SOGC (2002) recommends that the auscultated FHR be assessed (for 1 minute after a contraction) and recorded every 15 to 30 minutes in active labor and every 5 minutes in the active portion of second stage of labor. During the active phase of labor, EFM records should be reviewed and documented every 15 minutes and at least every 5 minutes in the second stage of labor (SOGC, 2002).

If risk factors are present on admission or appear during labor:

- During the active phase of the first stage of labor, the FHR should be determined and recorded at least every 15 minutes, preferably just after a uterine contraction when intermittent auscultation is used. If continuous electronic monitoring is used, the FHR tracing should be evaluated at least every 15 minutes. During the active phase of labor, EFM records should be reviewed and documented every 15 minutes (SOGC, 2002).

- During the second stage of labor, the FHR should be determined and recorded at least every 5 minutes if auscultation is used. If continuous electronic fetal monitoring is used the fetal heart rate tracing should be evaluated at least every 5 minutes (AAP & ACOG, 2002; AWHONN, 2000a; SOGC, 2002).

The appropriate use of EFM includes recording and interpreting the tracings. Nonreassuring findings should be noted and communicated to the physicians or CNM so that appropriate interventions can occur. When a change in the rate or pattern has been noted, it also is important to document a subsequent return to reassuring findings. Terms that describe the FHR patterns (e.g., early, late, variable or prolonged decelerations, accelerations, and variability) should be used in both medical record documentation and verbal communication among perinatal providers (AAP & ACOG, 2002).

(Box continues)

BOX 9-3 (cont.)

Suggestions for Maternal-Fetal Assessment and Documentation

During oxytocin induction or augmentation, the FHR should be evaluated every 15 minutes during the active phase of the first stage of labor and every 5 minutes during the second stage of labor (AAP & ACOG, 2002).

When EFM is used to record FHR data permanently, periodic documentation can be used to summarize fetal status as outlined by institutional protocols. During oxytocin induction or augmentation, at a minimum, the FHR should be documented before every dosage increase (Simpson, 2002). If the dosage is maintained at the same rate, a reasonable approach is for nurses to document the FHR at least every hour during oxytocin administration (Simpson, 2002).

Misoprostol (prostaglandin E1 [PGE1]) should be administered at or near the labor and birth suite, where the FHR can be monitored continuously (ACOG, 1999).

Cervidil (PGE$_2$) vaginal insert should be administered at or near the labor and birth suite, where the FHR can be monitored continuously while in place and for at least 15 minutes after removal (ACOG, 1999).

Prepidil (PGE$_2$ gel) should be administered at or near the labor and birth suite, where the FHR can be monitored continuously for 30 minutes to 2 hours after administration (ACOG, 1999).

Uterine Activity/Labor Progress

For women who are at no increased risk for complications, evaluation of the quality of uterine contractions and vaginal examinations should be sufficient to detect abnormalities in the progress of labor (AAP & ACOG, 2002). Uterine activity characteristics obtained by palpation should be documented (frequency, duration, intensity, relaxation between contractions) (SOGC, 2002). With EFM, the timing of FHR patterns interpretation should be done in association with uterine contractions. Uterine characteristics should be assessed and documented using palpation, a tocodynamometer, or an intrauterine pressure catheter to assist in assessment (SOGC, 2002).

During oxytocin induction or augmentation, at a minimum, uterine contractions should be assessed before every dosage increase. If the dosage is maintained at the same rate, a reasonable approach is for nurses to document uterine activity at least every hour during oxytocin administration (Simpson, 2002). Patient condition and institutional protocols should be considered in determining the frequency of uterine assessment and documentation.

Misoprostol should be administered at or near the labor and birth suite, where uterine activity can be monitored continuously (ACOG, 1999).

Cervidil should be administered at or near the labor and birth suite, where uterine activity can be monitored continuously while in place and for at least 15 minutes after removal (ACOG, 1999).

Prepidil should be administered at or near the labor and birth suite, where uterine activity can be monitored continuously for at least 30 minutes to 2 hours after placement (ACOG, 1999).

Vaginal examinations should be sufficient to detect abnormalities in the progress of labor (AAP & ACOG, 2002). Vaginal examinations include assessment of dilation and effacement of the cervix and station of the fetal presenting part (Simpson, 2002).

> ## BOX 9-3 (cont.)
>
> ### *Suggestions for Maternal-Fetal Assessment and Documentation*
>
> **During Regional Analgesia/Anesthesia**
>
> Women who receive epidural analgesia should be monitored in a manner similar to that used for any patient in labor. When regional epidural anesthesia/analgesia is administered during labor, maternal vital signs and the FHR should be monitored at regular intervals and documented by a qualified member of the healthcare team (AAP & ACOG, 2002; ASA, 1999).
>
> Before epidural anesthesia/analgesia is initiated, the nurse should assess and document maternal vital signs. The FHR is assessed before and after the procedure, either intermittently or continuously, and as possible during the procedure. Additional monitoring of the patient should be provided during epidural anesthesia/analgesia when the patient's condition warrants. A suggested protocol includes assessing the fetal heart rate after the initiation or re-bolus of a regional block, including patient controlled epidural anesthesia/analgesia. The FHR may be assessed every 5 minutes for the first 15 minutes. More or less frequent monitoring may be indicated based on consideration of factors such as type of anesthesia/analgesia, route and dose of medication used, the maternal-fetal response to medication, maternal-fetal condition, the stage of labor or institutional protocol (AWHONN, 2001).
>
> **Additional Parameters**
>
> - Assess character and amount of amniotic fluid, e.g., clear, bloody, meconium stained, and odor (AAP & ACOG, 2002)
> - Assess character and amount of bloody show/vaginal bleeding (AAP & ACOG, 2002)
> - Assess maternal affect and response to labor (JCAHO, 2003)
> - Assess level of maternal discomfort and effectiveness of pain management/pain relief measures (ACOG, 2002; JCAHO, 2003)
> - Assess labor support person/s' abilities (AWHONN, 2000b)
> - Over the course of labor, documentation may include, but need not be limited to, the presence of physicians or nurses, position changes, cervical status, oxygen and drug administration, blood pressure levels, temperature, amniotomy or spontaneous rupture of membranes, color of amniotic fluid and Valsalva's maneuver (AAP & ACOG, 2002)
>
> *Collaboration between perinatal care providers and review of current published guidelines as outlined above can facilitate development of institutional guidelines for practice.*
>
> *Note:* Adapted from: *Cervical ripening, induction and augmentation of labor:* (Practice Monograph) by K. R. Simpson, (2002), Copyright: Association of Women's Health, Obstetric, and Neonatal Nurses.

TABLE 9-1

Documentation of the FHR for Different Assessment Methods

AUSCULTATION	ULTRASOUND	SPIRAL ELECTRODE
Rate Rhythm	Rate	Rate
	Long-term variability	Long-term variability Short-term variability
	Periodic patterns Nonperiodic patterns	Periodic patterns Nonperiodic patterns
Increases and decreases Abrupt Gradual		

TABLE 9-2

Documentation of Uterine Activity for Different Assessment Methods

PALPATION	TOCODYNAMOMETER	INTRAUTERINE PRESSURE CATHETER
Frequency	Frequency	Frequency
Duration	Duration	Duration
Tone		Tone
Intensity		Intensity

on admission or develop during the course of labor, then the FHR should be assessed every 15 minutes, preferably just after a contraction, during the active phase of the first stage of labor and every 5 minutes during the second stage of labor (AAP & ACOG, 2002; AWHONN, 2000). The SOGC (2002) in Canada recommends assessment every 15 to 30 minutes during the active phase of labor regardless of risk status, and every 5 minutes once pushing is initiated. These assessments can occur via intermittent auscultation of the FHR or via continuous electronic fetal monitoring (AAP & ACOG, 2002; AWHONN, 2000). The use of regional anal-

gesia, oxytocin dosage rate and intervals between increases in oxytocin dosage rate are additional considerations when determining how often to assess and document maternal-fetal well being during labor. The Society of Obstetricians and Gynaecologists of Canada (SOGC, 2002) suggest documentation of the FHR every 30 minutes during the latent phase, every 15 to 30 minutes during the active phase and every 5 minutes during the second stage when using auscultation.

Clinical interventions based on comprehensive assessment of all of the characteristics of the FHR pattern depicted via EFM or the auditory characteristics noted during auscultation and the individual clinical situation of the mother and fetus including, but not limited to, gestational age and medications administered to the mother also are documented. If the clinical situation is such that more accurate data are needed about fetal status, an internal fetal spiral electrode (FSE) may be applied if feasible.

Additional assessments of fetal oxygenation using indirect and direct methods (see Chapter 8) also are documented in the medical record. For example, with scalp stimulation, the fetal response to the stimulation is documented (e.g., presence or absence of an acceleration). When fetal pulse oximetry is being used, fetal oxygen saturation ($FSpO_2$) data are usually recorded as a range of 5% (e.g., $FSpO_2$ = 40 to 45%). "At this time there are no standards or guidelines from ACOG or AWHONN for frequency of assessment and documentation of $FSpO_2$ data during labor. Therefore, existing standards and guidelines for fetal assessment during labor and the evidence about correlation between $FSpO_2$ values and fetal acid-basis status should guide development of unit protocols. Use of $FSpO_2$ monitoring implies a higher risk status for the fetus. Thus, if the $FSpO_2$ is $\geq$ 30%, the ACOG (1995) recommendations for how often to assess fetal status when risk factors for the fetus have been identified appear reasonable" (Simpson & Porter, 2001). If the $FSpO_2$ is < 30%, more frequent assessment are indicated. Based on data to suggest progressive deterioration in fetal oxygen and acid-base status when $FSpO_2$ is < 30% between contractions for more than 10 minutes, assessment and documentation of $FSpO_2$ at least every 5 minutes when $FSpO_2$ data are nonreassuring seems reasonable (Simpson & Porter, 2001).

If there are difficulties in obtaining an interpretable FHR tracing, documentation in the medical record about ongoing efforts to improve the tracing should be noted. A tracing of uterine activity is just as important as the FHR tracing. Identification of characteristics of FHR patterns is dependent on their relationship to uterine activity. In order to be able to make clinically appropriate decisions, both need to be determined as accurately as possible. Attention to obtaining an interpretable EFM tracing is often not noted when a retrospective review occurs as part of the quality monitoring process (Simpson & Knox, 2000) (see Chapter 5 for troubleshooting strategies to improve the FHM data). Prolonged periods of uninterpretable FHR and uterine activity tracing may imply that there was no one attending the mother and fetus. Sometimes a simple maternal position change or adjustment of the monitoring equipment will facilitate obtaining a continuous tracing. Documentation of troubleshooting efforts and results should be included in the medical record. If there is a need for more accurate assessment data, consideration should be given to placing an internal fetal spiral electrode (FSE) and/or intrauterine pressure catheter (IUPC) if clinically appropriate. The discussion between providers about the need for an FSE and/or IUPC, orders received, interventions initiated, data obtained as a result about maternal-fetal status and follow-up communication with the physician/CNM should be documented in the medical record.

EVALUATING THE QUALITY OF MEDICAL RECORD DOCUMENTATION

Periodic continuing education and institutional protocols, policies and procedures provide the foundation for expectations about medical record documentation. One way institutions can create a learning environment to decrease omissions and inaccuracies in medical record documentation is to conduct period chart audits. See Box 9-4 for an example of a medical record audit tool (Simpson, 1998).

Medical record audits provide data about the perinatal nurse's requisite knowledge base and clinical skills during the intrapartum period (Simpson, 1998). A well documented medical record should be comparable with the electronic monitoring tracing and includes appropriate ongoing assessment, intervention, and evaluation. This objective information can be used to verify clinical skills and plan ongoing continuing education to improve these skills and documentation.

BOX 9-4

Suggested Components of a Medical Record Audit

- Are the nurses' notes legible?
- Are the times noted on the admission assessment, the labor progress chart, and the initial EFM tracing consistent with each other within a reasonable time frame?
- Is there documentation of notification of the physician or CNM of admission within the time frame outlined in the policies and procedures?
- Is fetal well-being established before ambulation?
- Does the FHR baseline through EFM match the FHR baseline noted on the Labor Progress Chart?
- Does the FHR baseline variability through EFM match the FHR baseline variability noted on the Labor Progress Chart?
- If there is evidence of decreased FHR variability, is it noted on the Labor Progress Chart?
- If there is evidence of decreased FHR variability, are appropriate nursing interventions charted on the Labor Progress Chart?
- If there are FHR decelerations on the EFM tracing, are they correctly noted on the Labor Progress Chart?
- Are appropriate nursing interventions charted on the Labor Progress Chart during nonreassuring FHR patterns?
- Is there documentation of physician or CNM notification on the Labor Progress Chart during nonreassuring FHR patterns?
- If there are FHR accelerations noted on the Labor Progress Chart are they on the EFM tracing?
- Are maternal assessments noted on the Labor Progress Chart according to facility guideline?
- If there is evidence of a nonreassuring FHR pattern, is oxytocin dosage increased?
- If there is evidence of a nonreassuring FHR pattern, is misoprostol administered?
- If there is evidence of a nonreassuring FHR pattern, is Cervidil placed?
- If there is evidence of a nonreassuring FHR pattern, is oxytocin dosage decreased or discontinued?
- If there is evidence of a nonreassuring FHR pattern, is Cervidil removed?
- If there is evidence of uterine hyperstimulation, are appropriate nursing interventions charted on the Labor Progress Chart?
- If there is evidence of adequate labor, is oxytocin dosage increased?
- If there is evidence of uterine hyperstimulation, is oxytocin dosage increased?
- If there is evidence of uterine hyperstimulation, is misoprostol administered?
- Does the frequency of uterine contractions on the EFM tracing match what is noted on the Labor Progress Chart?
- Is the uterine activity monitor (external tocodynamometer or IUPC) adjusted to maintain an accurate baseline?
- Are oxytocin dosage increases charted when there is an inaccurate uterine baseline tracing or an uninterpretable FHR tracing?
- Are medications given when there is an uninterpretable FHR tracing before administration?
- Does documentation continue during the second stage of labor?
- Are women in the second stage of labor encouraged to push with contractions when the FHR is nonreassuring?
- If the FHR is nonreassuring during the second stage of labor, is oxytocin discontinued?

BOX 9-4 (cont.)

Suggested Components of a Medical Record Audit

- Does the time of birth match the end of the EFM tracing?
- If the woman had regional analgesia or anesthesia, is a qualified anesthesia provider involved in the decision to discharge her from PACU care?
- If the woman had regional analgesia or anesthesia, is the discharge from PACU care scoring evaluation documented?
- Are maternal assessments documented during the immediate postpartum period every 15 minutes for the first hour?
- Are newborn assessments documented during the transition to extrauterine life at least every 30 minutes until the newborn's condition has been stable for 2 hours?

Note: Adapted from "Using Guidelines and Standards from Professional Organizations as a Framework for Competence Validation" by K. R. Simpson, 1998, in K. R. Simpson and P. A. Creehan (Eds.), *AWHONN's Competence Validation for Perinatal Care Providers: Orientation, Continuing Education and Evaluation.* Philadelphia: Lippincott-Raven. Copyright: AWHONN.

☞ RISK MANAGEMENT AND COMMUNICATION OF FETAL HEART MONITORING INFORMATION

Along with emergency departments and perioperative services, perinatal units account for most of the claims of patient injuries and death (Knox et al., 1999). Many of these patient injuries related to human error are preventable. Fetal and neonatal injuries are more common than maternal injuries. Five common recurring clinical situations account for the majority of fetal and neonatal injuries (Knox et al., 1999):

◆ Inability to recognize and/or appropriately respond to both antepartum and intrapartum fetal compromise

◆ Inability to effect a timely cesarean birth (30 minutes from decision to incision) when indicated by fetal or maternal condition

◆ Inability to appropriately resuscitate a depressed baby

◆ Inappropriate use of oxytocin or misoprostol leading to uterine hyperstimulation, uterine rupture, and fetal distress and/or death

◆ Inappropriate use of forceps/vacuum/fundal pressure leading to fetal trauma and/or preventable shoulder dystocia

It is important to note that these same five clinical situations have been the source of the majority of legal claims related to fetal/neonatal injuries for more then 20 years when these data first began to be collected (Knox et al., 1999). Communication inadequacies and omissions can be associated with these recurring clinical situations. Failure to resolve a clinical conflict in a timely manner may contribute to patient injuries.

When cerebral palsy or other brain injury is diagnosed and the medical record indicates that there have been periods of a nonreassuring FHR pattern during labor without evidence of identification and timely intervention, there is a risk of liability exposure to the healthcare providers and the institution despite the fact that not all adverse or unexpected outcomes are preventable (Simpson & Knox, 2001). Under these circumstances, an argument can be made that the FHR was nonreassuring and that the lack of timely intervention is directly associated with the condition of the infant. In some cases experts who testify in medical malpractice cases for the defense and for the plaintiff offer differing opinions. Sometimes these opinions can appear to be completely dichotomous. The differences in opinion may include description and characterization and interpretation of the FHR patterns displayed, clinical implications, need for intervention and probable impact on the present condition of the plaintiff. It is sometime challenging for lay juries to sort out the technical language and determine which expert's opinion is closer to solid scientific principles and professional standards. Under these circumstances it may be difficult, if not impossible, for a jury to come to a reasonable decision about whether the healthcare providers involved met professional standards.

There are two key components to a successful risk management program: avoiding preventable adverse outcomes; and decreasing risk of liability exposure (Simpson & Knox, 2000). Although somewhat similar, these are two distinct concepts. Avoiding preventable adverse outcomes to the fetus during labor requires competent care providers who use consistent fetal heart rate monitoring language and who are in a practice environment with systems in place that permit timely clinical intervention. Decreasing risk of liability exposure includes methods to demonstrate evidence that appropriate timely care was provided and that accurately reflects maternal-fetal status before, during, and after interventions occurred. Risk management strategies that meet both components of a successful program are included in Box 9-5.

⬛ CONFLICT RESOLUTION

There are many challenges to achieving teamwork in the perinatal setting. Interpretation of maternal-fetal data and subsequent communication about that data between professional colleagues can sometimes result in conflict. It is helpful to acknowledge that no group of individuals can work together in an organization and always have the same expectations, goals, and identical perspectives. Conflict is an inevitable result when situations do not meet with individual expectations. While individual expectations may differ, usually there exists among caregivers a basic commitment to quality and to the best possible outcomes for mothers and babies. Mutual trust and respect and the capacity to engage in agreeable disagreement are the hallmarks of a professional unit. When involved in a clinical or administrative situation that can potentially cause conflict, consider that both parties probably have the best interests of the patient in mind, although there may be very different approaches proposed to achieve that goal (Simpson & Chez, 2001). At times, clinical practice issues arise when the "way we've always done it" conflicts with a new or an alternate approach.

Classic principles of conflict resolution (Mayer, 2000) can be used to successfully resolve the inevitable differences of opinion that occur in everyday clinical practice. If the conflict is not related to an emergent patient situation (e.g., there is at least some time for discussion), effective communication techniques can facilitate conflict resolution to the satisfaction of both parties, or at least to reach a workable compromise (Simpson & Chez, 2001). Taking time to really listen and understand the intent of the other person is a helpful starting point. While the other person is expressing himself or herself, give visual and verbal feedback to ensure that their concern is important and being taken seriously. For example, nodding of the head, or saying "I see, please go on . . ." or summarizing what it is the other person is concerned about by indicating "let me see if I am understanding you correctly . . ." Phrases such as, "I have a different perspective" usually work better in conflict resolution than, "You are wrong." Other successful strategies include a calm, collected attitude and careful consideration of the goal to be accomplished.

Communication in conflict resolution may not always be rational. This is especially true when dealing with difficult people, particularly those who exhibit hostile or aggressive behavior that is abusive, abrupt, intimidating or overwhelming (Mayer, 2000). Being confronted by this behavior often catches the other person by surprise and can generate feelings of helplessness. Under these circumstances, it is important to stand up for your-

---

BOX 9-5

Key Components of Risk Management Related to Fetal Heart Monitoring

1. Common EFM language in all professional communication and medical record documentation

2. Joint nurse, CNM, and physician education about FHM

3. Competent care providers

4. Collaboration and mutual respect between care providers

5. Clear definition for fetal well-being and assessment of fetal well-being on admission

6. Ongoing assessment and determination of fetal well-being during labor

7. Appropriate use of intrauterine resuscitation techniques

8. Accurate monitoring of the FHR and uterine activity through EFM or IA

9. Accurate interpretation of EFM and IA data

10. Organizational resources and systems to support clinically timely interventions when the FHR is nonreassuring

11. Continuation of FHM until birth

12. Neonatal resuscitation team in attendance at birth if there is any question of fetal compromise

13. Interdisciplinary case reviews for adverse outcomes

Note: Adapted from "Risk Management and EFM: Decreasing Risk of Adverse Outcomes and Liability Exposure," by K. R. Simpson and G. E. Knox, 2000 *Journal of Perinatal and Neonatal Nursing, 14*(3), 40–52. Copyright Lippincott, Williams & Wilkens.

---

self and command respect. Try to be calm, and then diffuse the situation in an assertive manner. For example, saying . . . "I am willing to discuss this with you when you are ready to speak to me with respect" may help stop the behavior and allow time for more respectful and rational discussion (Henrikson, 1999).

Selecting the best time and place for interaction is also essential (Mayer, 2000). Ideally, the setting should be private and away from patients, family members, or other colleagues. The focus of the discussion should remain on the issue, preferably on the potential impact on patient care. If the conversation deteriorates beyond personal capacity to handle it or the colleague becomes verbally abusive, ending the discussion until a later time

and informing a third party who has the ability to help or the responsibility to know about the interaction is helpful (Simpson & Chez, 2001). An important strategy for promoting positive long-term professional collaboration is the development of interdisciplinary specialty practice opportunities where colleagues can come together to work toward a common goal (Simpson & Knox, 1999). This can include the development of unit guidelines, joint learning from a case review or grand rounds, examining quality or research findings, designing unit projects, or discussion of conflict resolution. When colleagues come together to identify problems, define objectives, address alternatives, integrate changes, remain patient focused, disagree agreeably, negotiate, demonstrate mutual respect, recognize and praise positive attributes and actions, it can facilitate a professional culture for positive conflict resolution and promote mutual respect.

☞ CHAIN OF COMMAND

Some issues of conflict in the clinical setting cannot be resolved between the caregivers immediately involved and yet need to be resolved quickly. The nurse must initiate an appropriate course of action when, after careful deliberation, the issue is determined to be a matter of maternal/fetal well being or there is potential for the clinical situation to deteriorate rapidly, e.g., when a primary health care provider does not respond to a nonreassuring FHR pattern or deteriorating maternal condition. Decisive, timely nursing intervention may be necessary to avoid a potentially adverse outcome. Clinical knowledge and the use of the chain of command are ways to attempt to resolve differences of opinion in clinical practice settings. An example of chain of command is presented in Figure 9-2. Steps or levels in the chain of command are determined by the positions and availability of personnel in each individual institution. Generally, larger institutions and academic medical centers have more steps in the chain of command than community and rural hospitals. If discussions with the physician or CNM do not result in appropriate care for the clinical situation, the nurse has the responsibility to use the perinatal unit institutional chain of command to ensure appropriate and timely intervention (Simpson & Chez, 2001). At the first level, the staff nurse notifies the appropriately available immediate supervisory nurse as outlined in their institution's chain of command (e.g., charge nurse, nurse manager or nursing supervisor) to provide assistance and to review the conflict situation and possible actions and then documents in the medical record or variance report that this action has been taken as outlined in the institutional policies and protocols. In selected instances, it may be necessary to go further up the chain of command if the situation cannot be resolved. It is important to realize that this process may require more time than the situation can accommodate. Thus, invoking the complete use of the chain of command is generally more successful when there is an urgent situation (e.g., progressively nonreassuring FHR tracing) rather than an overt emergency (i.e., shoulder dystocia).

Institutions should support nurses who use the chain of command. Nurses may be reluctant to initiate this process because of intimidation, a perceived sense of personal or professional jeopardy, fear of retribution and/or lack of confidence in the institutional lines of authority and responsibility. Nurses and physicians need to know the institution's policy for chain of command. Data about the use of the chain of command can be collected and analyzed so that the process can be optimized and personnel can receive positive feedback for its appropriate use (Simpson & Chez, 2001). Chain of command should not be used as a routine method of conflict resolution. Clinical disagreements that result in initiation of the chain of command can be detrimental to nurse-physician relationships. Soon after a clinical disagreement that resulted in the use of the chain of command, all those involved should meet and calmly discuss what happened and why. Having an objective third party such as the risk manager present during this discussion may facilitate the interaction. Prospective plans should then be developed to avoid this situation in the future. A positive corporate culture supports use of the chain of command when necessary. When personnel are given the resources, support and guidance that are necessary to carry out the responsibilities of their positions, everyone generally benefits: the institution, their employees, the medical staff and the patients (Simpson & Chez, 2001).

☞ SUMMARY

Communication about fetal status is a critical aspect of perinatal nursing care. Verbal and written communication should be accurate, timely and concise. Common communication avenues include nurse to primary care provider, nurse to nurse, and nurse to patient and her family members/support person(s). A collaborative attitude and mutual respect are the foundations a healthy personal interaction. Over time, with patience and a joint commitment to the best possible outcomes for mothers and babies, respectful nonhierarchical communication styles among professional colleagues will be promoted and enhanced.

As a team, the perinatal care providers should select a common language to describe FHR patterns and common strategies for intervening based on those patterns. Patient safety related to FHM assessment is dependent on competent care providers, adequate and accurate monitoring of maternal-fetal status, and implementation of appropriate clinical interventions. Nurses, CNMs and physicians benefit from learning about FHM in joint continuing education classes. These joint continuing education classes enhance consistent communication of FHM data among these professionals and provide opportunites to discuss clinical controversies, and propose potential resolutions. Consistent and timely medical record documentation is important to effective communication and successful risk management. A single source of data entry at the point of care generally works best rather than charting events on multiple forms. One way to validate requisite knowledge and clinical skills is by medical record audits. Electronic information systems are becoming more common. These systems have benefits and limitations; more evidence is needed about how exclusive use of those systems affect healthcare provider interpretation of maternal-fetal status and the ability to store and retrieve medical data for future use.

Effective communication involves resolution of conflict that is often part of work among professionals with differing views and perspectives. Chain of command policies are helpful when conflict resolution efforts are not successful. The purpose of this chapter was to provide an overview of key issues related to communication of fetal heart monitoring information.

🖳 REFERENCES

American Academy of Pediatrics (AAP) & American College of Obstetricians and Gynecologists (ACOG). (2002). *Guidelines for perinatal care* (5th ed.). Elk Grove Village, IL: Authors.

American College of Obstetricians and Gynecologists (ACOG). (1995). *Fetal heart rate patterns: Monitoring, interpretation, and management* (Technical Bulletin No. 207). Washington, D.C.: Author.

ACOG. (1998). *Inappropriate use of the terms fetal distress and birth asphyxia* (Committee Opinion No. 197). Washington, D.C.: Author.

ACOG. (1999). *Induction of labor* (Practice Bulletin No. 10). Washington, D.C.: Author.

ACOG. (2002). *Analgesia and cesarean delivery rates* (Committee Opinion No. 269). Washington, D.C.: Author.

American College of Obstetricians and Gynecologist (ACOG) & Nurses' Association of the American College of Obstetricians and Gynecologists (NAACOG). (1986). *Joint ACOG/NAACOG statement on electronic fetal monitoring.* Washington, D.C.: Authors.

American Society of Anesthesiologists (ASA). (1999). Practice guidelines for obstetrical anesthesia: *A report by the American Society of Anesthesiologists.* Park Ridge, IL: Author.

Association of Women's Health, Obstetric and Neonatal Nurses (AWHONN). (2000a). *Fetal assessment* (Clinical Position Statement). Washington, D.C.: Author.

AWHONN. (2000b). *Professional nursing support of laboring women* (Clinical Position Statement). Washington, D.C.: Author.

AWHONN. (2001). *Nursing care of the woman receiving regional analgesia/anesthesia in labor* (Evidence-Based Clinical Practice Guideline). Washington, D.C.: Author.

Baggs, J. G., Ryan, S. A., & Phelps, C. E. (1992). The association between interdisciplinary collaboration and patient outcomes in a medical intensive care unit. *Heart and Lung, 21*(1), 18–24.

Baggs, J. G., Schmitt, M., Mushlin, A., Mitchell, P., Eldredge, D., & Hutson, A. (1999). Association between nurse-physician collaboration and patient outcomes in three intensive care units. *Critical Care Medicine, 27*(9), 1991–1998.

Benner, P., Sheets, V., Uris, P., Malloch, K., Sechwed, K., & Jamison, D. (2002). Individual practice and system causes of errors in nursing: A taxonomy. *Journal of Nursing Administration, 32*(10), 509–523.

Berry, M. C. (1999). Changes in the nursing environment create new liability exposures. *MMI Advisory, 15*(3), 1–4.

Chez, B. F. (1997). Electronic fetal monitoring: Then and now. *Journal of Perinatal and Neonatal Nursing, 10*(4), 1–4.

Feinstein, N., Sprague, A., & Trepanier, M. J. (2000). *Fetal heart rate auscultation.* Washington, D.C.: AWHONN.

Henrikson, M. (1999). Dealing with difficult people. *AWHONN Lifelines, 3*(3), 51–52.

Joint Commission on Accreditation of Healthcare Organizations (JCAHO). (2003). *Comprehensive accreditation manual for hospitals.* Chicago: Author.

Keenan, G. M., Cooke, R., & Hillis, S. L. (1998). Norms and nurse management of conflicts: Keys to understanding nurse-physician collaboration. *Research in Nursing and Health, 21*(1), 59–72.

Kendrick, J. M., & Simpson, K. R. (2001). Labor and birth. In K. R. Simpson & P. A. Creehan (Eds.), *AWHONN's perinatal nursing* (2nd ed., pp. 298–377). Philadelphia: Lippincott.

King, T. L., & Simpson, K. R. (2001). Fetal assessment during labor. In K. R. Simpson & P. A. Creehan (Eds.), *AWHONN's perinatal nursing* (2nd ed., pp. 378–416). Philadelphia: Lippincott.

Knaus, W. A., Draper, E. A., & Wagner, D. P. (1986). An evaluation of outcome from intensive care units in major medical centers. *Annals of Internal Medicine, 104*(3), 410–418.

Knox, G. E., Simpson, K. R., & Garite, T. J. (1999). High reliability perinatal units: An approach to the prevention of patient injury and medical malpractice claims. *Journal of Healthcare Risk Management, 19*(2), 24–32.

Kozak, L. J., Hall, M. J., & Owings, M. F. (2002). National hospital discharge survey 2002: Annual summary with detailed diagnosis and procedure data. *National Center for Health Statistics, 13*(153), 1–203.

Martin, J. A., Hamilton, B. E., Ventura, S. J., Menacker, F., & Park, M. A. (2002). Births: Final data for 2000. *National Vital Statistics Report, 50*(5), 1–104.

Mayer, B. S. (2000). *The dynamics of conflict resolution: A practitioner's guide.* San Francisco: Jossey-Bass.

National Institute of Child Health and Human Development (NICHD) Research Planning Workshop. (1997). Electronic fetal heart rate monitoring: Research guidelines for interpretation. *American Journal of Obstetrics and Gynecology, 177*(6), 1385–1390, and *Journal of Obstetric Gynecology and Neonatal Nursing, 26*(6), 635–640.

Peter, E. (2000). Ethical conflicts or political problems in intrapartum nursing care. *Birth: Issues in Perinatal Care, 27*(1), 46–48.

Risser, D. T., Rice, M. M., Salisbury, M. L., Simon, R., Jay, G. D., & Berns, S. D. (1999). The potential for improved teamwork to reduce medical errors in the emergency department: The MedTeams research consortium. *Annals of Emergency Medicine, 34*(3), 370–372.

Rommal, C. (1996). Risk management issues in the perinatal setting. *Journal of Perinatal and Neonatal Nursing, 10*(3), 1–31.

Sherwood, G., Thomas, E., Bennett, D. S., & Lewis, P. (2002). A teamwork model to promote safety in critical care. *Critical Care Nursing Clinics of North America, 14*(4), 333–340.

Simpson, K. R. (1991). *Attitudes of laboring women towards continuous electronic fetal monitoring.* Unpublished masters thesis, University of Missouri—St. Louis, School of Nursing.

Simpson, K. R. (1997). Electronic fetal heart rate monitoring: A primer for critical care nurses. AACN Clinical Issues, *Advanced Practice in Acute and Critical Care, 8*(4), 516–523.

Simpson, K. R. (1998). Using guidelines and standards from professional organizations as a framework for

competence validation. In K. R. Simpson & P. A. Creehan (Eds.), *AWHONN's competence validation for perinatal care providers: Orientation, continuing education and evaluation* (pp. 2–11). Philadelphia: Lippincott.

Simpson, K. R. (2001). EFM Competence validation: The pros and cons of traditional approaches. In C. A. Menihan & E. K. Zottoli (Eds.), *Electronic fetal monitoring: Concepts and applications* (pp. 239–250). Philadelphia: Lippincott.

Simpson, K. R. (2002). *Cervical ripening, induction and augmentation of labor* (Practice Monograph). Washington, D.C.: AWOHNN.

Simpson, K. R., & Chez, B. F. (2001). Professional and legal issues. In K. R. Simpson & P. A. Creehan (Eds.), *AWHONN's perinatal nursing* (2nd ed., pp. 21–52). Philadelphia: Lippincott.

Simpson, K. R., & Knox, G. E. (1999). Strategies for developing an evidence-based approach to perinatal care. *MCN: The American Journal of Maternal Child Nursing, 24*(3), 122–132.

Simpson, K. R., & Knox, G. E. (2000). Risk management and EFM: Decreasing risk of adverse outcomes and liability exposure. *Journal of Perinatal and Neonatal Nursing, 14*(3), 40–52.

Simpson, K. R., & Knox, G. E. (2001). Perinatal teamwork: Turning rhetoric into reality. In K. R. Simpson & P. A. Creehan (Eds.), *AWHONN's perinatal nursing* (2nd ed., pp. 53–67). Philadelphia: Lippincott .

Simpson, K. R., & Porter, M. L. (2001). Fetal oxygen saturation monitoring: Using this new technology for assessment during labor. *AWHONN Lifelines, 5*(2), 28–33.

Sleutel, M. R. (2000). Intrapartum nursing care: A case study of supportive interventions and ethical conflicts. *Birth: Issues in Perinatal Care, 27*(1), 38–45.

Society of Obstetricians and Gynaecologists of Canada (SOGC). (1995). Fetal health surveillance in labour. (Policy Statement). *Journal of the Society of Obstetricians and Gynaecologists of Canada, 17*(9), 865–901.

Society of Obstetricians, and Gynaecologists of Canada. (2002). Fetal health surveillance in labour (SOGC Clinical Practice Guidelines No. 112). *Journal of Obstetrics and Gynaecology in Canada, 112*(April), 1–7.

Stein, L. I. (1967). The doctor-nurse game. *Archives in General Psychiatry, 16*(6), 699–703.

Stein, L. I., Watts, D. T., & Howell, T. (1990). The doctor-nurse game revisited. *New England Journal of Medicine, 322*(8), 546–549.

Willis, E., & Parish, K. (1997). Managing the doctor-nurse game: A nursing and social science analysis. *Contemporary Nurse, 6*(3), 136–144.

CHAPTER 10

FHMPP Skill Stations

Faith Wight Moffatt

OVERVIEW

This chapter focuses specifically on the FHMPP Workshop skill stations. It is essential reading for all FHMPP Workshop participants but also may be a useful guide or refresher for others. FHMPP Workshop participants must complete the following skill stations:

◆ Leopold's maneuvers

◆ Auscultation of the fetal heart

◆ Fetal spiral electrode (FSE) and intrauterine pressure catheter (IUPC) placement

◆ Integration of fetal heart monitoring knowledge and practice

◆ Communication of fetal heart monitoring data

For each skill station, the objectives, principles, steps in skill performance, and requirements to pass successfully are identified. The reader is encouraged to refer back to relevant chapters of this text for more detail as needed.

FHMPP Workshop participants view videotapes, listen to audio tapes and use anatomical models to achieve learning objectives for each skill station. Each skill station of the FHMPP Workshop includes a practice session, which has elements similar to those that workshop participants will be required to address in the evaluation portion of the skill station. Your instructor will notify you about the amount of time allotted for completion of practice and evaluation portions for each skill station. It is important that you pay attention to the time allotted for each portion and complete your work in that time. To successfully complete the FHMPP Workshop, the participant must pass each skill station.

Workshop participants can prepare for the sessions by reading this chapter and familiarizing themselves with the objectives for the skill stations. If auscultation is not a regular part of your current clinical practice, you are encouraged to practice counting fetal heart rates (FHRs) using a watch and listening with a fetoscope, Doppler device or electronic fetal monitor (EFM) before the workshop. This may help you feel more comfortable counting the FHR in the auscultation skill station. Don't forget to bring a watch with a second hand for both the didactic workshop session and the auscultation skill station.

LEOPOLD'S MANEUVERS

This skill station focuses on performing Leopold's maneuvers to determine fetal lie, presentation and position and the site for FHR auscultation. Patient education about the procedure and comfort measures also are included.

Objectives

In this skill station, the participant will be asked to do the following:

1. Explain the purpose of Leopold's maneuvers
2. Describe patient comfort measures before the procedure
3. Perform the four steps of Leopold's maneuvers
4. Identify the optimal site for FHR auscultation on the basis of Leopold's maneuvers

Principles of Leopold's Maneuvers

1. Evaluation of uterine tone, irritability, tenderness, consistency and presence or absence of contractions can be obtained by palpation.
2. Estimated fetal weight and fetal movement can be assessed during an abdominal examination.
3. Fetal lie (longitudinal, transverse, oblique), presentation (cephalic, breech, shoulder) and position (anterior, posterior, transverse, right, left) may be evaluated with Leopold's maneuvers and confirmed by a vaginal examination.
4. Correct placement of the instrument used for auscultating FHR can be determined by completing Leopold's maneuvers.
5. Performing Leopold's maneuvers expedites location of FHR.

Steps in Skill Performance

1. Take measures to make the patient comfortable.
   a. Wash hands; warm them.
   b. Encourage the woman to empty her bladder.
   c. Expose the woman's abdomen from symphysis pubis to xiphoid process.
   d. Drape the woman appropriately.
   e. Position the woman with pillow under her head, knees flexed and arms at her sides.
   f. Place a small wedge under the woman's hips.
   g. Explain the purpose (to determine fetal lie, presentation, position and site for FHR auscultation) and steps of the Leopold's maneuvers you will be performing.
   h. Place your hands on the woman's abdomen during your explanation so that if her abdominal muscles become tense with your touch, they will relax by the time you perform the maneuvers.

2. Prepare for performing Leopold's maneuvers.
   a. Inspect the woman's abdomen for bulges (small parts), fetal movement and the long axis of the fetus.
   b. Use flat, palmar surface of hands, with fingers together for a gentle but firm examination.
   c. Stand at woman's right or left side, depending on your dominant side (e.g., if the nurse is right-handed, stand on the patient's right side; if left-handed, stand on the patient's left side).

3. Perform Leopold's maneuvers. (Figure 10-1)
   a. Beginning with the first maneuver, face the woman and place your hands at top and side of the fundus. Be attentive to the size, shape and consistency of what is in the fundus (note where longitudinal axis of the fetus is located).
   b. For the second maneuver, remain standing at the woman's side, facing her, with hands placed on either side at the middle of the abdomen. One hand will push the contents of the abdomen toward the other hand to stabilize the fetus for palpation. The hand that is palpating begins at the middle of the abdomen near the fundus and moves posterior toward the woman's back. Continue this process, progressing downward to the symphysis pubis. Determine which part of the fetus lies on the side of the abdomen. If firm, smooth and consistent, it is likely to be the back. If smaller, protruding and irregular, it is likely to be the small parts. Note the location of the small parts and the back. Reverse the hands and repeat the maneuver.
   c. For the third maneuver, remain facing the woman. With the middle finger and thumb, grasp the part of the fetus situated over the pelvic brim. With firm, gentle pressure, determine whether the head is the presenting part. This maneuver should confirm what you felt during the first two maneuvers. If the presenting part moves, it is not engaged in the pelvis. If the presenting part is fixed and difficult to move, it is likely to be engaged. The third maneuver also is known as Pallach's maneuver/grip.
   d. For the fourth maneuver, turn and face the woman's feet. Place your hands on the

Leopold's Maneuvers

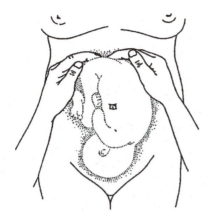

1st Maneuver
Assess part of fetus
in the upper uterus

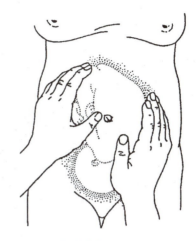

2nd Maneuver
Assess location
of the fetal back

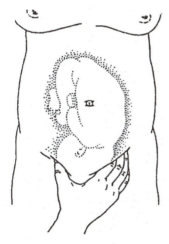

3rd Maneuver
Identify presenting part

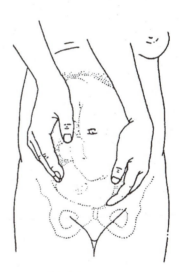

4th Maneuver
Determine the descent
of the presenting part

FIGURE 10-1

The Four Steps in Performing Leopold's Maneuvers
(Adapted from Oxorn, 1986; Simpson & Creehan, 1996)

sides of her uterus, below the umbilicus, pointing toward the symphysis pubis. Press deeply, with fingertips toward the pelvic inlet, and feel for the cephalic prominence. If the cephalic prominence is felt on the same side as the fetus's back, it will be the occiput (crown), and the head will be slightly extended. If the cephalic prominence is felt on the same side as the small parts, it is likely to be the sinciput (forehead), and the fetus will be in a vertex or well-tucked position. If the cephalic prominence is felt equally on each side, the fetus's head may be in a military position, which is common when the fetus is in a posterior position. Finally, move the hands toward the pelvic brim. If the hands come together around the presenting part, the presenting part is floating. If the hands stay apart, the presenting part is either dipping or engaged in the pelvis.

4. Share the information you learned with the woman, and ask if she would like to feel her fetus through palpation, if appropriate.
5. Locate and verify the FHR, which generally can be heard over the curved part of the fetus closest to the anterior wall of the uterus.

6. Document the findings of Leopold's maneuvers, the FHR and rhythm and appropriate nursing interventions.

Criteria for Passing

Participants are required to meet all of the following criteria to pass this skill station:

1. Explain the purpose of Leopold's maneuvers and describe patient comfort measures that should be taken before the procedure.
2. Perform all four steps of the Leopold's maneuvers:
   a. Assess and identify the part of fetus in the upper uterus.
   b. Assess the location of the fetal back.
   c. Identify the presenting part.
   d. Determine the descent of the presenting part.
3. Accurately indicate the optimal area for auscultation based on Leopold's maneuvers.

☞ AUSCULTATION OF THE FETAL HEART

This skill station focuses on auscultation skills to identify the FHR baseline rate, rhythm, increases or decreases from the baseline and nursing responses or interventions appropriate to the auscultated FHR.

Objectives

In this skill station, the participant will be asked to do the following:

1. Choose the appropriate timing of auscultation in relation to uterine contractions.
2. Identify accurate baseline FHR and rhythm.
3. Recognize changes from the baseline as either increases or decreases, as appropriate.
4. Select appropriate nursing responses and interventions to auscultated FHR and rhythm, including when, how and how often you will continue to assess the FHR.

Principles of Auscultation

1. Auscultation is a means of assessment that provides: data for interpretation of rate, rhythm and general increases or decreases in the FHR; and data for appropriate and timely interventions.
2. Use of auscultation requires the ability to integrate underlying physiology, elements of the maternal and fetal histories and physical assessment data with information gathered by auscultation.
3. Auscultation requires the development of auditory skills to establish baseline rates and identify changes in rate and rhythm.
4. Use of auscultation presumes knowledge and understanding of the indications, benefits and limitations of this method of fetal assessment.

Steps in Skill Performance

1. Perform Leopold's maneuver to locate the site for auscultation over the fetal back. (Verbalize only for this skill station).

2. Check maternal pulse and compare to auscultated FHR. (Verbalize only for this skill station.)
3. Palpate contractions to clarify relationship between FHR and uterine contractions. (Verbalize only for this skill station).
4. Count the FHR between uterine contractions for at least 30–60 seconds to identify a baseline rate and rhythm. Canadian guidelines recommend counting for at least 60 seconds.
5. Count the FHR immediately after a contraction and for a minimum of 30 seconds to assess changes in baseline rate. If distinct changes such as increases or decreases in the rate are noted, begin counting again to determine the change from baseline. Canadian guidelines recommend counting for at least 60 seconds. Counting the FHR for multiple, brief intervals may provide a clearer picture of the FHR decrease or increase. For example, count for 6 seconds and multiply by 10 to calculate the beats per minute; repeat this process for consecutive intervals.
6. Indicate appropriate nursing responses and interventions on the basis of your findings. Depending on the FHR and rhythm auscultated, interventions may include the following:
   a. Reposition the woman and then reassess the FHR, if needed.
   b. Increase frequency of auscultation to clarify FHR characteristics (such as whether the FHR is increasing or decreasing from the baseline).
   c. Auscultate with the next uterine contraction to further assess whether changes from the baseline are occurring, if it is not clear.
   d. Consider external EFM (to assess variability, type of deceleration).
   e. Consider other assessment techniques (e.g., fetal acoustic or scalp stimulation) to further clarify FHR characteristics, as indicated.
   f. Continue to promote maternal comfort and fetal oxygenation (e.g., position changes, anxiety reduction measures).
   g. Continue assessment with auscultation.
   h. Use fetoscope to auscultate (if using doppler device or ultrasonography) to validate irregular FHR rhythm.
   i. Notify woman's obstetric care provider of FHR rhythm, if needed.

7. Record the rate, rhythm and general increases or decreases in the FHR and nursing actions taken.

Criteria for Passing

Participants are required to meet all of the following criteria to pass this skill station:

1. Choose the appropriate timing of auscultation in relation to uterine contractions.

2. Accurately assess and document baseline FHR and rhythm for two different audiotaped cases of auscultated fetal heart sounds presented in this skill station.

3. Accurately document two appropriate responses/nursing interventions for the same two FHR cases as in requirement #2 that may include when, how and how often you will continue to assess the FHR.

☞ FSE AND IUPC PLACEMENT

This skill station focuses on the techniques of FSE and IUPC placement and acknowledges the total process from approaching the patient to obtaining accurate data.

Objectives

In this skill station, the participant will be asked to do the following:

1. Describe two relative contraindications and two potential risks to placing FSEs and IUPCs.
2. Demonstrate the correct sequence of steps for placing a FSE.
3. Demonstrate the correct sequence of steps for placing an IUPC and ensuring it functions properly.

Principles of FSE and IUPC Placement

1. Placement of a FSE or IUPC requires the skills and techniques of vaginal examination and EFM, as well as knowledge of indications, risks, limitations and contraindications associated with these devices.
2. Placing a FSE or IUPC is an invasive procedure; the practitioner should have knowledge and understanding of the following aspects of intrapartum care:

   ◆ Maternal and fetal anatomy, as assessed by vaginal examination

   ◆ Intrapartum changes

   ◆ Indications for direct measure of fetal heart rate or uterine contractions

   ◆ Relative contraindications to direct, invasive monitoring, including chorioamnionitis, active maternal genital herpes infection and human immunodeficiency virus (HIV) infection, certain fetal presentations and conditions that preclude vaginal examinations such as placenta previa or undiagnosed vaginal bleeding

   ◆ Potential risks of direct, invasive monitoring, including hemorrhage, abruption, uterine perforation and maternal and fetal infection

3. Electronic fetal cardiac and uterine pressure data provide another assessment perspective on which to base interpretation and appropriate, timely interventions.
4. The electrode usually is attached to the fetal scalp or buttock for direct measurement of the FHR by electrical activity. The spiral attaches approximately 2 mm into the presenting fetal part. The fetal lead detects the FHR electrical activity. The maternal reference electrode detects the maternal heart rate via her vaginal secretions or via placement of an external reference electrode. The external reference, when available, may be helpful when the signal is inadequate.
5. An IUPC offers a direct method of measuring uterine activity during labor; it is the only objective method of measuring uterine intensity or strength. It is measured in millimeters of mercury (mmHg) and is useful at any altitude.

Steps in Skill Performance

FSE Placement

Procedure

1. Explain procedure to the woman before application.
2. Wash hands. (Verbalize only for this skill station.)
3. Open electrode package and put on gloves. (Verbalize sterile technique.)
4. Remove wires from between drive tube and guide tube.
5. Pull electrode 1 in. back into guide tube so it does not extend beyond the end of the guide (see Figure 10-2).
6. Perform a vaginal examination to assess presenting part. Feel for firm bone and avoid the fetus's face, sutures, fontanels and genitalia (see Figures 10-3, 10-4a, 10-4b); maintain fingers on target areas.

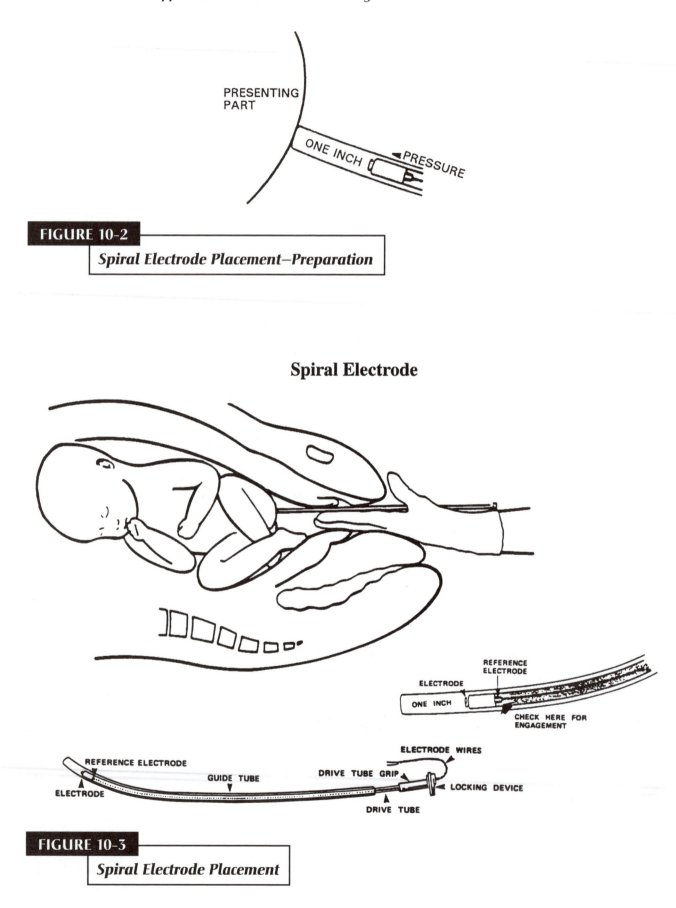

FIGURE 10-2

Spiral Electrode Placement—Preparation

Spiral Electrode

FIGURE 10-3

Spiral Electrode Placement

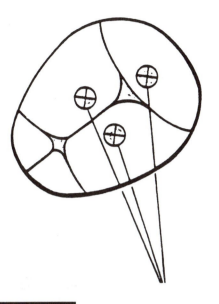

FIGURE 10-4a

Spiral Electrode Placement–Cephalic

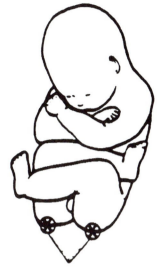

FIGURE 10-4b

Spiral Electrode Placement–Breech

7. Place the guide tube between two examining fingers and firmly place against the fetal presenting part at a right angle.
8. Advance the drive tube until it touches the presenting part.
9. Maintain pressure against the presenting part and turn clockwise (about 1½ times) until resistance is met.
10. Release the lock device and remove the guide tube.
11. Check placement of the electrode before withdrawing examining fingers.
12. Plug the cable into the monitor. (Verbalize only for this skill station.)
13. Document placement of the FSE. (Verbalize only for this skill station.)
14. Remove the FSE. To detach the electrode, rotate the electrode counterclockwise until it is free from the fetal presenting part. Do not pull the electrode from the fetal skin. Document that the electrode was removed intact.

IUPC Placement

Procedure

1. Prepare the IUPC according to the type of device and manufacturer's instructions.
2. Wash hands.

3. Set up the IUPC and put on gloves. (Verbalize sterile technique.)
   a. Assemble equipment and attach IUPC to adaptor cable. (Verbalize only for this skill station.)
   b. Calibrate to zero to assess normal atmospheric pressure, if using sensor tipped IUPC. Consult IUPC manufacturer's guidelines. (Verbalize only for this skill station.)
   c. Flush IUPC with syringe and calibrate to zero to assess normal atmospheric pressure, if fluid-filled. (Verbalize only for this skill station.)
4. Determine cervical site for catheter insertion and gently displace presenting part, if needed.
5. Insert guide (containing IUPC) between examining fingers.
6. Ensure catheter guide does not extend beyond fingers.
7. Insert IUPC through guide tube until catheter is between 30 cm and 45 cm markers identified on the catheter. Do not insert the IUPC into the uterus beyond the 45 cm mark. Do not force the IUPC. If resistance is met, stop advancing the IUPC, reposition fingers and IUPC, and continue insertion. If resistance is still met, discontinue insertion (see Figure 10-3).

8. Attach to cable and ensure proper functioning. (Verbalize only for this skill station).
9. Document placement of IUPC. (Verbalize only for this skill station.)

Criteria for Passing

Participants are required to meet both of the following criteria to pass this skill station:

1. Describe two relative contraindications and two potential risks to placement of FSEs and IUPCs.
2. Demonstrate all the steps, in the correct sequence, for FSE and IUPC placement procedures (as described above).

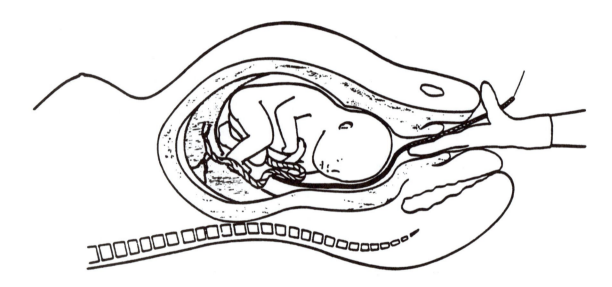

FIGURE 10-5

Intrauterine Pressure Catheter Placement

◼ INTEGRATION OF FETAL HEART MONITORING KNOWLEDGE AND PRACTICE

This skill station focuses on integrating all the information gathered, including history, assessments, physiology, monitoring modes, interpretation, interventions and evaluation. In the practice portion of this skill station, each participant will be given time to review and discuss patient histories and fetal monitor tracings. Verbal responses are appropriate for practice sessions; during testing, written responses to the fetal monitor tracings will be expected.

Objectives

In this skill station, the participant will be asked to do the following:

1. Demonstrate appropriate interpretation of the fetal monitor tracing.
2. Demonstrate knowledge of the physiologic mechanisms for the observed patterns.
3. Demonstrate knowledge of instrumentation factors affecting interpretation of the fetal monitor tracing.
4. Demonstrate an understanding of how physiologic mechanisms and interpretation influence the decision-making process.
5. Describe appropriate interventions or management steps for each case scenario.
6. Demonstrate knowledge of evaluation of fetal response to selected interventions.

Principles for Integrating FHR Monitor Data into Practice

1. A systematic review of the fetal monitor tracing provides the basis for determining appropriate responses or interventions to be initiated.
2. The fetal monitor tracing should be interpreted in light of the maternal and fetal histories and data from physical assessments.
3. The physiology of pregnancy and labor is dynamic. Integration of physiologic-based data must accommodate changes in physiologic states. Each maternal-fetal unit presents along a physiologic continuum. The nursing process forms the basis for the progression from assessment to interpretation, integration, decision-making, interventions and evaluation.

4. Key physiologic goals and supportive actions are as follows:
    a. Maximize uterine blood flow using the following interventions:
       1) Maternal position change
       2) Hydration
       3) Medication
       4) Anxiety/pain reduction
    b. Maximize umbilical circulation using the following interventions:
       1) Maternal position change
       2) Elevation of presenting part
       3) Amnioinfusion
    c. Maximize oxygenation using the following interventions:
       1) Maternal position change
       2) Maternal supplemental oxygen
       3) Maternal breathing techniques
       4) Correction or treatment of underlying disease
    d. Reduce uterine activity using the following interventions:
       1) Maternal position change
       2) Reduction/discontinuation of utertonic drugs
       3) Hydration
       4) Modified pushing
       5) Medication/tocolytics

5. Although there is not always universal agreement on whether specific patterns are reassuring or nonreassuring, there is a clear understanding that actions are indicated on the basis of the interpretation of certain fetal responses (e.g., variable decelerations, variability changes). Remember to respond to the likely physiologic etiology.

6. Additional actions should be considered based on evaluation of interventions and may include further assessments (e.g., scalp stimulation), troubleshooting of equipment, notification of woman's obstetric care providers and documentation.

7. Monitoring methods have improved over the years. However, every mode of fetal monitoring has certain limitations that may affect interpretation.

8. Evaluation includes reassessing maternal and fetal response to determine whether there is a need to continue, alter or discontinue interventions on the basis of observed responses.

Steps in Skill Performance

1. Review pertinent patient history.
2. Interpret the monitor tracing for FHR baseline, variability, periodic and nonperiodic changes.
3. Interpret the uterine activity patterns.
4. Describe possible physiologic mechanisms for patterns (e.g., inadequate oxygen reserves; inadequate uterine, placental or cord blood flow; fetal response to nervous system stimulation or movement; cord compression).

5. Identify instrumentation factors that may affect interpretation of the tracings.
6. Describe intervention and management steps that may be taken on the basis of findings from the history, interpretation of data and physiologic responses.
7. Evaluate fetal response to interventions.

Criterion for Passing

Participants are required to meet the following criterion to pass this skill station:

Complete the written examination for this skill station, correctly answering 80% of the items.

🖅 COMMUNICATION OF FETAL HEART MONITORING DATA

In this skill station, participants demonstrate proficiency in communicating and documenting maternal-fetal assessment information and initiating the chain of command.

Objectives

In this skill station, the participant will be asked to do the following:

1. Critique a videotaped scenario of nurse–primary health care provider communication, identifying important points the nurse in the video omitted.
2. Accurately interpret an EFM tracing and appropriately document the interpretation. Baseline FHR, FHR variability (including short-term variability if appropriate), periodic and nonperiodic FHR patterns and uterine activity must be identified and documented.
3. Document a plan of action or appropriate nursing response that takes into account communication principles, the role and responsibility of the nurse as patient advocate and what to do when a physician's or midwife's order is not consistent with what you believe to be in the best interest of the woman or her fetus or both.

Principles of Communication

1. Communication is the process by which we understand others and endeavor to be understood by them.
2. Communication is dynamic, constantly changing in response to the environment and the many factors within it.
3. The nurse caring for a maternity patient should possess effective communication skills.
4. Whether communication is verbal, nonverbal or recorded, it must be accurate, objective and concise.

Steps in Skill Performance

Communication with the Primary Health Care Provider

1. Clearly state the identity and location (name of hospital) of the nurse initiating the communication; then identify the patient being discussed.
2. Clarify the purpose of the conversation or call (e.g., to report an update of progress, obtain an order, ask questions, state concerns or request a primary health care provider's presence).
3. Provide a clear, concise review of the patient's history and her status. More detail is needed if the primary health care provider is covering for someone else or does not know the patient very well. If the primary health care provider requests actions that go against hospital policy, advise that it is not possible to do so, and offer an alternative when possible. For example, "I cannot give intravenous medication without an access to the vein. May I have an order for a heparin lock or infusion?" or "I cannot rupture membranes, but Dr. Jones is here. Would you like to talk with Dr. Jones?"
4. If the primary health care provider requests an action that seems inappropriate for the situation, state your discomfort and reason. If a conflict remains, tell the primary health care provider you will notify your supervisor first and initiate the chain of command.
5. Telephone orders should be in compliance with hospital protocol. Repeat the order back to the primary health care provider whenever possible. Write legibly and include the date and time. For example, "T.O. 4/15/03/ 8:35 am. Dr. Smith called to request pain medication for Ms. Thomas. Dr. Smith gave TO for 50 mg Demerol and 25 mg Phenergan via slow IVP. Medication order repeated back to Dr. Smith. Dr. Smith verified order."
6. Document the time of the conversation with the primary health care provider and the purpose or outcome in the patient record. For example, "Dr. Smith was notified of the

patient's vaginal examination and EFM pattern." In this case, the patient's record will contain documentation of the EFM pattern and vaginal examination that will coincide with that reported to the physician. The notes contain only action information, not details about the conversation. For example, "Dr. Smith requested to come for delivery." Each hospital should have a protocol for recording the actual conversation when necessary, such as a quality assurance report form or incident report. The nurse should be familiar with these protocols and forms.

Communication with the Woman in Labor and Her Support Person(s)

1. Explain events and procedures to the woman in labor in clear terms (at the level of the patient's understanding), without either extreme detail or brevity.
2. Ask whether the woman and her support person(s) have any questions, concerns, fears or requests.
3. Listen and respond to concerns, fears or requests. Answer questions and refer to the physician, certified nurse-midwife or other appropriate person when necessary.

Communication with Another Nurse

1. Clearly identify the patient(s) being discussed.
2. Convey urgent and stat requests or information directly, clearly and as calmly as possible.
3. Provide complete, clear patient care information and other information, such as the physician's or certified nurse-midwife's location and the support person's presence and demeanor.
4. Convey strategies that were particularly successful or unsuccessful for patient care continuity.

Guidelines for Recording Fetal Heart Monitoring Information

1. When documenting auscultation or palpation information, include the rate and rhythm

heard, as well as the occurrence of decreases or increases.
2. Documentation of EFM data includes the baseline range (unless uninterruptible), variability, accelerations, decelerations and uterine activity according to the capability of the equipment. For example, the FSE will provide data that differs from that of the ultrasound machine.
3. Documentation should reflect the trend of the pattern as opposed to each deceleration or acceleration.
4. Documentation should also describe the events so that they could be reasonably understood if the FHR tracing is mislabeled, lost (either a hard copy or a digital file) or incomplete.
5. Document the components of a pattern, such as the type of deceleration. If there is controversy regarding a deceleration pattern, a description may be helpful. If a description of the pattern is documented, include the shape, the range of the deceleration depth (nadir), duration of the nadir, recovery time from the end of the nadir to the baseline (or other rate) and baseline variability (long- and short-term variability).

Criteria for Passing

Participants are required to meet all of the following criteria to pass this skill station:

1. List four important points the nurse omitted in the videotaped scenario, "Nurse to Physician Reporting."
2. Accurately interpret an EFM tracing and appropriately document that interpretation. Baseline FHR, FHR variability (including short-term variability as appropriate), periodic and nonperiodic FHR patterns and uterine activity must be identified and documented.
3. Document a plan of action and appropriate nursing responses that take into account communication principles, the role and responsibility of the nurse as patient advocate and what to do when a physician's or midwife's order is not consistent with what you believe to be in the best interest of the woman or her fetus or both.

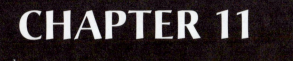

CHAPTER 11

Case Study Exercises

Rebecca L. Cypher

This chapter provides additional case study exercises as an adjunct to content presented in the FHMPP program. Included are a series of adaptations of actual case studies and electronic fetal monitoring (EFM) tracings from a variety of intrapartum clinical settings. This chapter is designed to promote and support critical thinking in the analysis of EFM tracings, in keeping with the framework used throughout the AWHONN FHMPP Workshop. The Systematic Approach to Interpretation Worksheet is provided to facilitate analysis of the case studies and EFM tracings.

For each case study exercise, readers are encouraged to a) review the brief history and data provided, b) analyze the EFM tracing and c) complete the Systematic Approach to Interpretation Worksheet. Answer keys for each exercise are provided at the end of each scenario. Readers should review their work and identify areas of strength and areas requiring more practice or review related to electronic fetal heart rate monitoring interpretation. In the clinical setting and in the FHMPP Workshop skill stations, longer EFM tracings may be available for interpretation and clinical decision-making purposes.

AWHONN Fetal Heart Monitoring Principles and Practices
Systematic Approach to Interpretation Worksheet

Case Study Exercise: _____

1. Contractions: *Frequency:* _____
   Duration: _____
   Intensity: _____
   Resting tone: _____

2. Baseline fetal heart rate: _____

3. Variability: Place a checkmark signifying the appropriate type of variability on the strip (LTV = long-term variability; STV = short-term variability).

LTV	Decreased (0–5 bpm)	_____
	Average (6–25 bpm)	_____
	Marked (> 25 bpm)	_____
	Unable to assess	_____
STV	Present	_____
	Absent	_____
	Unable to assess	_____

4. Accelerations and decelerations. When present, circle P if periodic or NP if nonperiodic.

Accelerations	P	NP
Early decelerations	P	
Variable decelerations	P	NP
Late decelerations	P	
Prolonged decelerations		NP

5. List possible underlying physiologic mechanisms or rationales for observed patterns.

6. List in order of priority the physiologic goal(s) for observed patterns.

7. List interventions to achieve the physiologic goals and actions needed related to instrumentation or further assessment.

Case Study Exercise A: Ruth

Age:	32 years old
Gravida/Para:	1/0
Gestational Age:	$39\frac{1}{7}$ weeks
Medical History:	Unremarkable
Surgical History:	Unremarkable
Psychosocial History:	Unremarkable
Current Obstetric History:	Normal prenatal laboratory results
	2nd trimester ultrasound findings consistent with date of last menstrual period (LMP)

Ruth presented to the labor and delivery unit at 8:00 A.M.; her membranes had spontaneously ruptured earlier that morning. The fluid was clear. Vaginal examination revealed that her cervix was 4 cm dilated and 90% effaced, and the fetus was vertex at −1 station. On admission, her vital signs were as follows: temperature: 97.8°F (36.5°C); blood pressure: 122/76 mmHg; pulse: 86 bpm; respiration: 22 breaths/minute.

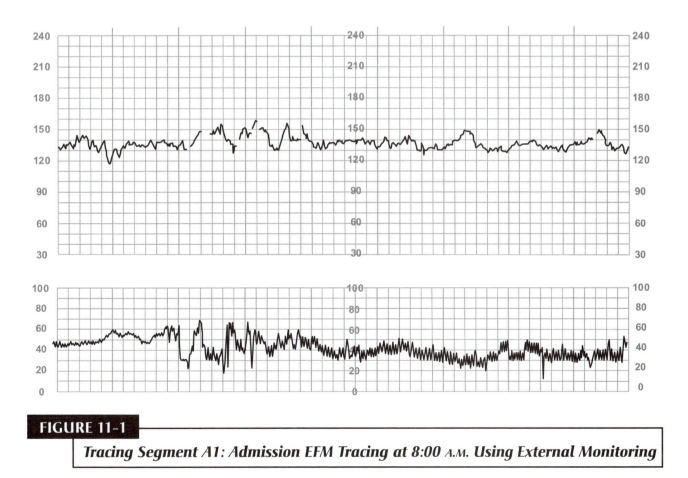

FIGURE 11-1

Tracing Segment A1: Admission EFM Tracing at 8:00 A.M. Using External Monitoring

AWHONN Fetal Heart Monitoring Principles and Practices Systematic Approach to Interpretation Worksheet

Case Study Exercise: Ruth A1

1. Contractions: *Frequency:*   **Irregular**
   Duration: **Unable to assess**
   Intensity: **Need to palpate**
   Resting tone: **Need to palpate**

2. Baseline fetal heart rate: **130–140 bpm**

3. Variability: Place a checkmark signifying the appropriate type of variability on the strip (LTV = long-term variability; STV = short-term variability).

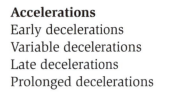

   LTV   Decreased (0–5 bpm)
   Average (6–25 bpm)   ✔
   Marked (> 25 bpm)
   Unable to assess

   STV   Present
   Absent
   Unable to assess   ✔

4. Accelerations and decelerations. When present, circle P if periodic or NP if nonperiodic.

   Accelerations   P   (NP)
   Early decelerations
   Variable decelerations
   Late decelerations
   Prolonged decelerations

5. List possible underlying physiologic mechanisms or rationales for observed patterns.
   a. **Fetal movement or response to environmental stimulus**
   b. **Direct sympathetic stimulation of the fetus**
   c. **Associated with nonacidotic, oxygenated fetus**

6. List in order of priority the physiologic goal(s) for observed patterns.
   a. **Maximize oxygenation**
   b. **Maximize uterine blood flow**
   c. **Maximize umbilical circulation**

7. List interventions to achieve the physiologic goals and actions needed related to instrumentation or further assessment.
   a. **Palpate contractions and adjust tocodynamometer (toco) to monitor contraction pattern more effectively**
   b. **Hydrate**
   c. **Continue to provide maternal comfort measures (e.g., position change, ambulation)**
   d. **Consider placing intrauterine pressure catheter (IUPC) if toco ineffective**
   e. **Continue routine assessments and interventions for labor**

Ruth's labor progressed slowly throughout the morning. Her husband and doula were with her and were very supportive. Ruth used a number of comfort measures including breathing, relaxation techniques and a birthing ball. At 11:30 A.M. she requested an epidural. Vaginal examination after the epidural revealed that her cervix was 5–6 cm dilated and swollen and the vertex at -1 station with + caput and molding.

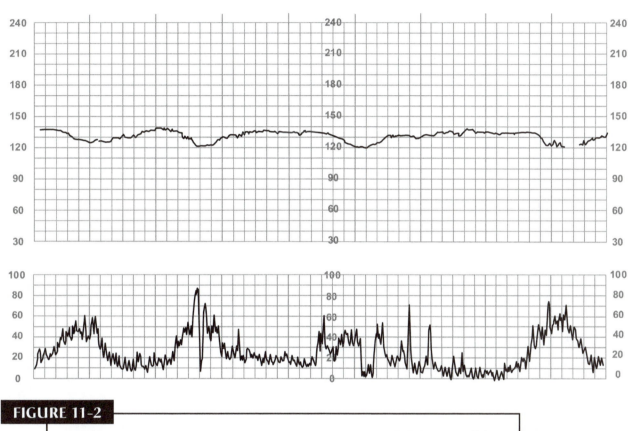

FIGURE 11-2

Tracing Segment A2: Labor and Delivery EFM Tracing at 12:25 P.M.
Using External Monitoring

AWHONN Fetal Heart Monitoring Principles and Practices Systematic Approach to Interpretation Worksheet

Case Study Exercise: Ruth A2

1. Contractions:　　*Frequency:*　**q 1½–3 min.**
　　　　　　　　　　Duration:　**60–70 sec.**
　　　　　　　　　　Intensity:　**Need to palpate**
　　　　　　　　　　Resting tone: **Need to palpate**

2. Baseline fetal heart rate: **130–135 bpm**

3. Variability: Place a checkmark signifying the appropriate type of variability on the strip (LTV = long-term variability; STV = short-term variability).

　　　　　LTV　　**Decreased (0–5 bpm)**　✔
　　　　　　　　　Average (6–25 bpm)
　　　　　　　　　Marked (> 25 bpm)
　　　　　　　　　Unable to assess

　　　　　STV　　Present
　　　　　　　　　Absent
　　　　　　　　　Unable to assess　✔

4. Accelerations and decelerations. When present, circle P if periodic or NP if nonperiodic.

　　　　　　　　Accelerations
　　　　　　　　Early decelerations　　Ⓟ
　　　　　　　　Variable decelerations
　　　　　　　　Late decelerations
　　　　　　　　Prolonged decelerations

5. List possible underlying physiologic mechanisms or rationales for observed patterns.
   a. **Reflex vagal response associated with cephalopelvic disproportion or persistent occiput position**
   b. **Possible loss of fetal reserves related to decreased long-term variability (variability)**

6. List in order of priority the physiologic goal(s) for observed patterns.
   a. **Maximize oxygenation**
   b. **Maximize uterine blood flow**
   c. **Maximize umbilical circulation**

7. List interventions to achieve the physiologic goals and actions needed related to instrumentation or further assessment.
   a. **Assess fetal heart rate response to fetal scalp stimulation**
   b. **Palpate contractions and adjust toco to monitor contraction pattern more effectively**
   c. **Consider placing IUPC**
   d. **Reevaluate management plan due to slow progress of labor**
   e. **Continue to assess decelerations and variability**

Case Study Exercise B: Eleanor

Age:	26 years old
Gravida/Para:	2/0101
Gestational Age:	$37^5/_7$ weeks
Medical History:	Unremarkable
Surgical History:	Appendectomy at age 15
Psychosocial History:	Unremarkable
Past Obstetric History:	Preterm delivery at 34 weeks of gestation due to severe preeclampsia
Current Obstetric History:	Normal prenatal laboratory results
	Rh negative
	Smokes 1 pack of cigarettes per day
	Three ultrasound examinations to evaluate growth: findings indicate appropriate interval growth

Eleanor was admitted to the labor and delivery unit with a complaint of leaking "clear fluid" for 24 hours. She stated her contractions had been more uncomfortable since her water broke but were more than 10 minutes apart. Vaginal examination revealed her cervix was 4 cm dilated and 75% effaced, and the fetus was vertex and at –1 station. On admission, her vital signs were as follows: temperature: 101.2°F (38.4°C); blood pressure: 132/84 mmHg; pulse: 90 bpm; respiration: 22 breaths/minute.

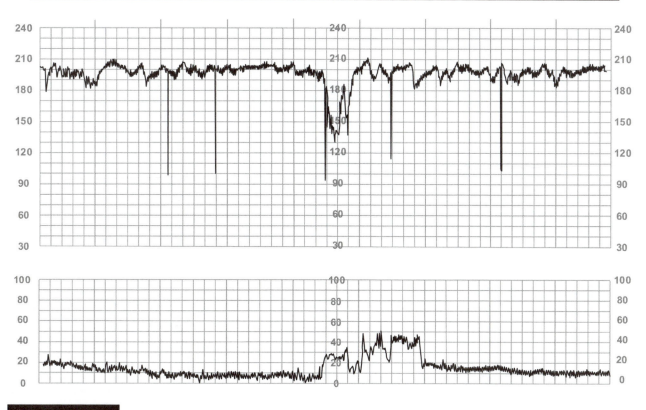

FIGURE 11-3

Tracing Segment B1: EFM Tracing Recorded 1 Hour after Admission Using a Fetal Spiral Electrode and External Toco

AWHONN Fetal Heart Monitoring Principles and Practices Systematic Approach to Interpretation Worksheet

Case Study Exercise: Eleanor B1

1. Contractions: *Frequency:*   **Unable to assess**
                         Duration: **Unable to assess**
                         Intensity: **Need to palpate**
                         Resting tone: **Need to palpate**

2. Baseline fetal heart rate: **190–205 bpm**

3. Variability: Place a checkmark signifying the appropriate type of variability on the strip (LTV = long-term variability; STV = short-term variability).

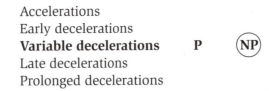

LTV	Decreased (0–5 bpm)	*STV*	**Present** ✔
	Average (6–25 bpm) ✔		Absent
	Marked (>25 bpm)		Unable to assess
	Unable to assess		

4. Accelerations and decelerations. When present, circle P if periodic or NP if nonperiodic.

        Accelerations
        Early decelerations
        Variable decelerations   **P**   **(NP)**
        Late decelerations
        Prolonged decelerations

5. List possible underlying physiologic mechanisms or rationales for observed patterns.
    a. **Maternal fever secondary to possible dehydration, infection or chorioamnionitis**
    b. **Endogenous catecholamine response resulting from anxiety**
    c. **Baroreceptor and parasympathetic responses resulting from umbilical cord compression or decreased amniotic fluid volume after rupture of membranes**
    d. **Compensatory response to hypoxemia**
    e. **Presence of fetal reserves demonstrated by + (present) STV**

6. List in order of priority the physiologic goal(s) for observed patterns.
    a. **Maximize umbilical circulation**
    b. **Maximize oxygenation**
    c. **Maximize uterine blood flow**

7. List interventions to achieve the physiologic goals and actions needed related to instrumentation or further assessment.
    a. **Administer maternal supplemental oxygen via snug face mask**
    b. **Change maternal position to maximize umbilical circulation and uterine blood flow**
    c. **Hydrate with plasma expander or IVF to increase maternal blood volume and maximize uterine blood flow**
    d. **Palpate contractions and adjust toco to assess uterine activity more effectively**
    e. **Notify woman's obstetric health care provider and neonatal team**
    f. **Consider placing IUPC for possible amnioinfusion if variable decelerations persist**
    g. **Consider administering antibiotics**
    h. **Provide support to decrease maternal anxiety and catecholamine response**
    i. **Evaluate fetal heart rate response to intervention**

Case Study Exercise C: Madison

Age:	24 years old
Gravida/Para:	1/0
Gestational Age:	$40\,^5/_7$ weeks
Medical History:	Unremarkable
Surgical History:	Unremarkable
Psychosocial History:	Single mother, father of baby involved and supportive
Current Obstetric History:	Normal prenatal laboratory results
	2nd trimester ultrasound findings consistent with date of LMP
	Blood pressure ranging from 96–120/68–78 mmHg during pregnancy
	5-lb weight gain in past week with proteinuria

Madison presented to the labor and delivery unit at 2:30 P.M. with complaints of contractions increasing in frequency and intensity since 9:00 A.M. Her membranes were intact. Vaginal examination revealed that her cervix was 4 cm dilated and 100% effaced, and the fetus was vertex and at +1 station. On admission, her vital signs were as follows: temperature: 98.2°F (36.7°C); blood pressure: 142/94 mmHg; pulse: 96 bpm; respiration: 20 breaths/minute.

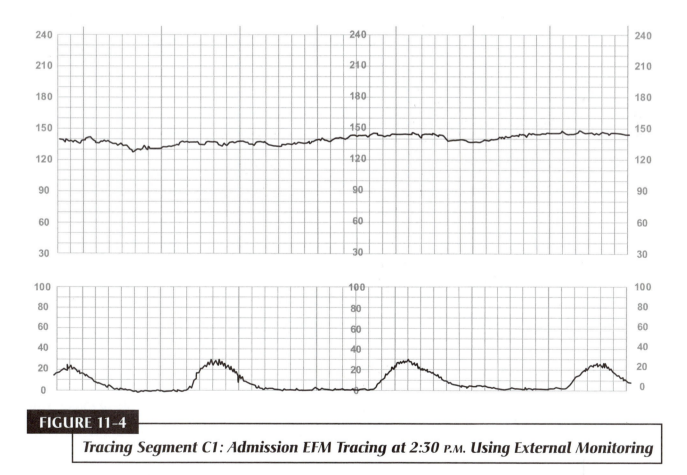

FIGURE 11-4

Tracing Segment C1: Admission EFM Tracing at 2:30 P.M. Using External Monitoring

AWHONN Fetal Heart Monitoring Principles and Practices Systematic Approach to Interpretation Worksheet

Case Study Exercise: Madison C1

1. Contractions: *Frequency:* **q 2 min.**
   Duration: **60–70 sec.**
   Intensity: **Need to palpate**
   Resting tone: **Need to palpate**

2. Baseline fetal heart rate: **140–145 bpm**

3. Variability: Place a checkmark signifying the appropriate type of variability on the strip (LTV = long-term variability; STV = short-term variability).

LTV	**Decreased (0–5 bpm)** ✔		*STV*	Present
	Average (6–25 bpm)			Absent
	Marked (> 25 bpm)			**Unable to assess** ✔
	Unable to assess			

4. Accelerations and decelerations. When present, circle P if periodic or NP if nonperiodic.

Accelerations	**Late decelerations** (P)
Early decelerations	Prolonged decelerations
Variable decelerations	

5. List possible underlying physiologic mechanisms or rationales for observed patterns.
   a. **Uteroplacental insufficiency resulting in late decelerations and associated with:**
      • **placental factors such as aging, infarcts or calcifications or**
      • **maternal factors such as maternal hypertension, supine positioning or decreased maternal oxygenation**
   b. **Loss of fetal reserves resulting in decreased LTV (and possibly STV)**

6. List in order of priority the physiologic goal(s) for observed patterns.
   a. **Maximize oxygenation**
   b. **Maximize uterine blood flow**
   c. **Reduce uterine activity**

7. List interventions to achieve the physiologic goals and actions needed related to instrumentation or further assessment.
   a. **Palpate uterus for contractions to confirm contraction pattern relative to the fetal heart rate tracing**
   b. **Administer maternal supplemental oxygen via snug face mask to maximize oxygenation**
   c. **Change maternal position to lateral recumbent to increase maternal cardiac output and maximize uterine blood flow**
   d. **Perform vaginal examination to determine labor progress, and consider placing internal monitors**
   e. **Notify the woman's obstetric health care provider**
   f. **Reduce uterine activity (e.g., consider tocolytic medication)**
   g. **Hydrate with plasma expanders—taking into consideration maternal status to avoid fluid overload—to increase maternal blood volume and maximize uterine blood flow**
   h. **Provide support to decrease maternal anxiety and catecholamine response**
   i. **Evaluate fetal heart rate response to interventions**
   j. **If pattern persists, prepare for operative delivery and possible resuscitative measures**

SECTION SIX

Advanced Fetal Heart Monitoring Principles and Practices

CHAPTER 12

Antenatal Fetal Assessment and Testing

Jana L. Atterbury
Gina M. Mikkelsen
Anne Santa-Donato

☞ INTRODUCTION

Maternity care changed dramatically during the last half of the 20th century, and the perinatal mortality rate decreased more than four-fold during that time as a result of the remarkable technologic and pharmacologic improvements in obstetric surveillance and care (CDC, NCHS, 2001). Many techniques have been used to identify a fetus that may be at risk for hypoxic injury or death, but, for many reasons, the perfect fetal screening test has not been developed (Manning, 1995). For most of the 20th century, a fetus could be indirectly assessed or directly visualized only during invasive procedures such as fetoscopy. Those direct fetal examinations required membrane rupture and were associated with a high pregnancy loss rate and, therefore, did not gain widespread acceptance (Sonek & Nicolaides, 1994). Instead, several unreliable maternal markers, including physical (e.g., fundal height); historical (e.g., risk assessment); or biochemical (e.g., estriol) characteristics, were used to estimate fetal well-being (Manning, 1995).

Since the 1970s, the fetus has become more accessible with the development of new technologies, such as electronic fetal heart rate (FHR) monitoring and high-resolution sonography (Vintzileos, 1995). Historically, the FHR and maternal perception of fetal movement were the only parameters used to assess fetal health; now, however, multiple fetal responses can be observed, quantified, and compared with established norms (Vintzileos, 2000). In addition, the effects of maternal conditions, such as diabetes or hypertension on the fetus can be described so that it is now possible to differentiate maternal from fetal risk (Manning, 1995).

Knowledge about fetal cardiovascular physiology and neurologic development has grown significantly through the rapid expansion of fetal research. Fetal physiologic parameters that can now be assessed include (a) observing gross motor activities (e.g., breathing, tone); (b) determining activity state (e.g., quiet sleep, active sleep); (c) monitoring eye lens motion; (d) measuring urine production; and (e) observing systolic-to-diastolic blood flow. However, the utility of any one or a combination of those and other variables to identify fetal hypoxia has not been established (Groome, Singh, Burgard, Neely, & Bartolucci, 1992b).

Throughout pregnancy, numerous pathophysiologic processes can place the fetus at risk for metabolic derangement, hypoxemia, and death. Early identification of those phenomena is an important first step in fetal surveillance (Vintzileos, 2000). Perinatal deaths are most often associated with congenital malformations (Vintzileos, Campbell, Ingardia, & Nochimson, 1983); asphyxia (Visser, Sadovsky, & Nicolaides, 1990b); and immune and nonimmune hydrops (Baskett, Allen, Gray, Young, & Young, 1987). Approximately 30% of the cases of cerebral palsy (CP) have been attributed to antepartum asphyxia, while fewer than 8% of CP cases are attributed to intrapartum events (Manning et al., 1997). Antepartum testing has been successful in reducing perinatal mortality when used for specific risk factors, either maternal (Landon, Langer, Gabbe, Schick, & Brustman, 1992; Kjos et al., 1995; Manning, Morrison, Lange, Harman, & Chamberlain, 1985; Nageotte, Towers, Asrat, & Freeman 1994a) or fetal (Alfirevic & Walkinshaw, 1995; Clark, Sabey, & Jolley, 1989; Devoe, Youssif, Gardner, Dear, & Murray, 1992).

☞ FETAL ANTEPARTUM SURVEILLANCE METHODS

The different methods used to evaluate fetal well-being are based on changes in fetal physiologic parameters in response to acute or chronic oxygen availability. If fetal oxygen consumption is reduced, the immediate fetal response is reduction of activities regulated by the central nervous system (CNS), including movement, tone, breathing, and heart rate reactivity (Figure 12-1). Oxygenated blood is shunted to the brain, heart, and adrenal glands, and if the insult is prolonged or repetitive, growth restriction or oligohydramnios can develop. The purpose of antepartum testing is to either validate fetal well-being or identify fetal hypoxemia by the presence or absence of one or more biophysical parameters and to intervene before permanent injury or death can occur whenever possible. The efficacy of antepartum surveillance to predict perinatal outcomes for different patient populations has not been established, but testing is usually indicated for conditions that place the fetus at risk for uteroplacental insufficiency and fetal demise. (ACOG, 1999). Also, for

nonreassuring findings, testing is recommended only when the fetus is considered viable and can be delivered (Ware & Devoe, 1994).

☞ FETAL MOVEMENT DETECTION

Maternal perception of fetal movement was one of the earliest tests of fetal well-being, and it remains an important assessment of fetal health. Although a variety of fetal movement counting methods (FMC, or kick counting) is used in clinical practice, neither the ideal number nor the optimal duration of FMC has been defined (AAP & ACOG, 2002).

Development of Fetal Gross Body Movements

The fetus moves spontaneously by about 7 weeks gestational age; 8 weeks after conception, movement is usually present in a normoxic fetus (Okado & Kojima, 1984). With neurologic maturation, fetal movement becomes more complex and coordinated, and more than 15 distinct movement patterns are present by midgestation (deVries, Visser, & Prechtl, 1982). Cycling between periods of high and low activity begins as early as 22 weeks (Groome, Owen, Singh, Neely, & Gaudier, 1992a), and synchronization of movement with fetal behavioral states begins early in the third trimester (Drogtrop, Ubels, & Nijhuis, 1990). Consequently, most term fetuses exhibit coordinated movement patterns that correspond to specific behavioral states (Groome & Watson, 1992). A comparison of ultrasound-detected fetal movements with maternally perceived fetal movements is presented in Table 12-1.

Fetal Movement Counting (FMC)

Decreases in maternally perceived fetal movements preceding fetal deaths have been reported over the past two decades (Sadovsky & Yaffe, 1973; Pearson & Weaver, 1976), and fetal movement screening has been associated with reduced fetal mortality rates (Moore & Piacquadio, 1989). Counting fetal movements during the second half

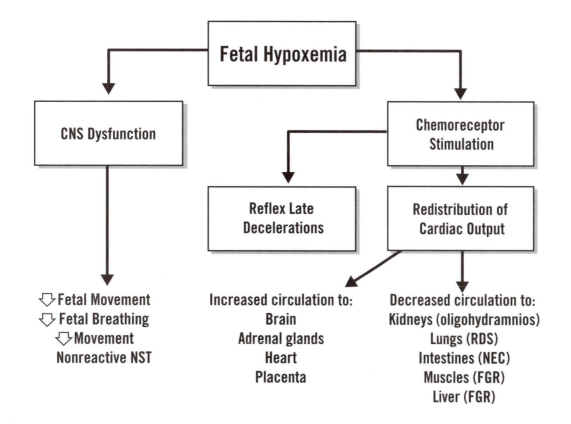

FIGURE 12-1

Fetal Acute and Chronic Responses to Hypoxemia and Effect on CNS-Regulated Activities

Source: Adapted from Manning, Harman, Menticoglou, & Morrison, 1991.

TABLE 12-1

Comparison of Maternally Perceived and Ultrasound-Visualized Movement Patterns

MATERNAL DESCRIPTION	ULTRASOUND VISUALIZED	MOTION TYPE	DURATION (SEC)	INTENSITY
Rollover, stretch	Whole fetal body	Rolling and stretching	3–30	Strong
Kick, jab, startle	Trunk and extremities	Simple or isolated	1–15	Strong
Flutter, weak kick	Lower extremities	Simple	< 1	Weak
Hiccup	Chest walls and extremities	High frequency	< 1	Weak

Source: Adapted from "Antepartum Fetal Assessment: Monitoring Fetal Activity," by W. F. Rayburn, 1982, *Clinics in Perinatology*, 9, p. 235. Adapted with permission.

of pregnancy is also a noninvasive, cost-effective method of assessing fetal well-being (Christensen & Rayburn, 1999).

Several different schemata for FMC have been proposed for quantifying maternally perceived movements and for identifying potentially hypoxic fetuses. FMC methods vary greatly according to the counting interval, number of movements considered reassuring, maternal activity during testing, and method of recording (Christensen & Rayburn, 1999). Typically, patients are instructed to count all fetal movements occurring in a specific time period and to contact the primary provider if a certain number of movements are not perceived during the prescribed counting interval (Rayburn, 1982).

A suggested approach to assessing fetal well-being includes daily fetal movement counts after the 28th week of pregnancy (AAP & ACOG, 2002). Maternal perception of 10 distinct fetal movements within a 2-hour period is considered reassuring; once movement is achieved, counts can be discontinued for that day (AAP & ACOG, 2002). Although the presence of fetal movement within a specified protocol is usually a reliable indicator of fetal well-being, the absence of fetal movement may or may not be predictive of adverse fetal outcomes (Devoe, et al., 1994; Gibby, 1988). Therefore, a nonreassuring finding should be followed by a biophysical means of fetal assessment (AAP & ACOG, 2002) such as a nonstress test (NST), biophysical profile (BPP), or modified biophysical profile.

Factors Influencing Fetal Movement

Fetal body movements and fetal movements perceived by the mother can be affected by several factors. The number of movements per week changes as the pregnancy progresses; total weekly movements increase two-fold from 20 to 32 weeks and then gradually decrease until term (Dawes, Houghton, Redman, &Visser, 1982; Sadovsky, Laufer, & Allen, 1979b). During the third trimester, a similar pattern occurs in amniotic fluid volume (that pattern corresponds to the fetal movement pattern described above). The amniotic fluid volume increases progressively until 32

weeks, remains stable until term, and then progressively decreases until 44 weeks, which results in restricted intrauterine space and concurrent reduction in total fetal movement. (Moore, 1995).

Fetal movement tends to decrease during periods of maternal physical activity and, conversely, may increase during maternal rest (Gibby, 1988). Chronic maternal anxiety and stress can also influence fetal movement. Mothers with high anxiety scores tend to have fetuses who demonstrate significantly less movement than fetuses whose mothers who have low anxiety scores (Groome, Swiber, Bentz, Holland, & Atterbury, 1995c).

Several additional factors can affect fetal motor activity, including the time of day, maternal tobacco and caffeine use, and glucose load (Devoe, Murray, Youssif, & Arnaud, 1993; Eller, Stramm, & Newman, 1992; Patrick, Campbell, Carmichael, Natale, & Richardson, 1982; Thaler, Goodman, & Dawes, 1980). Maternal perception of fetal movements can also be affected by maternal body size, anterior placental location, and polyhydramnios (Timor-Tritsch, Dierker, Hertz, & Rosen, 1979).

Fetal activity is diminished in the compromised fetus, and cessation of fetal movement has been documented preceding fetal demise (Christensen & Rayburn, 1999; Moore & Piacquadio, 1989). However, additional research is needed to determine the ideal system for performing FMC, the optimal criteria for a reassuring number of movements, the time needed for testing, the interval for repeat evaluation, the gestational age to begin testing, and, ultimately, the efficacy of FMC to prevent fetal mortality.

Doppler-Detected Fetal Movement

Tocodynamometry (toco) was adapted in the late 1970s to improve the quality and quantity of data concerning fetal movements and to provide direct comparison with FHR; the goal of toco was to more accurately assess fetal health (Timor-Tritsch, Dierker, Zador, Hertz, & Rosen, 1978b). The Timor-Tritsch device accurately identified and characterized fetal movement, but the signal was affected by maternal size, fetal position, and transducer placement (Devoe et al. 1994). Improved methods, known as cardiotocography

(CTG), actocardiography, or kinetocardiography, use a Doppler-based recording of the FHR, fetal activity, and uterine contractions to identify potentially hypoxic fetuses (Johnson, 1994).

Several studies suggest a strong positive correlation between movements recorded with Doppler-based systems and those observed with real-time ultrasound; however, the relationship between those technologies and FHR characteristics is unclear. Regardless of the movement detection algorithm, Doppler-based CTG has detected more than 95% of all body movements lasting more than 5 seconds and 100% of multiple movements seen during sonography (Besinger & Johnson, 1989; DiPietro, Costigan, & Pressman, 1999; Lowery et al., 1997). In addition, up to 80% of maternally perceived movements are recorded with CTG, but fewer than 20% of Doppler-recorded movements are detected by the mother. The large discrepancy may result from the ability of the Doppler-based device to detect small or single movements, or to detect movements lasting less than 20 seconds (Johnson, Jordan, & Paine, 1990; Lowery et al., 1997). CTG has not gained widespread use because the relationship between Doppler-derived fetal movements and FHR accelerations has not been consistently demonstrated (Baser, Johnson, & Paine, 1992; Devoe et al., 1994).

Reports concerning the reliability of antepartum CTG to reduce perinatal morbidity and mortality as well as maternal mortality were reviewed by the Cochrane Library (Table 12-2). Four randomized controlled trails (RCTs) with a combined study population of more than 1,500 women with high-risk pregnancies achieved the review criteria, but antenatal CTG had no effect on perinatal or maternal outcomes. Although in one study women with CTG experienced significantly fewer hospital admissions and shorter patient stays, the reviewers concluded that there was insufficient evidence to show that the use of antenatal CTG reduced fetal mortality (Pattison & McCowan, 2000).

Contraction Stress Test and the Oxytocin Challenge Test

The contraction stress test (CST) was the first antepartum surveillance method developed with the advent of electronic FHR monitoring; CST quickly became a primary fetal evaluation technique, replacing technically more difficult and prognostically less accurate biochemical (estriol) analyses (Lagrew, 1995). The goal of the CST is to identify a fetus that is at risk for compromise through observation of the fetal response to intermittent reduction in uteroplacental blood flow associated with contractions, and then to intervene if warning signs of fetal stress are present. Fetal acidemia is more likely to occur with chronic uteroplacental insufficiency, but it may not cause obvious changes in the fetal response during periods of no uterine activity. However, in a chronically stressed fetus, the additional acute stress of even small contractions can result in hypoxemia (Lagrew, 1995; Paul & Miller, 1995).

The CST as an antepartum test evolved from animal studies in which the flow of oxygenated blood into the intervillous space ceased during uterine contractions stronger than 30 mmHg, which, in turn, resulted in transient reductions of fetal PO_2 and caused late decelerations of the FHR. The mechanism for late decelerations during antepartum evaluation of a potentially and chronically stressed fetus is the same as that of an acutely stressed fetus during labor. During contractions, uteroplacental blood flow is reduced because of increased vascular resistance in uterine and umbilical vessels, and the flow of oxygenated blood into the intervillous space is reduced or halted (Olofsson, Thuring-Jonsson, & Marsal, 1996). With diminished fetal reserve and reduced O_2 availability, the fetal PO_2 can drop below critical levels, triggering chemoreceptor stimulation and signaling the brainstem to shunt oxygenated blood to the organs needed for survival. Peripheral hypertension stimulates the baroreceptors and causes a vagally mediated drop in heart rate.

During contractions, the resulting drop in the FHR appears as a late deceleration, and the FHR will not return to the previous baseline until intrauterine pressure relaxes and oxygenated blood re-enters the intervillous space. As the late deceleration pathway resolves, the fetal PO_2 rises and the FHR returns to normal. Intermittent and persistent reductions in oxygen availability with

TABLE 12-2

Summary of Selected Perinatal Clinical Practices Reviewed by the Cochrane Library

REVIEW (AUTHORS)	TRIALS	SUBJECTS	RESULTS (ODDS RATIO, 95% CI)[a]
Fetal manipulation for facilitating tests of fetal well-being (Tan & Sabapathy, 2001a)	2	1,090	No change in incidence of NR[b] tests (OR: 1.28,CI: 0.94–.074).
Maternal glucose administration for fetal well-being (Tan & Sabapathy, 2001b)	2	708	No change in incidence of NR tests; additional research is needed.
Ultrasound for fetal assessment in early pregnancy (Neilson, 2001)	9	—	Earlier detection multiple gestation (OR: 0.08, CI:0.04–0.16). Reduced rate of postdates inductions (OR: 0.61, CI: 0.52–0.72). No change in perinatal death rate (OR: 0.86, CI: 0.67–1.12). Improved assessment of GA,[c] earlier recognition of anomalies.
Cardiotocography for antepartum fetal assess- (Pattison & McCowan, 2000)	4	1,588	No significant change in perinatal morbidity or mortality. No increase in interventions.
Biophysical profile for fetal assessment in high-risk preganancies (Alfirevic & Neilson, 2001)	4	2,839	No difference in perinatal morbidity or mortality. Small increase of inductions in one study (OR: 2.1, CI: 1.14.0). Insufficient data to reach meaningful conclusions. Need for future RCTs.
Doppler ultrasound for fetal assessment in high-risk pregnancies (Alfirevic & Neilson, 2001)	11	7,000	Doppler umbilical artery waveform measurements were associated with reduced perinatal deaths (OR: 0.71, CI: 0.50–1.01) and fewer inductions (OR: 0.83, CI: 0.74–0.93) and admissions (OR: 0.56, CI: 0.43–0.72).
Fetal vibroacoustic stimulation (VAS) for - facilitationof tests of fetal well-being (Tan & Smyth, 2001)	7	4,325	VAS reduced incidence of NR NSTs (OR: 0.61, CI: 0.49–0.75) and overall testing time (WMD[d]: –4.55 min, CI: –5.96 – –3.14 min). Increased number of fetal movements (OR: 0.08, CI: 0.06–0.12). Future research should define optimal stimulus intensity and outcomes.

Source: Adapted from *The Cochrane Library,* Issue 4, 2001

[a] 95% CI = Confidence interval.

[b] NR = Nonreactive.

[c] GA = Gestational age.

[d] WMD = Weighted mean difference.

uterine contractions can cause the mechanism to occur repeatedly. Persistent late decelerations are recorded on the FHR tracing and represent a positive CST (Lagrew, 1995; Myers, Muellar-Huebach, & Adamsons, 1973; Poseiro, Mendez-Bauer, Pose, & Caldeyro-Barcia, 1969).

Progressive uteroplacental insufficiency and resultant chronic hypoxemia can cause a shift from aerobic to anaerobic metabolism in the fetus. With increasing central hypoxemia and acidemia, direct myocardial depression can occur and can blunt the myocardial response to stimulation. As a result, the fetal response to contractions may appear as shallow late decelerations with a loss of variability (Lagrew, 1995). Over time, the chronically stressed fetus can develop oligohydramnios, thus reducing the normal volume of amniotic fluid that surrounds and protects the umbilical cord. Therefore, the cord may be vulnerable, and if it is compressed during uterine contractions, variable decelerations may appear on the FHR tracing (ACOG, 1999).

🖳 CLINICAL APPLICATION OF THE CST

The CST correlates the fetal response to spontaneous or stimulated uterine contractions in order to assess fetal reserves. Early investigations of the CST revealed that repetitive late decelerations occurring during uterine contractions represented an early and potentially significant sign of fetal compromise (Christie & Cudmore, 1974; Freeman, 1975). Late decelerations also signified a change in fetal status developing before the loss of heart rate reactivity or accelerations and representing chronic central hypoxia. Therefore, the oxytocin challenge test OCT was thought to provide information for the detection of impending compromise that was superior to the use of FHR monitoring alone (Goupil et al., 1981).

Uterine Contractions

Antepartum evaluation using the CST requires uterine activity that mimics the stress of early labor. The minimum number of contractions needed to adequately test fetal health has not been

clearly established, but the criteria for evaluation of the CST were extrapolated from studies in the 1970s (Lagrew, 1995; Paul & Miller, 1995). Contraction intensity, measured by an intrauterine pressure catheter, provides a more accurate assessment of uterine activity relative to the FHR, but antepartum monitoring of uterine activity is limited to data that can be assessed with external tocodynamometry. A primary limitation of external uterine monitoring is that only the frequency and duration of contractions—and not the strength of contractions—can be assessed. However, the important assessment parameter for the CST is the FHR response to uterine contractions, regardless of the intensity.

Test Procedure

The CST is administered with the patient in the lateral recumbent (or semi-Fowler's) position, and the FHR and uterine activity are monitored for at least 10 minutes with external Doppler ultrasound and toco transducers (ACOG, 1999). During the initial period of monitoring, if three or more spontaneous contractions lasting at least 40 seconds occur in a 10–20 minute window, additional uterine stimulation is unnecessary (ACOG, 1999; AAP & ACOG 2002). Intravenous (IV) oxytocin infusion or nipple manipulation may be used to stimulate contractions if none are present within the first 10–20 minutes. Although nipple stimulation has been associated with uterine hyperstimulation (Schellpfeffer, Hoyle, & Johnson, 1985), similar rates of hyperstimulation, nonreassuring CST results, and successful tests with both IV oxytocin and nipple stimulation methods have been reported in the literature (Lipitz, Barkai, Rabinovici, & Mashiach, 1987; Oki, Keegan, Freeman, & Dorchester, 1987).

The procedure for the CST using nipple stimulation proposed by the American College of Obstetricians and Gynecologists (ACOG, 1999; AAP & ACOG, 2002) is as follows: One nipple is massaged gently through clothing until a contraction begins or for 2 minutes. If the contraction criteria are not met, the patient rests for 5 minutes, and the alternate nipple is stimulated. When nipple stimulation is unsuccessful (if contractions have not started), an IV infusion of oxytocin can be initiated at 0.5–1 mU/min and is increased every 15–20 minutes until at least three contractions occur in 10 minutes. The OCT is generally not recommended for pregnant women with a relative contraindication to uterine contractions, such as prematurity, a diagnosed placenta previa, a classical uterine incision scar, a history of extensive uterine surgery, or preterm rupture of membranes (Freeman, 1975; Ocak et al., 1992; AAP & ACOG, 2002).

Interpretation

The interval between CSTs is generally 7 days, although more frequent evaluation (including nonstress testing or BPPs) may be indicated for conditions such as postterm pregnancy, diabetes, intrauterine growth restriction, or hypertension (ACOG, 1999). The CST is interpreted by identifying the presence or absence of FHR decelerations and FHR reactivity in response to uterine contractions. According to AAP & ACOG (2002, p. 104), CST interpretation criteria can be categorized as follows:

◆ *Negative:* No late or significant variable decelerations are identified.

◆ *Positive:* Late decelerations are identified with 50% or more of contractions, even if the contraction frequency is less than three in 10 minutes.

◆ *Equivocal-suspicious:* Intermittent late (late decelerations with fewer than 50% of contractions) or significant variable decelerations are observed.

◆ *Equivocal-hyperstimulation:* Uterine contractions occur more frequently than every 2 minutes or last longer than 90 seconds with accompanying late decelerations.

◆ *Unsatisfactory:* Fewer than three contractions occur within 10 minutes, or there may be a tracing quality that cannot be interpreted.

Efficacy of the CST

The initial popularity of the CST arose from Freemanís (1975) review of 16 CST studies in which only one fetal death occurred within 7 days of test-

ing; similar results have been reported by more recent studies (Nageotte, Towers, Asrat, Freeman, & Dorchester, 1994b). Negative CSTs usually correlate with good fetal outcome. For example, the corrected stillbirth rate of 1.2 per 1,000 live births after a negative CST was significantly lower than the stillbirth rate of 8 per 1,000 for the general population (Lagrew, 1995). However, a false positive CST has been defined as the absence of fetal distress after testing (Freeman, Goebelsman, Nochimson, & Cerulo, 1976), and false-positive rates greater than 30% have been reported following the CST (Gauthier, Evertson, & Paul, 1979; Shalev, Zalel, & Weiner, 1993). Therefore, one of most significant limitations of the CST is its high false-positive rate, which can result in premature or unnecessary intervention (Druzin, Gabbe, & Reed, 2002). Follow-up of positive CST results should be individualized and based on evaluation of the patient's total clinical picture (ACOG, 1999).

☞ NONSTRESS TEST

The nonstress test (NST) evolved from early evidence that FHR accelerations were highly associated with fetal well-being (Lee, DiLoreto, & O'Lane, 1975) and that, conversely, the absence of FHR reactivity, including accelerations, was associated with an increased risk of perinatal mortality (Rochard et al., 1976). In a subsequent investigation, CSTs were always negative when two accelerations were recorded, and the criteria for NST reactivity (e.g., two accelerations in 20 minutes) evolved from that report (Evertson, Gauthier, Schifrin, & Paul, 1979). Compared with the CST, nonstress testing is technically easier to perform (Nageotte et al., 1994b); requires fewer resources (Keegan & Paul, 1980); and can be used in in-patient, out-patient, and home settings (Reece, Hagay, Garofalo, & Hobbins, 1992; Naef et al., 1994). As a result, nonstress testing became and remains a primary antepartum assessment of fetal well-being (Freeman, Anderson, & Dorchester, 1982).

Physiology of the Nonstress Test

The heart rate of a physiologically normal fetus with adequate oxygenation and a mature autonomic nervous system (ANS) accelerates in response to movement or other stimuli (Krebs, Petres, Dunn, & Smith, 1982). Several types of FHR accelerations have been described that may represent different physiologic mechanisms. Fetal movement is associated with accelerations that have a jagged appearance and that result from stimulation of the sympathetic nervous system (SNS) (Krebs et al., 1982). FHR accelerations occurring with a normal baseline rate and baseline variability are the components of a reactive NST and usually represent normal ANS function (Schifrin, 1995). Accelerations can occur after 20 weeks gestation but are less frequent and are of lower amplitude than those occurring later in pregnancy.

With greater autonomic maturity, the FHR has increasing cycles of high and low variation, and fetal movement and accelerations are clustered in periods of high FHR variation (Dawes et al., 1982; Guinn, Kimberlin, Wigton, Socol, & Frederiksen, 1998). The frequency and amplitude of accelerations increase with gestational age and evolve into distinct behavior states (Dawes et al., 1982; Groome et al., 1997a; Snijders, McLaren, & Nicolaides, 1990). Fetal movement and FHR accelerations are highly correlated and increase in a linear fashion with gestational age (DiPietro et al., 1999; Pillai & James, 1990), and more than 95% of accelerations have a synchronous onset or begin immediately after movement (Freeman, 1975; Lee et al., 1975).

The FHR response is reflective of the nature of fetal movement. For example, a larger increase in heart rate occurs with complex movements than with isolated fetal movements (Johnson, 1994). Although external Doppler-obtained assessment of FHR variability is less accurate than direct fetal electrocardiogram (ECG) assessment, heart rate variation with fetal movement is an important criterion for behavior states and demonstrates normal ANS function (Dawes et al., 1982; Nijhuis, Prechtl, Martin, & Bots, 1982). As FHR variability increases, so do the number of movements and the number and amplitude of accelerations (Dawes et al., 1982). The presence of accelerations, fetal movement, and variability usually preclude acidemia (Krebs et al., 1982; Ribbert, Snijders, Nicolaides, & Visser, 1990; Vintzileos &

Knuppel, 1994; Walkinshaw, Cameron, MacPhail, & Robson, 1992).

In contrast, the effects of hypoxia on NST results are unclear because the sequence of the FHR changes in the transition from normal fetal oxygenation to asphyxia is unclear. Progressive hypoxia may cause the loss of state changes before the FHR fails to accelerate (Visser, Bekedam, & Ribbert, 1990a). As fetal compromise continues, the rest cycles lengthen and eventually disappear, and FHR variability and fetal movement decrease. Subsequently, accelerations become smoother, less frequent, and finally disappear. Before fetal death, variability has been reported to decrease to less than 5 bpm, with absent movement and FHR accelerations (Visser et al., 1990b).

Clinical Application of the Nonstress Test

The ideal NST criteria have not been established, and early definitions for a reactive test range from a minimum of 1–5 accelerations with a duration of 10–15 seconds and an amplitude of 5–15 bpm above the baseline rate (Baser et al., 1992; Ware & Devoe, 1994; Vintzileos et al., 1983). There are no obvious improvements in the reliability of the NST to predict adverse perinatal outcome by using more than two accelerations or by requiring different acceleration duration or amplitude (Lee et al., 1975; Evertson et al., 1979; Vintzileos et al., 1987).

Test Procedure and Interpretation

The FHR is monitored with the external Doppler transducer until the criteria for two accelerations (spontaneous or acoustically stimulated) with an amplitude 15 bpm above the baseline and a duration of 15 seconds within a 20-minute period are recorded. A monitoring period of 40 minutes may be necessary to accommodate normal fetal sleep-wake cycles (ACOG, 1999; AAP & ACOG, 2002). A nonreactive NST is defined as fewer than two accelerations meeting the above criteria during a 40-minute period (ACOG, 1999; AAP & ACOG, 2002). Although the lateral tilt position is usually recommended during FHR monitoring, maternal semi-Fowler's position can shorten time to complete testing and has been associated with more reactive NSTs than supine positioning (Nathan, Haberman, Burgess, & Minkoff, 2000). However, aortocaval compression can occur when the maternal head is elevated less than 45°, and maternal symptoms of supine hypotension can occur before a drop in blood pressure is recorded. Therefore, maternal position during NST should be determined by the clinical situation and supine positioning with the head lower than 45° should be avoided (Moffatt & van der Hof, 1997).

Variable Decelerations during a NST

Variable decelerations occur in as many as one half to two thirds of NSTs (Meis et al., 1986; Timor-Tritsch, Dierker, Hertz, Deogan, & Rosen, 1978a) and have been associated with the strength of fetal movements (Timor-Tritsch, Dierker, Hertz, Deogan, & Rosen, 1978a) and umbilical cord compression (O'Leary, Andrinopoulos, & Giordano, 1980). The significance of variable decelerations during otherwise reactive NSTs has been the subject of debate because of differences in definitions for interpretation and perinatal outcomes among investigations (Druzin, Fox, Kogut, & Carlson, 1985; Glantz & D'Amico, 2001; Hoskins, Frieden, & Young, 1991; O'Leary et al., 1980). Decelerations occur in approximately 20% of fetuses, but single decelerations are more prevalent before 33 weeks (Guinn et al., 1998), and 2–3 decelerations are more common with advancing gestation (Dawes et al., 1982).

Perinatal outcomes following NSTs with variable decelerations may vary depending on the depth, duration, and frequency of FHR changes and the overall reactivity of the NST. Intrapartum nonreassuring FHR patterns tend to occur more often after a NST with three or more variable decelerations of more than 15 seconds' duration (Glantz & D'Amico, 2001; O'Leary et al., 1980). Prolonged decelerations of greater than 1 minute have been associated with oligohydramnios and stillbirth (Bourgeois, Thiagarajah, & Harbert, 1984; Druzin et al., 1985). NSTs with repetitive prolonged decelerations are associated with greater risks of non-

reassuring FHR patterns; cord complications (e.g., multiple nuchal, occult, body); and meconium (stained amniotic fluid) (Jaschevatzky et al., 1998). Oligohydramnios was reported to be present in study groups whose NSTs revealed variable decelerations (Glantz & D'Amico, 2001; Hoskins et al., 1991), and the risk of cesarean delivery for nonreassuring FHR patterns increased progressively with the worsening severity of decelerations and decreasing amniotic fluid volume (Hoskins et al., 1991). However, the greatest risks are associated with nonreassuring tracings, an amniotic fluid index lower than 5 cm, or postdates pregnancies (Clark et al., 1989; Dawes et al., 1982; Jaschevatzky et al., 1998; Walkinshaw et al., 1992). More important, a reactive NST with nonrepetitive variable deceleration lasting less than 30 seconds is not indicative of fetal compromise and usually requires no intervention (ACOG, 1999).

Efficacy of NSTs

A reactive NST with normal amniotic fluid volume is indicative of fetal well-being in 99% of pregnancies (Shalev et al., 1993; Vintzileos et al., 1987) and has a false-negative (i.e., stillbirth of a non-anomalous fetus or neonate within 1 week of a reactive NST) rate of less than 1% (Miller, Rabello, & Paul, 1996). However, the NST is much less reliable in predicting adverse perinatal outcomes, and false-positive (i.e., normal newborn after a nonreactive NST) results of greater than 90% have been reported (Miller et al., 1996; Mills, James, & Slade, 1990).

Many factors can affect the accuracy of the NST and can contribute to the high rate of false-positive results; of those, a significant influence is gestational age. Until cyclic changes of FHR and movement coalesce into behavior states with advancing gestational age and neurologic maturity, the FHR does not have the typical reactive appearance of a NST at term (Dawes et al., 1982; Guinn et al., 1998). The proportion of fetuses with reactive NSTs, defined as two accelerations (15 bpm lasting at least 15 seconds), increases progressively after 32 weeks (Vintzileos & Knuppel, 1994). Even with the criteria for reactivity of two accelerations of 10 bpm above baseline lasting 15 seconds, more than 15% of tests are nonreactive at 29 weeks (Guinn et al., 1998). The large proportion of nonreactive tests in premature fetuses is concerning because of the risk for potentially unnecessary intervention with false-positive tests. Antenatal testing may begin for patients at risk for stillbirth at 32–34 weeks' gestation and may be indicated at 26–28 weeks depending on the clinical circumstances. However, the implications of nonreassuring FHR patterns at an early gestational age is not clearly understood (AAP & ACOG, 2002).

Lower amplitude criteria for reactivity has been suggested to reduce the confounding affect of gestational age on NSTs (Castillo et al., 1989; Guinn et al., 1998). If the observation period is extended to 60 minutes, 100% of fetuses less than 32 weeks had reactive NSTs with the criteria of three 10-bpm amplitude accelerations in 30 minutes (Castillo et al., 1989). The presence of accelerations of any size is associated with normal acid-base status in both term and preterm fetuses (Vintzileos & Knuppel, 1994; Visser et al., 1990b). Criteria for a reactive NST that includes accelerations of 10 bpm above baseline, lasting at least 10 seconds during at least 30 minutes, may be used to evaluate NSTs before 32 weeks' gestation (Eganhouse & Burnside, 1992; Yanagihara et al., 2000).

Several conditions other than hypoxia can reduce heart rate reactivity, can interfere with fetal movement, and should be considered when interpreting NSTs (Manning, 1995). During quiet sleep, the FHR tracing has nonreactive features (such as diminished FHR variability and reduced fetal movement), but with a state change, the FHR can become reactive (with increased variability, presence of accelerations, and movement) (Nijhuis et al., 1982; Groome et al., 1999c). At term, the fetus is in a quiet sleep (QS) state about 30% of the time (Groome et al., 1999c). Thus, extending the observation period until a fetus becomes more active can reduce the incidence of nonreactive NSTs (Ware & Devoe, 1994). The FHR, fetal movement, and NST results are affected by maternal cigarette smoking and chronic maternal stress (Thaler et al., 1980; Groome et al., 1995c). Ingestion of substances such as caffeine, cocaine, morphine, sedatives, and alcohol has also been associated with false-positive NSTs (Devoe et al., 1993; Kopecky

et al., 2000; Rizk, Atterbury, & Groome, 1996; Vintzileos et al., 1987). In addition, glucose consumption has been reported to increase the FHR (Eller et al., 1992), and poor maternal nutritional status can decrease FHR reactivity (Onyeije & Divon, 2001).

🖙 FETAL STIMULATION

Various methods of fetal stimulation have been proposed to improve the reliability of antepartum surveillance and are used to differentiate nonreactive NSTs caused by hypoxia from those associated with fetal sleep states or narcosis. Three methods of fetal stimulation have been reviewed by the Cochrane Collaboration (2001), including vibroacoustic stimulation (VST), fetal manipulation, and glucose administration. Those methods are summarized in Table 12-3. Fetal manipulation (i.e., abdominal rocking, scalp stimulation) has been used during nonreactive NSTs in two trials, but with no demonstrated effect on the efficacy of antepartum testing (Tan & Sabapathy, 2001a). Glucose administration increases fetal breathing and has variable effects on fetal movement, but oral (e.g., orange juice) or intravenous glucose administration did not decrease the incidence of nonreactive NSTs in two trials with fewer than 1,000 participants (Tan & Sabapathy, 2001b). The reviewers concluded that there was no benefit on antepartum surveillance from either fetal manipulation or glucose administration, and further research with both methods was recommended (Tan & Sabapathy, 2001a; Tan & Sabapathy, 2001b).

Vibroacoustic Stimulation (VAS)

In 1925, Peiper described the response of fetuses to extrauterine sound; subsequently, multiple studies have explored fetal perception of sound or have used sound to evaluate fetal well-being. At approximately 24 weeks' gestation, the fetus abruptly develops a generalized startle response (which includes sudden movement of the extremities) to VAS; VAS evokes similar behavior in almost all normal fetuses after 28–29 weeks' gestational age (Groome, Gotlieb, Neely, & Waters, 1993). The expected fetal responses to VAS are FHR accelerations and increased gross body movements (Clark et al., 1989; Sarno, Ahn, Phelan, & Paul, 1990). Although some differences in specific FHR responses have been reported (Gagnon, Hunse, & Patrick, 1988; Jensen & Flottorp, 1982), a single startle response and acceleration of the FHR in response to VAS suggests a functional brainstem, regardless of gestational age (Groome, Mooney, Holland, Smith, & Atterbury, 1997b).

Before 30 weeks, a single prolonged acceleration is the usual fetal response to VAS; after that, general increases in rate and accelerations are the usual response (Gagnon et al., 1988). Premature fetuses with immature ANSs often have higher baseline heart rates than neurologically mature fetuses and, as a result, have cardio-acceleratory responses with lower amplitudes than at later gestational ages. An inverse relationship between baseline FHR and the amplitude of acceleration in premature fetuses has been described, and an increased baseline FHR may prevent an acceleration from reaching the criteria for a reactive NST. However, this relationship becomes clinically unimportant after approximately 30 weeks, as the fetus matures (Gagnon et al., 1988; Groome et al., 1993).

The fetal response to sound has been tested using different sound intensities, frequencies, and durations. Relatively high levels of sound are transmitted from the extrauterine to the intrauterine environment. The VAS significantly increases the baseline intrauterine sound level, exposing the fetus to sound intensity similar to that of the takeoff of a jet airplane (Smith, 1995). The primary device used to generate a stimulus for VAS is an artificial larynx (Clark et al., 1989; Miller-Slade et al., 1991; Sarno et al., 1990; Yao et al., 1990). The commercially available device produces 82-dB (decibels) (Sarno et al., 1990). Although the long-term sequelae of VAS stimulation on hearing or cognition are not clearly understood, fetuses clinically exposed to VAS have had no subsequently reported adverse effects at 4 years of age (Nyman, Barr, & Westgren, 1992). Different stimulus durations have been used, including 1-, 2-, 3-, and 5-second durations (Clark et al., 1989; Saracoglu, Gol, Sahin, Turkkani, & Oztopcu, 1999; Sarno et al., 1990). A significant increase in the amplitude and duration of accelerations has been associated with 3- and 5-second stimuli durations (Pietrantoni et al., 1991).

Several investigations have explored the reliability of antepartum testing with VAS compared to other surveillance methods. Significantly more visualized or palpated fetal movements occurred after VAS than without stimulation, and evoked accelerations were associated with more than 99% of reactive NSTs (Marden, McDuffie, Allen, & Abitz, 1997). Compared to standard NSTs, acoustic stimulation reduced the incidence of false-positive tests (Clark et al., 1989; Saracoglu et al., 1999; Serafini et al., 1984; Smith, Phelan, Platt, Broussard, & Paul, 1986b), and an impaired or absent response was a better predictor of perinatal outcomes than NSTs alone (Saracoglu et al., 1999; Trudinger & Boylan, 1980). In addition, VAS reduced the incidence of nonreactive NSTs by as much as 50% and decreased the average test duration by 10–20 minutes (Clark et al., 1989; Miller-Slade et al., 1990; Saracoglu et al., 1999).

Test Procedure and Interpretation

A commercially available artificial larynx should be used to perform acoustic stimulation as needed when FHR accelerations do not occur during an NST. The procedure includes positioning the artificial larynx on the maternal abdomen near the fetal head and applying the stimulus for up to 3 seconds. Acoustic stimulation can be repeated at approximately 1 minute intervals up to three times if the NST remains nonreactive (Druzin et al., 2002), for a total of approximately 9 seconds. A reactive NST using VAS is considered a valid indicator of fetal well-being (ACOG, 1999). However, if the NST is still nonreactive following VAS, the test should be followed up with a BPP or CST (Druzin et al., 2002).

No differences in perinatal outcome (i.e., fetal distress, meconium-stained amniotic fluid, Apgar scores lower than 7) have been reported following NSTs with spontaneous or stimulated accelerations (Sarno et al., 1990; Serafini et al., 1984; Smith, Phelan, Nguyen, Jacobs, & Paul, 1988). A Cochrane Collaboration (Tan & Smyth, 2001) review of the literature concerning fetal VAS (Table 12-2) revealed that VAS reduced the incidence of nonreactive antepartum NSTs and reduced the overall testing time. The reviewers were unable to draw conclusions about the efficacy of VAS because the prevalence of perinatal morbidity and mortality in the reviewed studies was too small. In addition, the reviewers observed that there is a paucity of literature concerning fetal hearing and neurologic development after sound stimulation, and that little is known about maternal anxiety and maternal satisfaction regarding testing. The reviewers concluded that VAS offered benefits by reducing the incidence of nonreactive NSTs, as well as the time to complete testing, but future research was recommended to define the optimum stimulus intensity, frequency, duration, and position and to determine the efficacy, reliability, safety, and perinatal outcomes associated with VAS (Tan & Smyth, 2001).

🖐 FETAL BIOPHYSICAL PROFILE

In response to the high proportion of false-positive nonstress and contraction stress tests, Manning, Platt, and Sipos (1980) proposed an assessment of fetal well-being that combined NST results with multiple physiologic parameters observed with real-time ultrasound. The biophysical profile (BPP) was based on previous reports that fetal

activity such as breathing when decreased with hypoxia or narcosis (Manning & Platt, 1979). Further, the BPP was based on the theory that acute and chronic hypoxia cause the reduction or cessation of fetal activities in a particular order, so that the absence of one parameter or more could represent the degree of fetal hypoxic stress (Manning, Morrison, Lange, & Harman, 1982).

The BPP provided improved prognostic information over antepartum FHR testing alone because fetal physiologic parameters associated with both chronic (amniotic fluid volume, gross body movements, and tone) and acute (heart rate reactivity and breathing movements) hypoxia were evaluated (Manning et al., 1980). Thus, the BPP includes the assessment of the following five components: (a) fetal breathing movement, (b) gross body movement, (c) fetal tone, (d) amniotic fluid volume, and (e) fetal heart rate reactivity (NST).

The fetal activities observed during the BPP result from complex processes within the CNS and ANS, and the presence of each suggests normal neurologic function and adequate oxygenation (Vintzileos et al., 1987). Fetal activity decreases or stops to reduce energy and oxygen consumption as fetal hypoxemia worsens, and it occurs in reverse order of normal development (Table 12-3). The fetal activities that appear earliest in pregnancy (e.g., tone and movement) are usually the last to cease, and activities that are last to develop

TABLE 12-3

*Embryology of the CNS Centers Responsible for Fetal Activities**

ACTIVITY	CENTER	GESTATIONAL AGE	HYPOXIA
Tone	Cortex—subcortical area	7.5–8.5 weeks	↑
Movement	Cortex—nuclei	9.0 weeks	
Breathing	Ventral surface—4th ventricle	20.0–21.0 weeks	
Fetal Heart Rate	Posterior hypothalamus, medulla	End 2nd trimester Onset 3rd trimester	

* The arrow suggests the order in which hypoxia affects fetal activities.

are usually the first to be suppressed (Vintzileos & Knuppel, 1994). The presence of short-term fetal activities (NST, breathing, movement, tone) indicates normal central oxygenation (Manning et al., 1993), whereas the clinical significance of absent activities is more difficult to determine because factors other than hypoxia can cause CNS depression (e.g., sedatives, narcotics, anesthetics) (Manning et al., 1982; Vintzileos et al., 1983).

Clinical Application of the BPP

Although multiple studies of the BPP have been undertaken worldwide, two groups of investigators are responsible for a large percentage of BPP research and for development of the BPP interpretation criteria (0, 1, or 2) (Manning et al., 1980; Vintzileos et al., 1983). In initial descriptions, an NST was performed first, and if nonreactive after 20 minutes, the FHR was monitored for an additional 20 minutes (Vintzileos & Knuppel, 1994). An ultrasound examination followed, and a score was assigned for each parameter detected during a 30-minute observation period. In addition to the BPP variables previously proposed (Manning et al., 1982), Vintzileos and associates (1983) added placental grading because of the increased incidence of intrapartum placental abruption (14.8%) and nonreassuring FHR patterns (44.4%) with Grade III placentae (Vintzileos et al., 1987). The scoring criteria for BPPs are listed in Table 12-4, and they illustrate a revised two-number scoring

TABLE 12-4

Biophysical Profile Scoring Criteria

FETAL PHYSIOLOGIC PARAMETER	NORMAL (SCORE = 2)	ABNORMAL (SCORE = 0)
Breathing movements	≥1 episode of ≥30 sec in 30-min observation period	Absent or episode ≤30 sec in 30 min observation period.
Gross body movements	≥3 discrete body or limb movements in 30 min (continuous movement is considered one movement)	≤2 episodes of body or limb movements in 30 min.
Tone	≥1 episode of active extension and return to flexion of limbs or trunk (opening and closing of hand is considered normal tone)	Either slow extension or return to partial flexion or limb movement in full extension or absent movement
Reactive fetal heart rate	≥2 accelerations ≥15 bpm lasting ≥15 sec associated with fetal movement in 20–30 minutes	2 accelerations or accelera-<15 bpm in 20 min.
Amniotic fluid volume	≥1 pocket of fluid ≥2 cm in two perpendicular planes	Either no pockets or a pocket, <2 cm in two perpendicular planes

Source: Adapted from Manning, Morrison, Lange, Harman, & Chamberlain, 1985.

method of 0 or 2, because the middle score of 1 did not improve the predictability of the BPP in clinical trails (Manning et al., 1985).

Test Procedure and Interpretation

During a real-time sonogram, the biophysical variables are monitored simultaneously until the normal criteria for each have been observed, or for a total observation period of 30 minutes. A system for BPP interpretation and management is summarized in Table 12-5. The average time to complete the BPP is approximately 10–20 minutes when performed by an experienced sonographer

(Manning et al., 1982; Manning, Baskett, Morrison, & Lange, 1981), and more than 98% of BPPs are completed within 30 minutes (Manning et al., 1990a). Normal fetal gross body movement is classified by at least three rolling movements of the extremities or trunk (Vintzileos et al., 1987), and fetal tone is defined by extension of the extremities with return to flexion or by opening and closing of the fetal hand (Manning et al., 1980).

Fetal breathing is the continuous movement of the chest or abdominal walls lasting at least 30 seconds, with breath-to-breath intervals shorter than 6 seconds. Amniotic fluid volume is determined by the presence of at least a 1- or 2-cm pocket

TABLE 12-5

Interpretation and Suggested Management for Biophysical Profile Scores

SCORE	INTERPRETATION	MANAGEMENT
10 / 10 8 / 10 (normal AFV) 8 / 8 (NST not done)	No acute or chronic asphyxia	No fetal indication exists for intervention. Conduct serial testing as indicated by condition.
8 / 10 (abnormal AFV)	No acute asphyxia; low risk of chronic hypoxia	Deliver if oligohydramnios present. Use serial testing if < 36 weeks. Twice weekly for diabetics.
6 / 10 (normal AFV)	Chronic asphyxia suspected	Deliver if fetus is ≥ 36 weeks and favorable conditions. Repeat test in 4–6 hours if > 36 weeks and L/S ratio < 2.0.
4 / 10 (normal AFV)	Chronic asphyxia suspected	Deliver if fetus is > 36 weeks. Repeat test same day if < 32 weeks.
2 / 10	Chronic asphyxia suspected	Extend observation period to 120 minutes. Deliver if repeat score is ≤ 4 regardless of gestational age.
0 / 10	Chronic asphyxia suspected	Deliver regardless of gestational age if persistent score ≤ 4.

Source: Adapted from Manning, Platt, & Chamberlain, 1980; Manning et al., 1990.
PNM = perinatal mortality
AFV = amniotic fluid volume
NST = nonstress test

measured in the vertical axis or by crowding of the fetal small parts (Manning, 1995; Vintzileos & Knuppel, 1994). Although the BPP and NST have similar reliability for the prediction of adverse outcomes when used as primary antepartum screening tests (Manning, Lange, Morrison, & Harman, 1984), the BPP is most often used as a follow-up examination as summarized in Table 12-6. The timing of the NST may vary and may be done first along with determination of fetal breathing movement (Vintzileos et al., 1987), or after a BPP with at least one abnormal parameter (Manning et al., 1995).

The usual interval between BPP examinations is 1 week (Manning, Harman, Menticoglou, & Morrison, 1991), but more frequent testing may be used for specific high-risk conditions, such as twice weekly examinations for high-order multiple gestation or insulin-dependent diabetes (Elliot & Finberg, 1995), or daily examinations for severe preeclampsia or preterm premature rupture of membranes (Chari, Friedman, O'Brien, & Sibai, 1995; Lewis et al., 1999). In addition, the optimal gestational age at which to initiate antepartum surveillance with the BPP has not been established, and recommendations range from 24–25 weeks (Manning, 1995) to 32–34 weeks (Miller et al., 1996; ACOG, 1999). As with all antepartum testing methods, the interpretation of the BPP score is determined by the maternal and fetal clinical situation, and a management approach based on specific pregnancy complications has been recommended (Vintzileos & Knuppel, 1994).

Nursing Role in BPP Testing

The BPP was developed in an antepartum testing center where the majority of ultrasound examinations was performed by nurses with special training (Manning et al., 1981). In addition, an increasing number of nurses have completed additional training to conduct a fetal assessment with real-time Doppler sonography, and the BPP interpretation by specially trained nurses is equal to or better than that of medical subspecialists (Gegor, Paine, Costigan, & Johnson, 1994). The BPP is an ultrasound examination of limited scope that may be performed by nurses who have com-

pleted additional education and who can demonstrate competence to perform limited obstetric ultrasound (AWHONN, 1998). Furthermore, nurses should verify that performing limited obstetric ultrasound is within their scope of practice as defined by state or provincial licensing bodies and is consistent with individual facility regulations (AWHONN, 1998). Nurses who use advanced-practice skills, such as sonography, are professionally responsible for documentation of specialized training used to determine initial competence, are responsible for maintenance of competence, and may participate in establishing local policies and procedures (Gegor et al., 1994; Raines, 1996).

Efficacy of the BPP

A BPP score of 10/10, with a reactive NST and with normal amniotic fluid volume, is associated with normal fetal oxygenation and development more than 99.9% of the time (ACOG, 1999). In addition, the false-negative rate (i.e., stillbirth within 1 week of a normal BPP) in more than 86,000 patients was 0.7 to 2.3 stillbirths per 1,000 births, and feto-maternal hemorrhage was the most frequent cause of false-negative BPPs (Dayal et al., 1999). However, the predictive value of the BPP is not clearly understood because of differences in study methodologies, participants, and sample size and because of a lack of standard criteria for BPP interpretation and divergent outcome definitions. Although multiple cohort and case-control studies of the BPP have reported encouraging results, the BPP has been studied in a surprisingly small number of RCTs (Alfirevic & Neilson, 2001). Moreover, the outcome of more than 150,000 fetuses assessed with BPP has been reported, but fewer than 3,000 of those were enrolled in an RCT. Adverse outcomes were infrequent in both descriptive and experimental BPP studies, and power analyses either were not calculated or were not reported (Table 12-7).

The relationship between acidemia and fetal activity during BPP has been studied extensively and provides insight into the effects of acidemia on fetal CNS function. In addition to the comparison of antepartum BPP scores with umbilical cord gas results, cordocentesis has been used to des-

TABLE 12-6

Comparison of Study Populations, Test Types, and Results of Randomized Controlled Trials of Fetal Surveillance Methods

STUDY	POWER ANALYSIS	POWER	POPULATION (PREGNANCIES)	GROUP STUDY	GROUP CONTROL	TEST TYPE	RESULTS
Alfirevic & Walkinshaw (1995)	Yes	No	145 >41 weeks	Modified BPP[a] (n = 72)	NST (n = 72)	Venous PH and BE	No differences in pH, base excess, or neonatal outcomes.
Bracero, Morgan, & Byrne (1999)	Yes	No	410 high-risk	Computer NST (n = 205)	Visual NST (n = 205)	BPP	Computer group had fewer BPPs. No outcome differences.
Lewis et al. (1999)	Yes	No	135 women 23–34 weeks PPROM	NST (n = 69)	BPP (n = 66)	BPP	Both tests too insensitive to predict infection.
Manning, Lange, Morison, & Harman (1984)	No	—	735 high-risk	NST (n = 360)	BPP (n = 375)	BPP	No outcome differences.
Marden, McDuffie, Allen, & Abitz (1997)	No	—	577 >31 weeks	FAST[b] (n = 197)	NST Sham (n = 360)	BPP	More movement visualized and palpated with FAST. No outcome differences.
Nageotte, Towers, Asrat, Freeman, & Dorchester (1994b)	Yes	No	1,307 high-risk NR BPP	CST[c] (n = 628)	BPP (n = 679)	BPP	Women in CST group had more interventions; no differences in outcome.
Nathan, Haberman, Burgess, & Minkoff (2000)	Yes	Yes	108 referred 32–42 weeks	Sitting first (n = 131)	Supine first (n = 158)	BPP	No adverse outcomes. Semi-Fowler's position was more likely to have reactive NST.

(table continues)

TABLE 12-6 (cont.)

Comparison of Study Populations, Test Types, and Results of Randomized Controlled Trials of Fetal Surveillance Methods

STUDY	POWER ANALYSIS	POWER	POPULATION (PREGNANCIES)	GROUP STUDY	GROUP CONTROL	TEST TYPE	RESULTS
Platt et al. (1985)	No	—	149 high-risk	BPP (*n* = 688)	NST (*n* = 960)	CST	No differences exist in outcomes. had larger PPV for prediction of outcomes.
Sarinoglu, Dell, Mercer, & Sibai (1996)	No	—	192 high-risk > 28 weeks NR NST[d]	FSR[e] (+) (*n* = 159)	FSR[e] (−) (*n* = 41)	BPP	All women with + FSR had BPP score ≥6. All women with BPP <6 had FSR −.
Tyrell et al. (1990)	No	—	500 high-risk > 28 weeks	Routine Monitoring[g] (*n* = 250)	Selective Monitoring[g] (*n* = 250)	BPP	No difference exists in perinatal or maternal outcomes.

[a] Biophysical profile.
[b] Fetal acoustic stimulation.
[c] Contraction stress test.
[d] Nonreactive nonstress.
[e] Fetal startle response.
[f] Routine monitoring included growth scans, NST, kick counts.
[g] Selective monitoring included weekly biophysical profile and umbilical and uterine artery Doppler velocimetry.

TABLE 12-7

Comparison of Nonstress Tests and Biophysical Profile Prediction of Perinatal Outcomes

STUDY	NONSTRESS TEST								BIOPHYSICAL PROFILE							
	ABNORMAL OUTCOMES				DEATH				ABNORMAL OUTCOMES				PERINATAL DEATH			
	SENS. (%)	SPEC. (%)	PPV (%)	NPV (%)	SENS. (%)	SPEC. (%)	PPV (%)	NPV (%)	SENS. (%)	SPEC. (%)	PPV (%)	NPC (%)	SENS. (%)	SPEC. (%)	PPV. (%)	NPV (%)
Baskett et al. (1984)	20.5	90.6	24.9	88.2	57.6	87.1	3.3	99.6	88.1	44.1	6.1	99.0	57.6	89.5	4.1	99.7
Devoe et al. (1998)	15.0	30.0	88.0	28.0	88.9	49.1	11.6	99.8	21.0	96.0	48.8	89.0	93.6	99.2	68.1	99.2
Landon, Langer, Gabbe, Schick, & Brustman (1992)	33.3	93.8	40.0	91.2	100.0	93.8	10.0	100.0	50.0	97.6	80.0	92.3	80.0	94.2	40.0	100.0
Manning et al. (1990)	88.1	43.7	16.5	96.7	88.1	43.7	16.5	96.7	47.7	69.0	87.2	36.3	64.4	70.0	16.9	96.7
Mills, James, & Slade (1990)	—	—	—	—	28.5	77.8	0.0	99.3	—	—	—	—	30.0	98.7	33.3	99.6
Platt et al. (1985)	13.9	95.8	33.3	88.1	33.3	94.9	6.7	99.3	31.8	99.5	87.5	92.6	66.7	97.1	25.0	99.5

(table continues)

TABLE 12-7 (cont.)

Comparison of Nonstress Tests and Biophysical Profile Prediction of Perinatal Outcomes

| STUDY | NONSTRESS TEST | | | | | | | | BIOPHYSICAL PROFILE | | | | | | | |
| | ABNORMAL OUTCOMES | | | | DEATH | | | | ABNORMAL OUTCOMES | | | | PERINATAL DEATH | | | |
	SENS. (%)	SPEC. (%)	PPV (%)	NPV (%)	SENS. (%)	SPEC. (%)	PPV (%)	NPV (%)	SENS. (%)	SPEC. (%)	PPV (%)	NPC (%)	SENS. (%)	SPEC. (%)	PPV. (%)	NPV (%)
Shalev, Zalel, & Weiner (1993)	100.0	84.2	57.1	100.0	100.0	14.2	72.8	100.0	100.0	84.2	57.1	100.0	100.0	14.2	72.8	100.0
Vintzileos et al. (1987)	100.0	92.0	71.0	100.0	100.0	95.3	17.8	100.0	23.8	89.6	28.4	100.0	100.0	80.0	12.0	100.0
Walkinshaw, Cameron, MacPhail, & Robson (1992)	19.2	88.0	28.0	82.0	50.0	68.9	9.3	95.6	42.0	78.0	32.0	83.3	50.0	68.9	9.3	95.5

Sens. = sensitivity
Spec. = specificity
PPV = positive predictive value
NPV = negative predictive value

cribe fetal acid-base status before term (Shalev et al. 1993; Sonek & Nicolaides, 1994). Regardless of the criteria used, a normal BPP (e.g., score of 8 or greater) is associated with normal acid-base status.

The BPP and cord pH are highly correlated, and the pH tends to be higher when the BPP score is increased (Manning et al., 1995; Vintzileos et al., 1987). In contrast, a significant inverse relationship between a worsening fetal cord pH and the absence of FHR reactivity, fetal breathing, movement, and tone—in that order—has been described (Vintzileos & Knuppel, 1994). FHR reactivity and breathing are reduced with an umbilical cord pH lower than 7.20, and movement and tone are decreased with a pH lower than 7.10. In addition, both a progressively lower pH and base excess values have been reported as individual biophysical parameters were abolished; the average pH and base excess decreased significantly as individual fetal activities were abolished (Vintzileos et al., 1987; Vintzileos & Knuppel, 1994; Manning et al., 1993).

In addition to fetal-neonatal blood gases, the BPP has also been evaluated for its ability to predict other perinatal variables associated with fetal hypoxia (Table 12-8), such as nonreactive NSTs. The predictive ability of the BPP is reported to be improved by the combination of variables, and the risk of abnormal outcomes is increased with an enlarged number of abnormal variables (Devoe et al., 1992). A relationship has been described between abnormal BPP scores and cases of cerebral palsy (Manning et al., 1997). In addition, the BPP has been reported to significantly reduce the perinatal mortality rate when compared to an untested population from 7.69 to 1.86 (Manning, 1995).

Modified BPP

Amniotic fluid volume may reflect a normal decline near or beyond term or may be indicative of fetal hypoxia. Hypoxic fetuses demonstrate "brain sparing," where there is a physiologic redistribution of cardiac output that allows the greatest oxygenation of the fetal brain while decreasing blood flow to other vital organs, including the kidneys (Manning, 1995). That response may precede a

decrease in renal function and then a decrease in fetal urine, which is the primary component of amniotic fluid in the third trimester. Oligohydramnios may be a reflection of acute or chronic fetal asphyxia and increased risk for poor perinatal outcomes. Those concepts led to the development of the so-called modified BPP, which combines the NST and an ultrasound-obtained amniotic fluid volume index as a test of uteroplacental function (Nageotte et al., 1994a). The amniotic fluid index (AFI) represents the sum of the measurements (in centimeters) of the deepest umbilical cord free pockets of amniotic fluid in all four abdominal quadrants (ACOG, 1999).

The modified BPP consists of an NST and a measurement of AFI as indicators of short-term fetal well-being and long-term placental function, respectively (ACOG, 1999). A modified BPP is considered normal when the NST is reactive and the AFI is greater than 5 centimeters (ACOG, 1999). The modified BPP has the advantage of requiring less time to complete, and it is associated with similar perinatal outcomes when compared with antepartum tests (Nageotte et al., 1994b; Shah, Brown, Salyer, Fleischer, & Boehm, 1989).

SUMMARY

A great deal remains unknown about the benefits and risks of antepartum surveillance. Adverse perinatal outcomes are infrequent, which is an important factor in the overall positive predictive ability of each of the antepartum tests described in this chapter. The indications for testing vary among studies, but testing is usually reserved for maternal or fetal conditions associated with risks for uteroplacental insufficiency and stillbirth. Numerous lists of indications for antepartum testing have been proposed, although the efficacy of any test to predict long-term perinatal outcomes for complicated or normal pregnancies has not been determined. The optimal gestational age at which testing should begin continues to be the subject of research, and prematurity has confounding effects on the predictive value of surveillance. Different protocols for testing, including the intervals between tests and management of nonreac-

TABLE 12-8

Comparison of Prediction of Acidemia by Biophysical Profile

STUDY	BPP CRITERIA	STUDY POPULATION OF WOMEN)	ACIDEMIA CRITERIA	PREDICTION OF ACIDEMIA			
				SENS. (%)	SPE. (%)	PPV (%)	NPV (%)
Landon, Langer, Gabber, Schick, & Brustman (1992)	≤6 / 10[a]	Diabetics NR NST (134)	Arterial cord pH < 7.20	33.3	93.8	40.0	86.1
Manning et al. (1993)	≤6 / 10[a]	High-risk antepartum (493)	Venous cord pH < 7.20	100.0	92.3	3.0	97.0
Sassoon, Castro, Davis, Bear, & Hobel (1990)	≤6 / 10[a]	Low-risk Laboring (95)	Arterial cord pH < 7.20 or 7.15	20.0	78.0	9.0	89.0
Vintzileos et al. (1987)	≤7 / 12[b]	Low-risk cesarean (124)	Arterial cord pH < 7.20	90.0	96.1	81.9	98.0

[a] Manning, Morrison, Lange, Harman, & Chamberlain. (1985)
[b] Vintzileos, Campbell, Ingardia, & Nochimson. (1983)

NR NST = nonreactive nonstress test
Sens. = sensitivity
Spec. = specificity
PPV = positive predictive value
NPV = negative predictive value

tive results have been recommended, but the most efficacious schema have not been described.

The use of low- and high-technology fetal assessment methods has led to a decrease in perinatal death and complications in pregnancies with identified risk factors for uteroplacental insufficiency. One goal of fetal testing is to reduce the frequency of preventable stillbirths secondary to hypoxic insults. However, half of all unexpected fetal deaths occur in women with low-risk pregnancies without identifiable risk factors that would make them candidates for antepartum fetal testing. Although antepartum surveillance is yet of unproven value, it is a widely integrated and accepted clinical practice and has been consistently associated with substantially lower rates of fetal death in both untested (presumably lower-risk) pregnancies and pregnancies with similar complicating factors that were managed before the advent of currently employed techniques of antepartum surveillance.

The search for the perfect antepartum test is ongoing and includes research to improve existing technologies or to develop new technologies. Computerized systems for interpretating antepartum FHR tracings and BPPs have been developed and may improve the prognostic ability of current antepartum tests while reducing the time needed for completion (Bracero et al., 1999). Doppler velocimetry is one of the newer methods of antepartum testing that may improve the ability to diagnose fetal growth restriction and fetal hypoxia by detecting abnormal blood flow patterns in uterine and umbilical vessels using Doppler ultrasound (Yoon et al., 1993). As nursing responsibilities increase and nurses' roles expand relative to caring for high-risk women during the antepartum period, ongoing assessment and evaluation, patient care, education, research, and application of evidence-based interventions will improve the outcomes for both women and their newborns.

REFERENCES

Alfirevic, Z. & Neilson, J. P. (2001). Biophysical profile for fetal assessment in high risk pregnancies (Cochrane Review). *The Cochrane Library* [Online], 4. Oxford: Update Software

Alfirevic, Z. & Walkinshaw, S. A. (1995). A randomized controlled trial of simple compared with complex fetal monitoring after 42 weeks of gestation. *British Journal of Obstetrics and Gynecology, 102,* 638–643.

American Academy of Pediatrics (AAP) & American College of Obstetricians and Gynecologists (ACOG). (2002). *Guidelines for perinatal care* (5th ed.). Elk Grove Village, IL: Authors.

American College of Obstetricians and Gynecologists (ACOG). (1999). *Antepartum fetal surveillance* (Practice Bulletin No. 9). Washington, D.C.: Author.

Association of Women's Health, Obstetric and Neonatal Nurses. (1998). *Clinical competencies and education guide: Limited ultrasound examinations in obstetric and gynecologic/infertility settings.* Washington, D.C.: Author.

Baser, I., Johnson, T. R., & Paine, L. L. (1992). Coupling of fetal movement and fetal heart rate accelerations as an indicator of fetal health. *Obstetrics and Gynecology, 80*(1), 62–66.

Baskett, T. F., Allen, A. C., Gray, J. H., Young, D. C., & Young, L. M. (1987). Fetal biophysical profile and perinatal death. *Obstetrics and Gynecology, 70*(3 Pt. 1), 357–360.

Besinger, R. E., & Johnson, T .R. (1989). Doppler recordings of fetal movement: Clinical correlation with real-time ultrasound. *Obstetrics and Gynecology, 74*(2), 277–280.

Bourgeois, F. J., Thiagarajah, S., & Harbert, G. M. (1984). The significance of fetal heart decelerations during nonstress testing. *American Journal of Obstetrics and Gynecology, 150*(2), 213–216.

Bracero, L. A., Morgan, S., & Byrne, D. W. (1999). Comparison of visual and computerized interpretation of nonstress test results in a randomized controlled trial. *American Journal of Obstetrics and Gynecology, 181*(5 Pt. 1), 1254–1258.

Castillo, R. A., Devoe, L. D., Arthur, M., Searle, N., Metheny, W. P., & Ruedrich, D. A. (1989). The preterm nonstress test: Effects of gestational age and length of study. American Journal of Obstetrics and Gynecology, 160(1), 172–175.

Centers for Disease Control and Prevention, National Center for Health Statistics. National Vital Statistics System (CDC, NCHS). (2001). Infant mortality rates, fetal mortality rates, and perinatal mortality rates, according to race: United States, selected years 1950–99. Deaths: Final data for 1999. In *National vital statistics reports,* 49, Table 23. Washington, D.C.: Government Printing Office.

Chari, R. S., Friedman, S. A., O'Brien, J. M., & Sibai, B. M. (1995). Daily antenatal testing in women with severe preeclampsia. *American Journal of Obstetrics and Gynecology, 173*(4), 1207–1210.

Christensen, F. C., & Rayburn, W. F. (1999). Fetal movement counts. *Obstetrics and Gynecology Clinics of North America, 26*(4), 607–621.

Christie, C. B., & Cudmore, D. W. (1974). The oxytocin challenge test. *American Journal of Obstetrics and Gynecology, 118*(3), 327–330.

Clark, S. L., Sabey, P., & Jolley, K. (1989). Nonstress testing with acoustic stimulation and amniotic fluid volume assessment: 5973 tests without unexpected fetal death. *American Journal of Obstetrics and Gynecology, 160*(3), 694–697.

Daniels, S. M., & Boehm, N. (1991). Auscultated fetal heart rate accelerations: An alternative to the nonstress test. *Journal of Nurse Midwifery, 36*(2), 88–94.

Dawes, G. S., Houghton, C. R., Redman, C. W., & Visser, G. H. (1982). Pattern of normal fetal heart rate. *British Journal of Obstetrics and Gynaecology, 89*(4), 276–284.

Dayal, A. K., Manning, F. A., Berck, D. J., Mussalli, G. M., Avila, C., Harman, C. R., & Menticoglou, S. (1999). Fetal death after normal biophysical profile score: An eighteen-year experience. *American Journal of Obstetrics and Gynecology, 181*(5 Pt. 1), 1231–1236.

Devoe, L., Boehm, F., Paul, R., Frigoletto, F., Penso, C., Goldenberg, R., Rayburn, W., & Smith, C. (1994). Clinical experience with the Hewlett-Packard M-1350A fetal monitor: Correlation of Doppler-detected fetal body movements with fetal heart rate parameters and perinatal outcome. *American Journal of Obstetrics and Gynecology, 170*(2), 650–655.

Devoe, L. D., Murray, C., Youssif, A., & Arnaud, M. (1993). Maternal caffeine consumption and fetal behavior in normal third-trimester pregnancy. *American Journal of Obstetrics and Gynecology, 168*(4), 1105–1112.

Devoe, L. D., Youssif, A. A., Gardner, P., Dear, C., & Murray, C. (1992). Refining the biophysical profile with a risk-related evaluation of test performance. *American Journal of Obstetrics and Gynecology, 167*(2), 346–352.

deVries, J. I., Visser, G. H., & Prechtl, H. F. (1982). The emergence of fetal behaviour: I. Qualitative aspects. *Early Human Development, 7*(4), 301–322.

DiPietro, J. A., Costigan, K. A., & Pressman, E. K. (1999). Fetal movement detection: Comparison of the Toitu actograph with ultrasound from 20 weeks gestation. *Journal of Maternal-Fetal Medicine, 8*(6), 237–242.

Drogtrop, A. P., Ubels, R., & Nijhuis, J. G. (1990). The association between fetal body movements, eye movements, and heart rate patterns in pregnancies between 25 and 30 weeks of gestation. *Early Human Development, 23*(1), 67–73.

Druzin, M. L., Fox, A., Kogut, E., & Carlson, C. (1985). The relationship of nonstress test to gestational age. *American Journal of Obstetrics and Gynecology, 153*(4), 386–389.

Druzin, M. L, Gabbe, S. G. & Reed, K. L. (2002). Antepartum fetal evaluation. In Gabbe, S. G., Neibyl, J. R., & Simpson, J. L. *Obstetrics: Normal and problem pregnancies* (4th ed.). New York: Churchill Livingstone. 151–162

Eganhouse, D. J. & Burnside, S. M. (1992). Nursing assessment and responsibilities in monitoring the preterm pregnancy. *JOGNN, 25,* 355–363.

Eller, D. P., Stramm, S. L., & Newman, R. B. (1992). The effect of maternal intravenous glucose administration on fetal activity. *American Journal of Obstetrics and Gynecology, 167*(4 Pt. 1), 1071–1074.

Elliot, J.P., & Finberg, H.J. (1995). Biophysical profile testing as an indicator of fetal well-being in high-order multiple gestations. *American Journal of Obstetrics and Gynecology, 172*(2 Pt. 1), 508–512.

Evertson, L. R., Gauthier, R. J., Schifrin, B. S., & Paul, R.H. (1979). Antepartum fetal heart rate testing. I. Evolution of the nonstress test. *American Journal of Obstetrics and Gynecology, 133*(1), 29–33.

Freeman, R. K. (1975). The use of the oxytocin challenge test for antepartum clinical evaluation of uteroplacental respiratory function. *American Journal of Obstetrics and Gynecology, 121*(4), 481–489.

Freeman, R. K., Anderson, G., & Dorchester, W. (1982). A prospective multi-institutional study of antepartum fetal heart rate monitoring. II. Contraction stress test versus nonstress test for primary surveillance. *American Journal of Obstetrics and Gynecology, 143*(7), 778–781.

Freeman, R. K., Goebelsman, U. W., Nochimson, D., & Cerulo, C. (1976). An evaluation of the significance of a positive oxytocin challenge test. *Obstetrics and Gynecology, 47*(1), 8–13.

Gagnon, R., Hunse, C., & Patrick, J. (1988). Fetal responses to vibratory acoustic stimulation: Influence of basal heart rate. *American Journal of Obstetrics and Gynecology, 159*(4), 835–839.

Gauthier, R. J., Evertson, L. R., & Paul, R .H. (1979). Antepartum fetal heart rate testing. II. Intrapartum fetal heart rate observation and newborn outcome following a positive contraction stress test. *American Journal of Obstetrics and Gynecology, 133*(1), 34–39.

Gegor, C. L., Paine, L. L, Costigan, K., & Johnson, T. R. (1994). Interpretation of biophysical profiles by nurses and physicians. *Journal of Obstetric, Gynecologic, and Neonatal Nursing, 23*(5), 405–410.

Gibby, N. W. (1988). Relationship between fetal movement charting and anxiety in low-risk pregnant women. *Journal of Nurse-Midwifery, 33*(4), 185–188.

Glantz, C., & D'Amico, M. L. (2001). Lack of relationship between variable decelerations during reactive nonstress tests and oligohydramnios. *American Journal of Perinatology, 18*(3), 129–35.

Goupil, F., Legrand, H., Vaquier, J., Breart, G., Milliez, J., Rochart, F., & Sureau, C. (1981). Antepartum fetal heart rate monitoring. II. Deceleration patterns. *European Journal of Obstetrics, Gynecology, and Reproductive Biology, 11*(4), 239–249.

Groome, L. J., Gotlieb, S. J., Neely, C. L., & Waters, M. D. (1993). Developmental trends in fetal habituation to vibroacoustic stimulation. *American Journal of Perinatology, 10*(1), 46–49.

Preliminary report. *Journal of Maternal-Fetal Medicine, 4,* 173–178.

Groome, L. J., Mooney, D. M., Holland, S. B., Bentz, L. S., Atterbury, J. L., & Dykman, R. A. (1997a). The heart rate deceleratory response in low-risk human fetuses: Effect of stimulus intensity on response topography. *Developmental Psychobiology, 30*(2), 103–113.

Groome, L. J., Mooney, D. M., Holland, S. B., Smith, L. A., & Atterbury, J. L. (1997b). Heart rate response in individual human fetuses to stimulation with a low-intensity sound. *Journal of Maternal–Fetal Investigation, 7,* 105–110.

Groome, L. J., Owen, J., Singh, K. P., Neely, C. L., & Gaudier, F. L. (1992a). Spontaneous movement of the human fetus at 18–22 weeks of gestation: Evidence of early organization of the active rest cycle. *Journal of Maternal-Fetal Investigation, 2,* 27–32.

Groome, L. J., Singh, K. P., Burgard, S. L., Neely, C. L., & Bartolucci, A. A. (1992b). The relationship between heart rate and eye movement in the human fetus at 38–40 weeks of gestation. *Early Human Development, 30,* 93–99.

Groome, L. J., Swiber, M. J., Bentz, L. S., Holland, S. B., & Atterbury, J. L. (1995c). Maternal anxiety during pregnancy: Effect on fetal behavior at 38 to 40 weeks of gestation. *Developmental and Behavioral Pediatrics, 16,* 391–396.

Groome, L. J., Swiber, M. J., Holland, S. B., Bentz, L. S., Atterbury, J. L., & Trimm, R. F. III (1999c). Spontaneous motor activity in the perinatal infant before and after birth: Stability in individual differences. *Developmental Psychobiology, 35,* 25–34.

Groome, L. J., & Watson, J. E. (1992 [AQ: Note no b in text.). Assessment of in utero neurobehavioral development. I. Fetal behavioral states. *Journal of Maternal-Fetal Investigation, 2,* 183–194.

Guinn, D. A., Kimberlin, D. F., Wigton, T. R., Socol, M. L., & Frederiksen, M. C. (1998). Fetal heart rate characteristics at 25 to 28 weeks' gestation. *American Journal of Perinatology 15*(8), 507–510.

Hoskins, I. A., Frieden, F. J., & Young, B. K. (1991). Variable decelerations in reactive nonstress tests with decreased amniotic fluid index predict fetal compromise. *American Journal of Obstetrics and Gynecology, 165*(4 Pt. 1), 1094–1098.

Jaschevatzky, O. E., Marom, D., Ostrovsky, P., Ellenbogen, A., Anderman, S., & Ballas, S. (1998). Significance of sporadic deceleration during antepartum testing in term pregnancies. *American Journal of Perinatology, 15*(5), 291–294.

Jensen, O. H., & Flottorp, G. (1982). A method for controlled sound stimulation of the human fetus. *Scandinavian Audiology, 11*(3), 145–150.

Johnson, T. R. (1994). Maternal perception and Doppler detection of fetal movement. *Clinics in Perinatology, 21*(4), 765–777.

Johnson, T. R., Jordan, E. T., & Paine, L. L. (1990). Doppler recordings of fetal movement. II. Comparison with maternal perception. *Obstetrics and Gynecology, 76*(1), 42–43.

Keegan, K. A. Jr., & Paul, R. H. (1980). Antepartum fetal heart rate testing. IV. The nonstress as a primary approach. *American Journal of Obstetrics and Gynecology, 136*(1), 75–80.

Kopecky, E. A, Ryan, M. L., Barrett, J. F., Seaward, P. G., Ryan, G., Koren, G., & Amankwah, K. (2000). Fetal response to maternally administered morphine. *American Journal of Obstetrics and Gynecology, 183*(2), 424–430.

Krebs, H. B., Petres, R. E., Dunn, L. J., & Smith, P. J. (1982). Intrapartum fetal heart rate monitoring: VI. Prognostic significance of accelerations. *American Journal of Obstetrics and Gynecology, 142*(3), 297–305.

Lagrew, D. C. (1995). The nonstress test. *Clinical Obstetrics and Gynecology, 38*(1), 11–25.

Landon, M. B., Langer, O., Gabbe, S. G., Schick, C., & Brustman, L. (1992). Fetal surveillance in pregnancies complicated by insulin-dependent diabetes mellitus. *American Journal of Obstetrics and Gynecology, 167*(3), 617–621.

Lee, C. Y., DiLoreto, P. C., & O'Lane, J. M. (1975). A study of fetal heart rate acceleration patterns. *Obstetrics and Gynecology, 45*(2), 142–146.

Lewis, D. F., Adair, C. D., Weeks, J. W., Barrilleaux, P. S., Edwards, M. S., & Garite, T. J. (1999). A randomized clinical trial of daily nonstress testing versus biophysical profile in the management of preterm premature rupture of membranes. *American Journal of Obstetrics and Gynecology, 181*(6), 1495–1499.

Lipitz, S., Barkai, E., Rabinovici, J., & Mashiach, S. (1987). Breast stimulation test and oxytocin challenge test in fetal surveillance: A prospective randomized study. *American Journal of Obstetrics and Gynecology, 157*, 1178–1181.

Lowery, C. L., Russell, W. A. Jr., Baggot, P. J., Wilson, J. D., Walts, R. C., Bentz, L. S., & Murphy, P. (1997). Time quantified detection of fetal movements using a new fetal movement algorithm. *American Journal of Perinatology 14*(1), 7–12.,

Mahomed, K., Gupta, B. K., Matikiti, L., & Murape, T. S. (1992). A simplified form of cardiotocography for antenatal fetal assessment. *Midwifery, 8*(4), 191–194.

Manning, F. A. (1995). Dynamic ultrasound based fetal assessment: The fetal biophysical profile score. *Clinical Obstetrics and Gynecology, 38*(1), 26–44.

Manning, F. A., Baskett, T. F., Morrison, I., & Lange, I. (1981). Fetal biophysical profile scoring: A prospective study in 1,184 high-risk patients. *American Journal of Obstetrics and Gynecology, 140*(3), 289–294.

Manning, F. A., Bondagji, N., Harman, C. R., Casiro, O., Menticoglou, S., & Morrison, I. (1997). Fetal assessment based on the fetal biophysical profile score: Relationship of last BPS result to subsequent cerebral palsy. *Journal of Gynecologic Obstetric Biologic Reproduction, 26*(7), 720–729.

Manning, F. A., Harman, C. R., Menticoglou, S., & Morrison, I. (1991). Assessment of fetal well-being with ultrasound. *Obstetric and Gynecology Clinics of North America, 18*(4), 891–905.

Manning, F. A., Harman, C. R., Morrison, I., Menticoglou, S. M., Lange, I. R., & Johnson, J. M. (1990). Fetal assessment based on fetal biophysical profile scoring: IV. An analysis of perinatal morbidity and mortality. *American Journal of Obstetrics and Gynecology, 162*(3), 703–709.

Manning, F. A., Lange, I. R., Morrison, I., & Harman, C. R (1984). Fetal biophysical profile score and the nonstress test: A comparative trial. *Obstetrics and Gynecology, 64*(3), 326–331.

Manning, F. A., Morrison, I., Lange, I. R., & Harman, C. R. (1982). Antepartum determination of fetal health: Composite biophysical profile scoring. *Clinics in Perinatology, 9*(2), 285–296.

Manning, F. A., Morrison, I., Lange, I. R., Harman, C. R., & Chamberlain, P. F. (1985). Fetal assessment based on fetal biophysical profile scoring: Experience in 12,620 referred high-risk pregnancies. I. Perinatal mortality by frequency and etiology. *American Journal of Obstetrics and Gynecology, 151*(3), 343–350.

Manning, F. A., & Platt, L. D. (1979). Maternal hypoxemia fetal breathing movements. *Obstetrics and Gynecology, 53*(6), 758–760.

Manning, F. A., Platt, L. D., & Sipos, L. (1980). Antepartum fetal evaluation: Development of a fetal biophysical profile. *American Journal of Obstetrics and Gynecology, 136*(6), 787–795.

Manning, F. A., Snijders, R., Harman, C. R., Nicolaides, K., Menticoglou, S., & Morrison, I. (1993). Fetal biophysical profile score. VI. Correlation with antepartum umbilical venous fetal pH. *American Journal of Obstetrics and Gynecology, 169*(4), 755–763.

Marden, D., McDuffie, R. S., Allen, R., & Abitz, D. (1997). A randomized controlled trial of a new fetal acoustic stimulation test for fetal well-being. *American Journal of Obstetrics and Gynecology, 176*(6), 1386–1388.

Meis, P. J., Ureda, J. R., Swain, M., Kelly, R. T., Penry, M., & Sharp, P. (1986). Variable decelerations during nonstress tests are not a sign of fetal compromise. *American Journal of Obstetrics and Gynecology, 154*(3), 586–590.

Miller, D. A., Rabello, Y. A., & Paul, R. H. (1996). The modified biophysical profile: Antepartum testing in the 1990s. *American Journal of Obstetrics and Gynecology, 174*(3), 812–817.

Miller-Slade, D., Gloeb, D. J., Bailey, S., Bendell, A., Interlandi, E., Kline-Kaye, V., & Kroesen, J. (1991). Acoustic stimulation-induced fetal response compared to traditional nonstress testing. *Journal of Obstetric, Gynecologic, and Neonatal Nursing, 20*(2), 160–167.

Mills, M. S., James, D. K., & Slade, S. (1990). Two-tier approach to the biophysical assessment of the fetus. *American Journal of Obstetrics and Gynecology, 163*(1 Pt. 1), 12–17.

Moffatt, F. W., & van den Hof, M. (1997). Semi-Fowler's positioning, lateral tilts, and their effects on nonstress tests. *Journal of Obstetric, Gynecologic, and Neonatal Nursing, 26*(5), 551–557.

Moore, T. R. (1995). Assessment of amniotic fluid volume in at-risk pregnancies. *Clinical Obstetrics and Gynecology, 38*(1), 78–91.

Moore & Piacquadio (1989) A prospective evaluation of fetal movement screening to reduce the incidence of antepartum fetal death. *American Journal of Obstetrics and Gynecology, 160*(5 Pt. 1): 1075–80.

Myers, R. E., Muellar-Huebach, E., & Adamsons, K. (1973). Predictability of the state of fetal oxygenation from a quantitative analysis of the components of late deceleration. *American Journal of Obstetrics and Gynecology, 115*(8), 1083–1094.

Naef, R. W. III, Morrison, J. C., Washburne, J. F., McLaughlin, B. N., Perry, K. G. Jr., & Roberts, W. E. (1994). Assessment of fetal well-being using the nonstress test in the home setting. *Obstetrics and Gynecology, 84*(3), 424–426.

Nageotte, M. P., Towers, C. V., Asrat, T., & Freeman, R. K. (1994a). Perinatal outcome with the modified biophysical profile. *American Journal of Obstetrics and Gynecology, 170*(6), 1672–1676.

Nageotte, M. P., Towers, C. V., Asrat, T., Freeman, R. K., & Dorchester, W. (1994b). The value of a negative antepartum test: Contraction stress test and modified biophysical profile. *Obstetrics and Gynecology, 84*(2), 231–234.

Nathan, E. B., Haberman, S., Burgess, T., & Minkoff, H. (2000). The relationship of maternal position to the results of brief nonstress tests: A randomized clinical trial. *American Journal of Obstetrics and Gynecology, 182*(5), 1070–1072.

Neilson, J. P. (2001). Ultrasound for fetal assessment in early pregnancy (Cochrane Review). *The Cochrane Library* [On-line]), 4. Oxford

Neilson, J. P., & Alfirevic, Z. (2001). Doppler ultrasound for fetal assessment in high risk pregnancies (Cochrane Review). *The Cochrane Library* [On-line], 4. Oxford

Nijhuis, J. G., Prechtl, H. F., Martin, C. B. Jr., & Bots, R. S. (1982). Are there behavioural states in the human fetus? *Early Human Development, 6*(2), 177–195.

Nyman, M., Barr, M., & Westgren, M. (1992). A four-year follow-up of hearing and development in children exposed in utero to vibro-acoustic stimulation. *British Journal of Obstetrics and Gynecology, 99*(8), 685–688.

Ocak, V., Demirkiran, F., Sen, C., Colgar, U., Ocer, F., Kilavuz, O., & Uras, Y. (1992). The predictive value of fetal heart rate monitoring: A retrospective analysis of 2,165 high-risk pregnancies. *European Journal of Obstetrics, Gynecology, and Reproductive Biology, 44*(1), 53–58.

Okado, N., & Kojima, T. (1984). Ontogeny of the central nervous system: Neurogenesis, fibre connection, synaptogenesis, and myelination in the spinal cord. In H. F. Prechtl (Ed.), *Continuity of neural functions from prenatal to postnatal life* (pp. 31–45). Oxford: Spastics International Medical Publications.

Oki, E. Y., Keegan, K. A., Freeman, R. K., & Dorchester, W. L. (1987). The breast-stimulation contraction stress test. *Journal of Reproductive Medicine, 32*(12), 919–932.

O'Leary, J. A., Andrinopoulos, G. C., & Giordano, P. C. (1980). Variable decelerations and the nonstress test: An indication of cord compromise. *American Journal of Obstetrics and Gynecology, 137*(6), 704–706.

Olofsson, P., Thuring-Jonsson, A., & Marsal, K. (1996). Uterine and umbilical circulation during the oxytocin challenge test. *Ultrasound in Obstetrics and Gynecology, 8*(4), 247–251.

Onyeije, C. I., & Divon, M. (2001). The impact of maternal ketonuria on fetal test results in the setting of postterm pregnancy. *American Journal of Obstetrics and Gynecology, 184*(4), 713–718.

Paine, L. L., Benedict, M. L., Strobino, D. M., Gegor, C. L., & Larson, E. L. (1992). A comparison of the auscultated acceleration test and the nonstress test as predictors of perinatal outcome. *Nursing Research, 41*(2), 87–91.

Paine, L. L., Johnson, T. R., Turner, M. H., & Payton, R. G. (1986a). Auscultated fetal heart accelerations.

II. An alternative to the nonstress test. *Journal of Nurse Midwifery, 31*(2), 73–77.

Paine, L. L., Payton, R. G, & Johnson, T. R. (1986b). Auscultated fetal heart accelerations. Part I. Accuracy and documentation. *Journal of Nurse Midwifery, 31*(2), 68–72.

Paine, L. L., Zanardi, L. R., Johnson, T. R., Rorie, J. A., & Barger, M. K. (2001). A comparison of two time intervals for the auscultated acceleration test. *Journal of Nurse Midwifery, 46*(2), 98–102.

Patrick, J., Campbell, K., Carmichael, L., Natale, R., & Richardson, B. (1982). Patterns of gross fetal body movements over 24-hr observation intervals during the last 10 weeks of pregnancy. *American Journal of Obstetrics and Gynecology, 142*(4), 363–371.

Pattison, N., & McCowan (2000). Cardiotocography for antepartum fetal assessment (Cochrane Review). *The Cochrane Library* [On-line], 4. Oxford: Update Software. Available

Paul, R. H., & Miller, D. A. (1995). Nonstress test. *Clinical Obstetrics and Gynecology, 38*(1), 3–10.

Pearson, J. F., & Weaver, J. B. (1976). Fetal activity and fetal wellbeing: An evaluation. *British Medical Journal, 1*(6021), 1305–1307.

Pietrantoni, M., Angel, J. L., Parsons, M. T., McClain, L., Arango, H. A., & Spellacy, W. N. (1991). Human fetal response to vibroacoustic stimulation. *Obstetrics and Gynecology, 78*(5 Pt. 1), 807–811.

Pillai, M., & James, D. (1990). Are the behavioral states of the newborn comparable to those of the fetus? *Early Human Development, 22*(1), 39–49.

Platt, L. D., Walla, C. A., Paul, R. H., Trujillo, M. E., Loesser, C. V., Jacobs, N. D., & Broussard, P. M. (1985). A prospective trial of the fetal biophysical profile versus the nonstress test in the management of high-risk pregnancies. *American Journal of Obstetrics and Gynecology, 153*(6), 624–633.

Poseiro, J. J., Mendez-Bauer, C., Pose, S. V. & Caldeyro-Barcia, R. (1969). *Effect of uterine contractions on maternal blood flow through the placenta* (Scientific Publications No. 185, pp. 161–171). Washington, D.C.: Pan American World Health Organization.

Raines, D. A. (1996). Fetal surveillance: Issues and implications. *Journal of Obstetric, Gynecologic, and Neonatal Nursing, 25*(7), 559–564.

Rayburn, W. F. (1982). Antepartum fetal assessment: Monitoring fetal activity. *Clinics in Perinatology, 9*, 231–252.

Reece, E. A., Hagay, Z., Garafalo, J., & Hobbins, J. C. (1992). A controlled trial of self-nonstress test versus assisted nonstress test in the evaluation of fetal well-being. *American Journal of Obstetrics and Gynecology, 166*(2), 489–492.

Ribbert, L. S., Snijders, R. J., Nicolaides, R. H., & Visser, G. H. (1990). Relationship of fetal biophysical profile and blood gas values at cordocentesis in severely growth-restricted fetuses. *American*

Journal of Obstetrics and Gynecology, 163(2), 569–571.

Rizk, B., Atterbury, J. L., & Groome, L. J. (1996). Reproductive risks of cocaine. *Human Reproduction Update, 2*(1), 43–55.

Rochard, F., Schifrin, B. S., Goupil, F., Legrand, H., Blottiere, J., & Sureau, C. (1976). Nonstressed fetal heart rate monitoring in the antepartum period. *American Journal of Obstetrics and Gynecology, 126*(6), 699–706.

Sadovsky, E., Laufer, N., & Allen, J. W. (1979b). The incidence of different types of fetal movement during pregnancy. *British Journal of Obstetrics and Gynecology, 86*(1), 10–14.

Sadovsky, E., & Yaffe, H. (1973). Daily fetal movement recording and fetal prognosis. *Obstetrics and Gynecology, 41*(6), 845–850.

Saracoglu, F., Gol, K., Sahin, I., Turkkani, B., & Oztopcu, C. (1999). The predictive value of fetal acoustic stimulation. *Journal of Perinatology, 19*(2), 103–105.

Sarinoglu, C., Dell, J., Mercer, B. M., & Sibai, B. M. (1996). Fetal startle response observed under ultrasonography: A good predictor of a reassuring biophysical profile. *Obstetrics and Gynecology, 88*, 599–602.

Sarno, A. P., Ahn, M. O., Phelan, J. P., & Paul, R. H. (1990). Fetal acoustic stimulation in the early intrapartum period as a subsequent predictor of fetal condition. *American Journal of Obstetrics and Gynecology, 162*(3), 762–767.

Sassoon, D. A., Castro, L. C., Davis, J. L, Bear, M., & Hobel, C. J. (1990). The biophysical profile in labor. *Obstetrics and Gynecology 76*, 360–365.

Schellpfeffer, M. A., Hoyle, D., & Johnson, J. W. (1985). Antepartum uterine hypercontractility secondary to nipple stimulation. *Obstetrics and Gynecology, 65*(4), 588–591.

Schifrin, B. S. (1995). Antenatal fetal assessment: Overview and implications for neurologic injury and routine testing. *Clinical Obstetrics and Gynecology, 38*(1), 132–141.

Serafini, P., Lindsay, M. B., Nagey, D. A., Pupkin, M. J., Tseng, P., & Crenshaw, C. (1984). Antepartum fetal heart rate response to sound stimulation: The acoustic stimulation test. *American Journal of* Obstetrics and Gynecology, 148(1), 41–45.

Shah, D. M., Brown, J. E., Salyer, S. L., Fleischer, A. C., & Boehm, F. H. (1989). A modified scheme for biophysical profile scoring. *American Journal of Obstetrics and Gynecology, 160*(3), 586–591.

Shalev, E., Zalel, Y., & Weiner, E. (1993). A comparison of the nonstress test, oxytocin challenge test, Doppler velocimetry, and biophysical profile in predicting umbilical vein pH in growth-retarded fetuses. *International Journal of Gynecology and Obstetrics, 43*(1), 15–19.

Smith, C. V. (1995). Vibroacoustic stimulation. *Clinical Obstetrics and Gynecology, 38*(1), 68–77.

Smith, C. V., Phelan, J. P., Nguyen, H. N., Jacobs, N., & Paul, R. H. (1988). Continuing experience with the fetal acoustic stimulation test. *Journal of Reproductive Medicine, 33*(4), 365–368.

Smith, C. V., Phelan, J. P., Platt, L. D., Broussard, P., & Paul, R. H. (1986b). Fetal acoustic stimulation testing. II. A randomized clinical comparison with the nonstress test. *American Journal of Obstetrics and Gynecology, 155*(1), 131–134.

Snijders, R. J., McLaren, R., & Nicolaides, K. H. (1990). Computer-assisted analysis of fetal heart rate patterns at 20–41 weeks' gestation. *Fetal Diagnosis and Therapy, 5*(2), 79–83.

Sonek, J., & Nicolaides, K. (1994). The role of cordocentesis in the diagnosis of fetal well-being. *Clinics in Perinatology, 21*(4), 743–764.

Tan, K. H., & Sabapathy, A. (2001a) Fetal manipulation for facilitating tests of fetal wellbeing (Cochrane Review). *The Cochrane Library* [On-line], 4. Oxford.

Tan, K. H., & Sabapathy, A. (2001b). Maternal glucose administration for facilitating tests of fetal wellbeing (Cochrane Review). *The Cochrane Library* [On-line], 4. Oxford

Tan, K. H., & Smyth, R. (2001c). Fetal vibroacoustic stimulation for facilitation of tests of fetal wellbeing (Cochrane Review). *The Cochrane Library* [On-line], 4. Oxford.

Thaler, I., Goodman, J. D., & Dawes, G. S. (1980). Effects of maternal cigarette smoking on fetal breathing and fetal movements. *American Journal of Obstetrics and Gynecology, 138*(3), 282–287.

Timor-Tritsch, I. E., Dierker, L. J., Hertz, R. H., Deogan, N. C., & Rosen, M. G. (1978a). Studies of antepartum behavioral state in the human fetus at term. *American Journal of Obstetrics and Gynecology, 132*(5), 524–528.

Timor-Tritsch, I. E., Dierker, L. J., Hertz, R. H., & Rosen, M. G. (1979). Fetal movement: Brief review. *Clinical Obstetrics and Gynecology, 22*(3), 583–592.

Timor-Tritsch, I. E., Dierker, L. J., Zador, I., Hertz, R. H., & Rosen, M. G. (1978b). Fetal movements associated with fetal heart rate accelerations and decelerations. *American Journal of Obstetrics and Gynecology, 131*(3), 276–280.

Trudinger, B. J., & Boylan, P. (1980). Antepartum fetal heart rate monitoring: Value of sound stimulation. *Obstetrics and Gynecology, 55*(2), 265–268.

Tyrell, S. N., Lilford, R. J., MacDonald, H. N., Nelson, E. J., Porter, J., & Gupta, J. K. (1990). Randomized comparison of routine vs. highly selective use of Doppler ultrasound and biophysical profile scoring to investigate high-risk pregnancies. *British Journal of Obstetrics and Gynaecology, 97*, 909–916.

Vintzileos, A. M. (1995). Antepartum fetal surveillance. *Clinical Obstetrics and Gynecology, 38*(1), 1–2.

Vintzileos, A. M. (2000). Antenatal assessment for the detection of fetal asphyxia: An evidenced-based approach using indication-specific testing. *Annals of the New York Academy of Sciences, 900*, 137–150.

Vintzileos, A. M., Campbell, W. A., Ingardia, C. J., & Nochimson, D. J. (1983). The fetal biophysical profile and its predictive value. *Obstetrics and Gynecology, 62*(3), 271–278.

Vintzileos, A. M., Gaffney, S. E., Salinger, L. M., Kontopoulos, V. G., Campbell, W. A., & Nochimson, D. J. (1987). The relationships among the fetal biophysical profile, umbilical cord pH, and Apgar scores. *American Journal of Obstetrics and Gynecology, 157*(3), 627–631.

Vintzileos, A. M., & Knuppel, R. A. (1994). Multiple parameter biophysical testing in the prediction of fetal acid-base status. *Clinics in Perinatology, 21*(4), 823–848.

Visser, G. H., Bekedam, D. J., & Ribbert, L. S. (1990a). Changes in antepartum heart rate patterns with progressive deterioration of the fetal condition. *International Journal of Biomedical Computing, 25*(4), 239–246.

Visser, G. H., Sadovsky, G., & Nicolaides, K. H. (1990b). Antepartum heart rate patterns in small-for-gestational age third-trimester fetuses: Correlations with blood gas values obtained at cordocentesis. *American Journal of Obstetrics and Gynecology, 162*(3), 698–703.

Walkinshaw, S., Cameron, H., MacPhail, S., & Robson, S. (1992). The prediction of fetal compromise and acidosis by biophysical profile scoring in the small for gestational age fetus. *Journal of Perinatal Medicine, 20*(3), 227–232.

Ware, D. J., & Devoe, L. D. (1994). The nonstress test: Reassessment of the "gold standard." *Clinics in Perinatology, 21*(4), 779–796.

Wu, B. T. (1991). Use of fetal heart rate in the scoring system in intrapartum fetal monitoring (Chinese). *Chinese Journal of Obstetrics and Gynecology (Chung-Hua Fu Chan Ko Tsa Chin), 26*(3), 140–143.

Yanagihara, T., Ueta, M., Hanaoka, U., Tanaka, Y., Kuno, A., Kanenishi, K., Yamshiro, C., Tanaka, H., & Toshiyuki, H. (2000). Late second-trimester nonstress test characteristics in preterm delivery before 32 weeks gestation. *Gynecologic and Obstetric Investigation, 51*, 32–35.

Yao, Q. W., Jakobsson, J., Nyman, M., Rabaeus, H., Till, O., & Westgren, M. (1990). Fetal response to different intensity levels of vibroacoustic stimulation. *Obstetrics and Gynecology, 75*(2), 206–209.

CHAPTER 13

Fetal Arrhythmias and Dysrhythmias

Keiko L. Torgersen

☛ FETAL CARDIAC EMBRYOLOGY AND PHYSIOLOGY

The fetal cardiovascular system, including the heart, blood vessels and cells, all originate from the mesodermal germ layers (Sadler, 1990). There are essentially three stages of development: 1) The heart initially begins to develop as a paired tubular structure that forms a single, slightly bent heart tube by day 22 of development and connects with the developing arch system, vitelline and umbilical veins (Bharti & Lev, 1994); it is very primitive in nature (Moore, 1988). 2) Formation of the atrioventriculobulbar loop that forms the common atrium and early ventricles occurs around day 26 (Sadler, 1990). 3) Absorption of the bulbus cordis and sinus venosus forms the four-chamber heart (Bharti & Lev, 1994). It is during the second stage of development, at approximately 28 days, cardiac contractions are thought to begin in the ventriculobulbar portion of the heart, and a heartbeat begins (Gow & Hamilton, 1992).

Two theories describe the development of the fetal cardiac conduction system, specifically the sinoatrial (SA) node. The first suggests that the SA node comes from the sinus venosus musculature when the embryo is about 7–10 mm in length, usually between day 31 and day 35 (Drose, 1998; Moore, 1988). The second suggests the SA node appears as a new formation on the ventrolateral surface of the superior vena cava (Gow & Walls, 1947). Debate also exists regarding the atrioventricular (AV) node, which appears when the embryo is about 8–9 mm in length. The most recent theory is that the proximal end develops from the sinus venosus and the distal end develops from the atrial canal (Bharti & Lev, 1994). Additionally, another debate exists regarding the formation of the bundle branch (Anderson & Taylor, 1972; Fields, 1951). The debate involves "whether the bundle branches originate in situ from the ventricular trabeculae, originate from the proliferation of tissue from the AV bundle, or originate in situ from the junction of the anterior and posterior parts of the ventricular septum" (Drose, 1998, p. 7). However, there is agreement that the AV bundle and the left bundle branch appear when the embryo is about 10–11 mm in length and the right bundle branch appears when the embryo is about 13 mm in length.

The concepts of impulse formation and the process of conduction are essential to understanding arrhythmic and dysrhythmic patterns

(Cabaniss, 1993). When myocardial cells are at rest, they maintain a stable electrical charge across the cell membrane. Once an electrical impulse arrives and reduces the transmembrane charge to a threshold level, the entire cell will depolarize. After depolarization, the entire cell will then actively repolarize (Bianchi, Crobleholme & D'Alton, 2000; Cabaniss, 1993; Tanel & Rhodes, 2001). The unique automaticity—e.g., the spontaneous depolarization of cells—of the fetal heart is present early in gestation in all parts of the developing heart (Bianchi et al., 2000; Kamino, Hirota & Fujii, 1981). This automaticity occurs because the heart has specialized cells that can rhythmically and gradually reduce the charge to threshold and start the impulses spontaneously (Cabaniss, 1993). The rhythmic contraction of the heart begins around day 21–22 after conception and is present before the conduction system is fully established; it is functionally mature at approximately 16 weeks of gestation (Ho & Anderson, 1990).

The fetal heart rate (FHR) changes throughout gestation, starting slowly, at around 80 beats per minute (bpm), increasing to the range of the 170s by day 63 and then decreasing to the range of the 140s at 15 weeks of gestation (Shenker, Astle, Reed & Anderson, 1986). After 34 weeks of gestation, the FHR patterns are related to fetal rest and activity (Case & Fyfe, 1990). The specialized cells of the cardiac conduction system exist in the SA node, the AV node, the bundle of His and the Purkinje fibers (Cabaniss, 1993). The SA node is the pacemaker of the heart. The electrical signal travels down the specialized conduction tissue through the atria to the AV node. At the AV node, the conduction of the signal is slowed down. The signal then passes through the bundle of His to the Purkinje fibers, at which time the ventricle contraction is initiated (Shaffer & Wiggins, 1998).

Electrical activity actually begins before the contractile apparatus of the fetal heart completely differentiates. Electrical activity is supplied via the autonomic nervous system, specifically the sympathetic and parasympathetic nervous systems. Sympathetic innervation usually is present by day 10 and occurs via the first thoracic sympathetic ganglia. Innervation is in the SA node, the AV node and within the arterioles of the fetal circulation.

Parasympathetic innervation, present by day 80 of gestation, originates from the cardiac ganglia located on the surface and in the outflow tract of the fetal heart. In addition, sensory innervation of the fetal heart originates from the distal ganglia of the vagus nerves, although there is little clinical evidence to show at what stage of development this begins to function (Kirby, 1998).

When the parasympathetic nervous system is stimulated, the FHR decreases as a result of the vagal effect on the SA node. The SA node, as main pacemaker of the heart, is innervated by the right vagus nerve and maintains an inherent heart rate of 120–160 bpm. Stimulation of the vagal nerve will slow the SA node rate of firing, producing a decrease in the FHR. As the impulse moves through the SA node, the next stop is the AV node. The AV node is innervated by the left vagus nerve but differs in rate from the SA node and carries an inherent heart rate of 50–70 bpm. The electrical impulse leaves the AV node and travels to the AV junction. The AV junction consists of the bundle of His, the Purkinje fiber system or the ventricular myocardium. The bundle of His (AV junction) has an inherent rate of less than 40 bpm. Should the bundle of His provide the "heart rate" of the fetus, the fetus will not be viable because of the extremely low rate. The sympathetic nervous system, widely distributed throughout the fetal myocardium, increases the strength of the myocardial contraction, increases the FHR, increases arterial blood pressure and is often seen as the responsible agent for supraventricular dysrhythmias such as supraventricular tachycardia (SVT), atrial flutter or atrial fibrillation (Gewitz & Philips, 1999; Uckan & Townsend, 1999). In contrast, the parasympathetic nervous system decreases the FHR due to vagal stimulation on the SA node that decreases the rate of firing and the rate of impulse transmission from the atrium to the ventricle. It is also responsible for the transmission of impulses that creates beat-to-beat variability of the FHR (Polin & Fox, 1999; Uckan & Townsend, 1999).

Notably, sympathetic innervation is incomplete at term. However, parasympathetic innervations are fully developed during fetal life. All of these (sympathetic/parasympathetic innervations) play a role in what is seen on the fetal and electrocardiography (ECG) tracings (Uckan & Townsend, 1999).

📠 INCIDENCE

In situations of abnormal metabolism, such as fetal hypoxia, the entire cardiac impulse process may occur at other sites within the heart, resulting in abnormal fetal heart patterns (Cabaniss, 1993). Approximately 2–14% of all pregnancies exhibit fetal dysrhythmic patterns (Chan, Woo, Ghosh, Tang & Lam, 1990; Copel, Buyon & Kleinman, 1995; DeVore, Siassi & Platt, 1984; Southall et al., 1980). Of those, approximately 90% are considered benign, requiring little to no intervention. However, 10% are potentially life-threatening; they may result from cardiac structural or conduction defects or underlying maternal or fetal disease (Bianchi et al., 2000; Drose, 1998).

📠 DEFINITIONS

Although the terms "dysrhythmia" and "arrhythmia" are often used interchangeably to describe FHR patterns, they represent two different categories of patterns. Specifically, arrhythmia means a FHR without rhythm and describes the sporadic, irregular beats typical of the frequent fetal events heard or recorded on the FHR tracing. Arrhythmias are associated with variability of the R-R intervals but with normal P waves that occur in a regular fashion preceding each QRS complex. Arrhythmia is described as "any irregularity of fetal cardiac rhythm or any regular rhythm that remains outside the general range of 100–160 bpm" (Kleinman, Nehgme & Copel, 1999, p. 301). Arrhythmias occur unassociated with uterine activity.

A dysrhythmic pattern, on the other hand, is a fetal heart rhythm associated with disordered impulse formation, impulse conduction or a combination of both (Cabaniss, 1993). In essence, the pattern will demonstrate an abnormal P-QRS relationship as evidenced by early P waves or bizarre-looking QRS complexes or both. Arrhythmias and dysrhythmias both derive their names from the anatomical site of variant impulse formation, conduction or both (Figure 13-1).

📠 ETIOLOGY AND FACTORS THAT IMPACT CARDIAC SIGNAL

Arrhythmic or dysrhythmic patterns usually result from a malfunction(s) in the mechanism that creates the normal electrical impulse formation and/or impulse conduction in the heart. The problems can be a result of automaticity, excitability or conductivity.

Automaticity is the spontaneous, diastolic depolarization of normally specialized cells, e.g., the AV node, SA node, bundle of His or Purkinje fibers. That means there would be a problem with the spontaneous diastolic depolarization of the AV node, SA node, bundle of His or the Purkinje fibers. Excitability is the readiness of the cardiac cells to respond to a stimulus or irritation of the cardiac cells; therefore, the problem would be with the inability of cells to receive the impulse resulting in another area of the heart becoming the pacemaker (impulse center) of the heart. Conductivity refers to the capacity of the cardiac cells to conduct a current through the cardiac cells. This would create a problem with the cells conducting the impulse charge, or current, coming into the cells to the appropriate area of the heart.

Etiologies associated with these patterns may include conduction system defects, cardiomyopathy, cardiac tumors, cardiac structural disease, maternal collagen disease or infections such as cytomegalovirus or Coxsackie B viruses. Most dysrhythmias will convert to a normal sinus rhythm shortly after birth; however, further assessment may be warranted in some cases.

Arrhythmic or dysrhythmic patterns may also be a result of fetal cardiac anomalies or fetal heart damage. Identification and diagnosis of many fetal cardiac abnormalities is difficult because most occur in fetuses without well-defined risk factors. Overall, the incidence of congenital cardiac anomalies/fetal heart damage is low, affecting only about 10% of fetuses that demonstrate fetal arrhythmias/dysrhythmias (Bianchi et al., 2000; Drose, 1998). Some such cardiac anomalies are incompatible with postnatal life, and parents often choose to terminate such pregnancies. Regardless if an anomaly is found, in the presence of arrhyth-

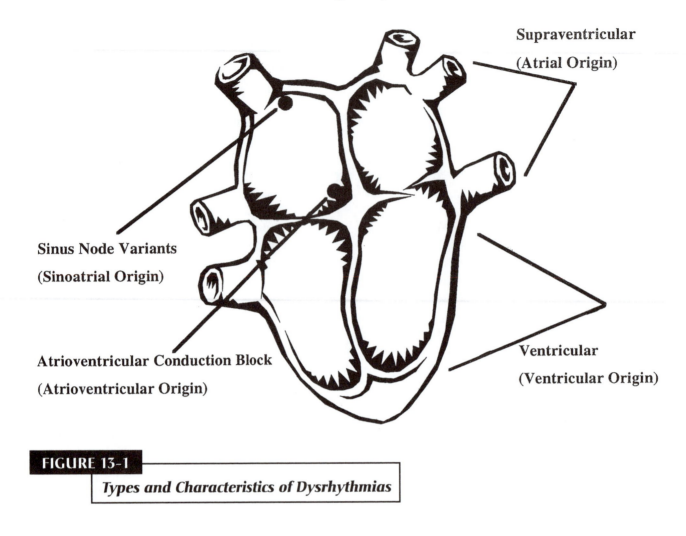

Supraventricular
(Atrial Origin)

Sinus Node Variants
(Sinoatrial Origin)

Atrioventricular Conduction Block
(Atrioventricular Origin)

Ventricular
(Ventricular Origin)

FIGURE 13-1

Types and Characteristics of Dysrhythmias

mic or dysrhythmic patterns, all fetal systems should be closely evaluated and monitored to rule out chromosomal abnormalities, and parental counseling should be initiated.

☞ DURATION

It is unclear how long a dysrhythmia may last before it should be considered abnormal (Allan et al., 1983). It is suggested that normal dysrhythmic variations last only a few seconds, whereas a dysrhythmia lasting longer than several minutes is pathologic (Allan, Crawford, Anderson & Tynan, 1984). Cameron et al. (1988) suggested several classifications, including time frames, for assessing dysrhythmic patterns. The classifications include patterns of bradycardia of 100 bpm for

more than 10 seconds and patterns of atrial or ventricular premature, or ectopic, beats that occur more than once in every 10 beats.

☞ RECORDING THE FETAL CARDIAC COMPLEX

As with adult hearts, the depolarization and repolarization of the fetal cardiac muscle cells creates electrical activity that can be recorded. The most common method of monitoring this activity is by ECG (Kleinman et al., 1999). The fetal heart produces an ECG tracing similar to the adult heart. The P wave represents atrial depolarization (atrial contraction) that forces blood through the AV valves, i.e., the tricuspid and mitral valves. The depolarization of the ventricles (ventricular contraction) is represented by the QRS complex that represents the closure of the AV valves and blood flowing through the pulmonic and aortic valves. Finally, the T wave represents the heart muscle relaxing or ventricular repolarization. The ECG is an important tool for assessing arrhythmias and dysrhythmias, as it provides valuable information concerning FHR and atrial and ventricular relationships and can help identify the origin or mechanism of a variety of abnormal FHR patterns (Kleinman et al., 1999; Shaffer & Wiggins, 1998).

Other tools, however, should also be considered before using ECG, including auscultation of the FHR and internal or external fetal heart monitoring. More technologically advanced methods are also available, such as fetal magnetocardiography (FMCG), Motion-mode (M-mode) fetal echocardiography (EchoCG) or Doppler flow studies. In all cases, maternal pulse and FHR should be assessed at the same time to distinguish the two. Concurrent assessment ensures the FHR monitor records the true FHR and not the maternal pulse.

Auscultation

Auscultation of the FHR involves listening to the audible characteristics of the FHR. As noted in chapter 5, auscultation of the FHR can be achieved using a fetoscope, a Pinard-type stethoscope or a Doppler device (Feinstein, Sprague & Trépanier, 2000). For a dysrhythmic pattern, the fetoscope or a Pinard-type stethoscope is preferred, as it allows the practitioner to hear actual heart sounds and verify the presence of a dysrhythmic FHR pattern. The Doppler device uses sound wave technology, such as ultrasonography, and cannot be used to reliably verify the presence of a dysrhythmic FHR pattern (Feinstein et al., 2000).

External and Internal Electronic Fetal Monitoring

The FHR can also be recorded externally using ultrasonography or internally using a direct fetal ECG electrode, more commonly referred to as the fetal spiral electrode (FSE). The internal mode with FSE monitors the R wave of the fetal ECG complex; the external mode with ultrasonography or Doppler device monitors a signal that is generated by the movement of the heart.

The limitations of this technology should be recognized when monitoring a fetus with unusual FHR patterns. The practitioner should be able to assess for and rule out electrical or mechanical interference, also known as artifact. Because of technological limitations, the fetal monitor can record inaccurate or incomplete data. In addition, a fetal monitoring computer's capability is limited to its programming, and the device cannot recognize numbers outside programmed ranges, that is, a FHR less than 50 bpm or greater than 240 bpm. When the device encounters rates outside of this range, it generally halves rates above 240 bpm and doubles those below 50 bpm. Therefore, the audible rate can be greater than or less than the recorded rate; in other words, a disparity exists between what is seen and what is heard.

Each fetal monitor also contains a "logic" function, also referred to as the "artifact eliminator," which is key to the monitor's ability to discern a dysrhythmic pattern. When the logic or artifact eliminator function is activated, i.e., turned on, the true FHR will not be recorded if consecutive R-R intervals increase or decrease at a rate greater than 25 bpm to 28 bpm depending on the model. Therefore, it is important to ensure the logic or artifact eliminator function is turned off to obtain a true and accurate reading of the FHR.

The use of FSE is significantly limited for sustained rapid FHR rates, as seen with SVT, atrial flutter, atrial fibrillation and ventricular tachycardia. Because of the rapid rate and the fixed R-R interval in these dysrhythmic patterns, it can be difficult to assess the short-term variability. Therefore, using the FSE will provide little to no additional information regarding baseline variability (Feinstein & McCartney, 1997).

Regardless of the monitoring mode, the practitioner should also assess the tracing for electrical or mechanical interference (artifact). This is done by checking the security of the connection on the monitoring device and listening for skipped beats not picked up by external modes of monitoring.

Chapter 5 includes a more detailed discussion of internal and external methods of fetal assessment.

Doppler Velocimetry

Doppler velocimetry has been used to diagnose dysrhythmias and arrhythmias. It is a noninvasive method of looking at and quantifying placental resistance to blood flow (Burner, Gabbe, Levy & Arger, 1993). This technique allows the practitioner to analyze arterial waveforms in the fetal heart for evidence of increased peripheral resistance, as is sometimes seen with dysrhythmic patterns. It is most reliable in fetuses predisposed to intrauterine growth restriction (IUGR), such as those with maternal hypertensive disorders, collagen vascular diseases or other diseases where vasospasms play a major role (King & Simpson, 2001). Despite its ability to identify increased peripheral resistance, Doppler velocimetry is not as reliable for diagnosing dysrhythmic patterns and, therefore, is not used as frequently as other technological advances.

Fetal Echocardiogram

A more useful diagnostic tool to assess dysrhythmic fetal heart patterns is the fetal echocardiogram. If a sustained dysrhythmia is recognized, fetal ECG is recommended for direct imaging of cardiac wall motion to assess for rhythm, cardiac structure, cardiac function, fetal well-being, and to determine if hydrops is present.

Fetal Magnetocardiography

Fetal magnetocardiography (FMCG) is a noninvasive diagnostic tool used to analyze electrophysical changes of the heart as early as 20 weeks of gestation. Compared with other common methods, FMCG provides more information that can be used to influence therapeutic decisions and thus contribute to optimal pre- and postnatal management. However, its clinical applicability and correlation with methods, such as ECG, high-resolution two-dimensional imaging, M-mode, pulsed-wave Doppler and color Doppler imaging, have not been demonstrated (Kleinman et al., 1999). If no dysrhythmias are found after the cardiac study with FMCG, further follow up provides no added benefit.

M-Mode EchoCG

M-mode EchoCG uses real-time imaging techniques to observe and time electromechanical events of the fetus' cardiac activity (Kleinman et al., 1999). This evaluation often follows a two-dimensional examination (Shaffer & Wiggins, 1998) and is considered essential in differentiating some arrhythmias (DeVore et al., 1984). At the present time, the use of M-mode EchoCG is the most accurate method for confirmation or identification of the dysrhythmic pattern and for assessment of the effects on the fetus (DeVore et al., 1984; Shaffer & Wiggins, 1998; Strasburger, 2000). Following the EchoCG, weekly follow-up evaluations with auscultation are recommended to assess for runs of tachycardia. M-mode imaging is helpful in evaluating contractility in abnormalities that affect heart wall motion by looking at the timing of atrial and ventricular events in the cardiac conduction cycle. Then, analysis of the AV contraction sequence can provide an accurate picture of the precise cardiac rhythm (Kleinman et al., 1983; Shaffer & Wiggins, 1998). M-mode EchoCG has also been found to be helpful in assessing and evaluating valve motion and FHR (Drose, 1998).

Color-coded M-mode EchoCG provides an added dimension by showing flow information in color. This method provides important physiologic data that may help discern structural cardiac damage (Copel, Morotti, Hobbins & Kleinman, 1991), as well as analyzing the electromechanical activity of the fetal heart (Kleinman et al., 1999).

Some factors may limit the data from the M-mode EchoCG. These factors include poor resolution due to maternal obesity, polyhydramnios, and rib shadowing and difficulty obtaining a reproducible view due to fetal movement and position change in utero (Strasburger, 2000).

Pulsed Doppler EchoCG

Pulsed Doppler EchoCG provides information about electromechanical events as well as views of the heart chambers and the great vessels. The use of pulsed Doppler EchoCG has been found to enhance the ability to detect cardiac malformations in utero (Reed, Sahn, Marx, Anderson & Shenker, 1987). This feature can provide the parents with reassurance about the fetal heart, even though the incidence of structural heart defects causing dysrhythmic patterns is relatively low. The cardiac specialist also can view the fetal heart in two- and three-dimensional views to assess cardiac rhythm, rate, and determine dysrhythmias from normal cardiac function. Most of these tools are only available at tertiary care medical centers or medical facilities specializing in fetal or pediatric cardiology.

☞ FETAL ARRHYTHMIAS

The literature describes three main types of rhythm disturbance encountered in the fetus: 1) irregular heart rhythms, 2) tachyarrhythmias (fast heart rhythms) and 3) bradyarrhythmias (slow heart rhythms) (Crosson & Benner, 1999; Kleinman et al., 1999; Sharland, 2001). The most common arrhythmia is an irregular heart rhythm; however, it is usually a benign pattern (Kleinman, 1986; Sharland, 2001; Silverman, Enderlein, et al., 1985). An irregular heart rhythm can occur secondary to isolated extrasystoles or premature beats that can be either atrial or ventricular in origin (Kleinman, 1986; Silverman, Enderlein, et al., 1985). The premature atrial beat can also be conducted to the ventricles, causing ventricular contraction, or, if it occurs early in diastole, it may not be conducted (i.e., nonconducted) and result in a "missed beat" (Crosson & Brenner, 1999; Kleinman et al., 1999; Sharland, 2001).

Sinus Node Variants

Most sinus node variants are patterns of baseline change (see Chapter 6). Most are common phenomena that usually have no effect on the well-being of the fetus, as there is usually no change in the true fetal ECG, i.e., a change reflected in the rate but not in the cardiac rhythm or conduction cycle.

Intermittent periods of bradycardia are considered benign when they are accompanied by long-term variability that is average or within normal limits or by short-term variability (Feinstein & McCartney, 1997; Parer, 1997). However, a sustained bradycardia requires further assessment and evaluation.

Sinus Bradycardia

Sinus bradycardia is a FHR less than 110 bpm sustained for greater than 10 minutes (Figure 13-2). Some sources define sinus bradycardia, from the standpoint of an arrhythmia, as a FHR less than 100 bpm (Crosson & Brenner, 1999; Shaffer & Wiggins, 1998; Sharland, 2001; Strasburger, 2000). The ECG will illustrate normal P waves occurring in routine relationship preceding each QRS complex. Sinus bradycardia reflects abnormal fetal or maternal condition, such as maternal or fetal compromise (Feinstein & McCartney, 1997; Parer, 1997; Tucker, 2000). This is due to parasympathetic stimulation or the withdrawal of sympathetic stimulation. Sinus bradycardia between 90 and 120 bpm often demonstrates average variability and is considered benign or reassuring/normal baseline rate for many healthy fetuses. (Feinstein & McCartney, 1997; Freeman, Garite, & Nageotte, 1991; Parer, 1997; King & Simpson, 2001).

Sinus bradycardia can also occur under other specific physiologic and pathologic stimuli. The most common etiology is head compression, which stimulates the vagus nerve and thus lowers the FHR. Other less frequent causes include hypothermia, hypoxia and a response to certain drugs, such as beta-blocking agents. Persistent sinus bradycardic rates of less than 100 bpm are considered unusual and are associated with IUGR, increased vagal tone, maternal beta-blocker therapy, prolonged QT syndrome or severe fetal hydrops (Allan et al., 1984; Ferrer, 1998; Meijboom et al., 1994; Shaffer & Wiggins, 1998; Sharland, 2001; Southall et al., 1979).

Sinus Tachycardia

Tachycardias, also referred to as tachyarrhythmias, are the second most common type of fetal

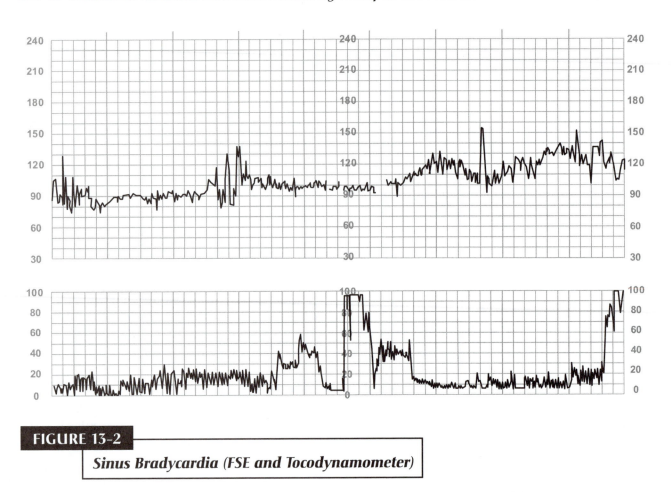

FIGURE 13-2

Sinus Bradycardia (FSE and Tocodynamometer)

arrhythmia. (Shaffer & Wiggins, 1998). They can be classified as either arrhythmias, such as sinus tachycardia or as dysrhythmias, such as SVT, atrial flutter, atrial fibrillation or (rarely) ventricular tachycardia (Crosson & Brenner, 1999; Kleinman et al., 1999; Shaffer & Wiggins, 1998; Sharland, 2001; Strasburger, 2000). Sinus tachycardia is classified as a sinus node variant, which is an arrhythmia of the FHR; the remaining tachyarrhythmias are classified as dysrhythmias of the FHR and are discussed later in this chapter.

Sinus tachycardia is defined as a FHR greater than 160 bpm sustained for greater than 10 minutes (Figure 13-3). Some sources define sinus tachycardia, as related to an arrhythmia, as a FHR greater than 180 bpm (Crosson & Brenner, 1999; Shaffer & Wiggins, 1998; Sharland, 2001; Strasburger, 2000). The ECG will demonstrate normal P waves (normal atrial contraction) occurring in routine fashion preceding each QRS complex (normal

ventricular contraction), much like sinus bradycardia. In contrast to SVT, sinus tachycardia shows some variability within the baseline rate at a rate of around 5–15 bpm (Shaffer & Wiggins, 1998).

Unlike sinus bradycardia, sinus tachycardia is produced by the withdrawal of parasympathetic stimulation of the sinus node or sympathetic stimulation (Crosson & Brenner, 1999; Shaffer & Wiggins, 1998). Sinus tachycardia may result from a variety of physiologic and pathologic stimuli. The most common causes are responses to continuous fetal activity, maternal fever or certain medications, e.g., betasympathomimetic drugs, such as terbutaline, or parasympatholytic medications, such as atropine, hydralazine (Apresoline) or hydroxyzine hydrochloride (Atarax) (Crosson & Brenner, 1999; Kleinman et al., 1999; Sharland, 2001; Strasburger, 2000). Other causes may be underlying fetal abnormalities such as a compensatory response to hypoxia, secondary to barore-

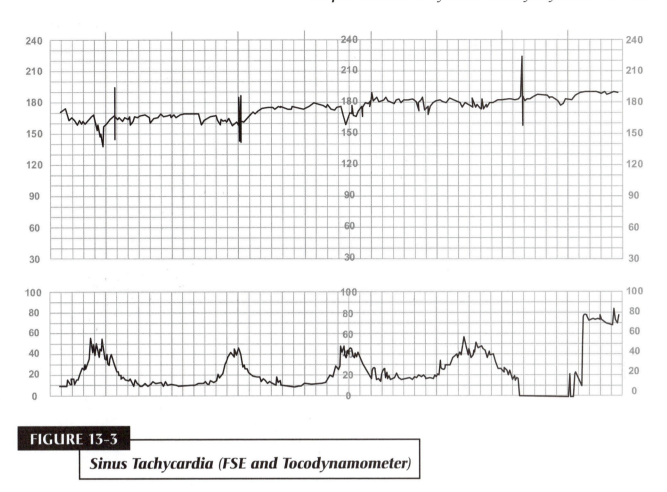

FIGURE 13-3

Sinus Tachycardia (FSE and Tocodynamometer)

ceptors or chemoreceptor stimulation (Shaffer & Wiggins, 1998); acidosis; myocarditis; maternal drug ingestion or hormone or catecholamine transfer (Mucklow, 1986; Pickoff, 1998).

Sinus tachycardia usually does not exceed 200–210 bpm (Crosson & Brenner, 1999; Shaffer & Wiggins, 1998; Strasburger, 2000). However, when it does exceed 210 bpm, it is difficult to differentiate from SVT, secondary to the rapid rate. Also because of the very rapid heart rate, it may be difficult to assess short-term variability, making the differentiation between sinus tachycardia and SVT even more challenging (Crosson & Brenner, 1999; Shaffer & Wiggins, 1998; Strasburger, 2000).

Marked Sinus Arrhythmia

Marked sinus arrhythmia is a normal phenomenon enhanced by a limited number of physiologic and pathologic stimuli, such as respirations, hypoxia and certain medications, such as ephedrine. Marked sinus arrhythmia occurs when there is an alternating stimulation and removal of parasympathetic nervous system activity in response to fetal hypoxemia. Marked sinus arrhythmia is also often seen as a result of the partial pressure of oxygen (PO_2) and partial pressure of carbon dioxide (PCO_2) relationship that is mediated by the baroreceptors and chemoreceptors (Cabaniss, 1993; Crosson & Brenner, 1999; Kleinman et al., 1999).

This arrhythmic pattern can demonstrate changes in the FHR varying as much as 120 bpm within 5-second intervals. This pattern is most frequently seen with increased uterine activity and is commonly referred to as marked long-term variability (Cabaniss, 1993). However, unless repetitive decelerations accompany this pattern, there is usually no significant change noted in fetal oxygenation (Reiss, Gabbe & Petrie, 1996)

(Figure 13-4). Marked sinus arrhythmia is believed to be produced by stimulation of the parasympathetic nervous system alternating with the withdrawal of parasympathetic activity, i.e., producing a sympathetic response. The most common cause is a parasympathetic response to fetal hypoxemia (Cabaniss, 1993; Murray, 2001). This pattern is seen most often with increased uterine activity. Marked sinus arrhythmia is commonly associated with bradycardia and can be seen preceding prolonged and nonreassuring variable decelerations (King & Simpson, 2001; Tucker, 2000).

Treatment for sinus bradycardia, sinus tachycardia, and marked sinus arrhythmia is addressed in Chapter 7.

◼ FETAL DYSRHYTHMIAS

As noted earlier, fetal dysrhythmias are classified, or named, based on their origin and are referred to as supraventricular, ventricular or AV dysrhythmias. Supraventricular dysrhythmias are often referred to as "premature beat," "extrasystole" or "tachyarrhythmia" patterns and occur more commonly than "premature" ventricular dysrhythmic patterns (Cabaniss, 1993; Crosson & Brenner, 1999; Kleinman et al., 1999). Unlike the sinus node variants, dysrhythmic patterns show actual changes in the fetal ECG. Atrial depolarization occurs early in the cardiac contraction phase and usually results in a P wave occurring early in relation to the QRS complex (Crosson & Brenner, 1999; Murray, 2001; Shaffer & Wiggins, 1998; Sharland, 2001; Strasburger, 2000). An irregular pattern or "skipped" beat(s) can be heard with ultrasonography or a fetoscope. Typically these patterns are considered benign and require no intervention other than observation. Regardless of the pattern, the dysrhythmias tend to disappear in late labor, particularly during uterine contractions, during pushing or passive descent of

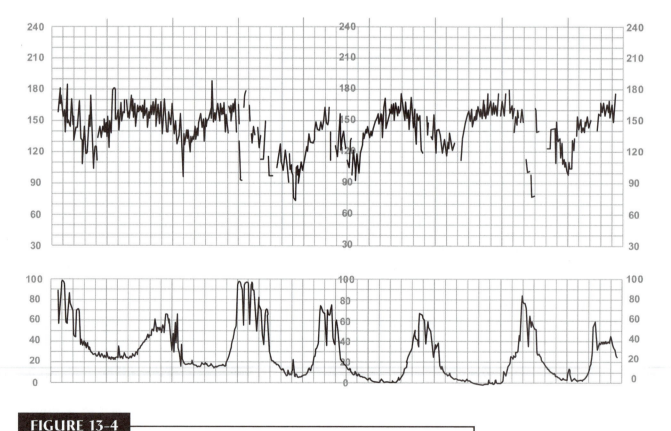

FIGURE 13-4

Marked Sinus Arrhythmia (FSE and Tocodynamometer)

the fetus in the second stage of labor, during variable decelerations or soon after birth. These patterns usually are not associated with any underlying cardiac disease (Cabaniss, 1993; Copel et al., 1995; Kleinman et al., 1999). Atrial dysrhythmias can precipitate SVT in susceptible fetuses, which is the major clinical reason for evaluating fetuses with extrasystoles (dysrhythmias) (Kleinman et al., 1999). The prognosis of fetal tachycardia depends on the presence of associated physiology, the type of fetal heart pattern, the presence of fetal hydrops, the heart rate and the availability and relative success of treatment (Sharland, 2001; Strasburger, 2000).

Supraventricular Dysrhythmias

Supraventricular dysrhythmias are patterns that originate above the ventricles, i.e., in the atria, hence the term "supraventricular." Supraventricular patterns include, but are not limited to, premature atrial contractions (PACs), PACs with bigeminy, trigeminy or both and tachyarrhythmias, such as SVT, atrial flutter and atrial fibrillation.

PACs

Premature atrial contractions (Figure 13-5 A, B) may be associated with redundancy or an aneurysm of the foraminal flap (Fyfe, Meyer & Case, 1988; Steward & Wladimiroff, 1988), as well as maternal use of caffeine, cigarettes or alcohol (Nyberg & Emerson, 1990; Strasburger, 2000). They can be either conducted (i.e., PAC followed by a ventricular contraction, then a compensatory pause followed by normal sinus rhythm) or nonconducted (i.e., PAC followed by compensatory pause) (Shaffer & Wiggins, 1998). They are characterized by the early discharge of an atrial focus, as seen by a premature P wave followed by a narrow, normal-appearing QRS complex. Often a PAC is followed by an incomplete compensatory pause, produced by the incomplete depolarization of the fetal heart (Crosson & Brenner, 1999; Kleinman et al., 1999; Shaffer & Wiggins, 1998). The fetal tracing will illustrate vertical spikes above and below the FHR baseline, often creating an illusion of three parallel horizontal lines. The

upper line, often above 180 bpm, is produced by the premature beat. The lower line is produced by the incomplete compensatory pause and is usually only a short distance from the FHR baseline, which forms the middle line on the tracing. The middle line may be observed for variability, accelerations or decelerations (Cabaniss, 1993). These patterns occur more frequently than premature ventricular contractions (PVCs) but, as noted earlier, usually do not suggest any underlying cardiac disease. However, 1% of fetuses with persistent PACs can develop SVT in as little as 36 hours (Kleinman, 1986).

Etiologies for PAC development include maternal ingestion of caffeine, alcohol or nicotine; maternal hyperthyroidism; trisomy 18 and drug exposure (Cabaniss, 1993; Strasburger, 2000). If supraventricular dysrhythmic patterns occur intrapartally, they typically disappear during labor, making intrauterine therapy unnecessary. Congenital cardiac malformations have been reported in up to 2% of fetuses with isolated extrasystoles (Beall & Paul, 1986; Reed, 1991).

Premature atrial contractions also can occur in patterns identified as PACs with bigeminy (occurring every other beat), PACs with trigeminy (occurring every third beat) or a combination of both (PACs with bigeminy and trigeminy) (Fyfe, Meyer & Case, 1993; Reed, 1989). They can also occur in conjunction with other dysrhythmic or arrhythmic patterns (Reed, 1989), for example, sinus tachycardia accompanied by PACs with bigeminy.

PAC with Bigeminy, Trigeminy or Both

Atrial bigeminy occurs when a premature atrial depolarization or contraction occurs with every other beat. The pattern will be one normal beat (normal P-QRS relationship) and one premature beat, or PAC (Cabaniss, 1993; Shaffer & Wiggins, 1998) (Figure 13-6 A, B). Such a pattern is the most frequent type of intrapartum fetal dysrhythmia (Cabaniss, 1993; Strasburger, 2000). If it occurs with bigeminy alone, the monitor tracing gives the appearance of two horizontal parallel lines. The upper line will reflect the rate between the normal and premature beats, and the lower line will reflect the partial (or incomplete) compensatory pause.

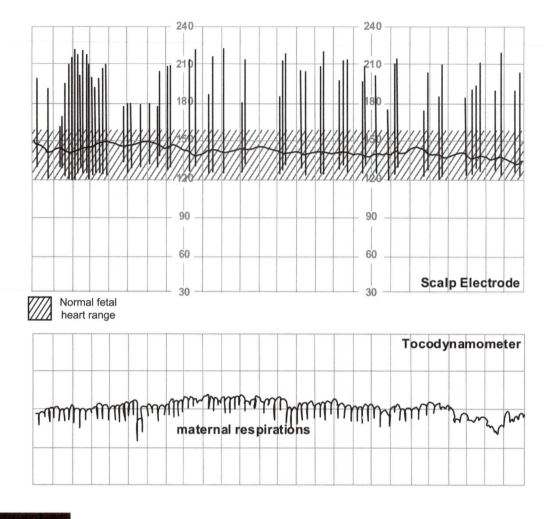

The baseline FHR will be obscured because of the pattern; therefore, it will not be seen during the bigeminal pattern. This pattern (PAC with bigeminy) may also be seen in conjunction with a slight slowing of the baseline FHR or with shallow variable decelerations (Cabaniss, 1993).

Atrial trigeminy occurs when a premature atrial depolarization or contraction occurs with every third beat. The pattern will be two normal beats (normal P-QRS relationship) and one premature beat, or PAC. (Figure 13-7 A, B) The fetal tracing will show vertical spikes with long upward strokes and short downward strokes (Cabaniss, 1993). The upward stroke represents the premature beat, and the downward stroke represents the partial (incomplete) compensatory pause; the baseline FHR will be seen intermittently between the premature beats. If an atrial dysrhythmia occurs with both bigeminy and trigeminy, the bigeminal pattern often dominates the appearance, and the tracing will show uninterrupted parallel vertical lines, often with the baseline obscured (Cabaniss, 1993; Murray, 2001; Strasburger, 2000).

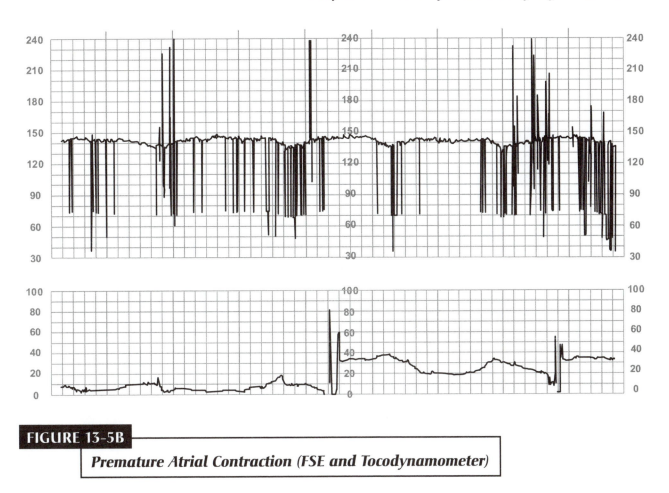

FIGURE 13-5B

Premature Atrial Contraction (FSE and Tocodynamometer)

Nonconducted PACs

Nonconducted PACs occur with the discharge of an atrial focus that is too premature to move through the AV junctional tissue. The premature depolarization—because it partially penetrates the AV junction—is followed by a pause until the AV junction recovers sufficiently to admit the next sinus node discharge (Cabaniss, 1993; Kleinman et al., 1999). The ECG will show an early P wave, often occurring in the apex or descending limb of the previous T wave, followed by a pause that is terminated by the next sinus beat (Cabaniss, 1993). The upper line represents the normal baseline rate, and the lower line represents the pause produced by the nonconducted premature beat. The baseline FHR is visible on the tracing (Figure 13-8 A, B) (Cabaniss, 1993). Multiple missed beats may produce a slow ventricular rate, which can be difficult to distinguish from complete heart block (Sharland, 2001).

SVT

Among the few dysrhythmic patterns that are cause for concern is SVT (Figure 13-9). It is also the second most frequent cause of fetal tachycardia, after maternal infection (Kleinman et al., 1999; Shaffer & Wiggins, 1998; Strasburger, 2000). The pattern of SVT usually presents between 15 and 40 weeks of gestation, yet it is seen most commonly around 30–32 weeks of gestation (Allan et al., 1984; Cuneo & Strasburger, 2000; Ferrer, 1998). It is a sustained, rapid, regular dysrhythmia of atrial origin in excess of 180–210 bpm and may be paroxysmal (i.e., occurring suddenly or in waves/spasms) or continuous. At rates lower than 210 bpm, the FHR pattern may show some variability within the baseline rate at a rate of around 5–15 bpm (Shaffer & Wiggins, 1998). Supraventricular tachycardia is often characterized by a fixed R-R interval with P waves preceding each QRS complex, as identified by ECG. This

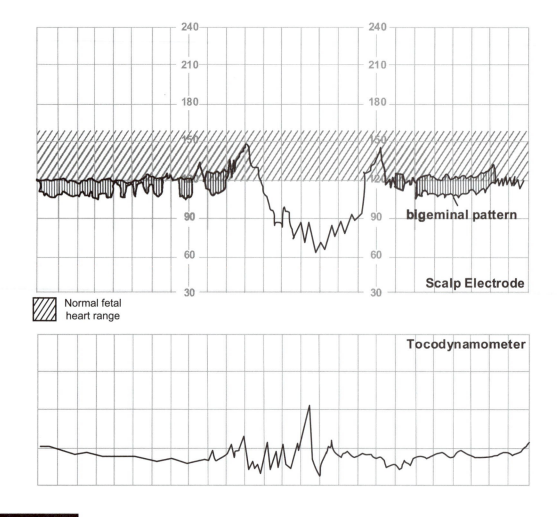

Normal fetal heart range

bigeminal pattern

Scalp Electrode

Tocodynamometer

FIGURE 13-6A

PAC with Bigeminy (FSE and Tocodynamometer)
Note: From *Fetal Monitoring Interpretation,* by M. L. Cabaniss, 1993, p. 477.
Copyright © 1993 Lippincott-Raven. Reprinted with permission.

pattern is usually initiated by PVCs, but 1% of PACs, especially persistent PACs, can also develop into SVT in as little as 36 hours (Crosson & Brenner, 1999). Supraventricular tachycardia may contribute to increased birth weight, heavier placenta and neonatal diuresis of a few days' duration, often related to hydrops (Crosson & Brenner, 1999). Lastly, SVT may also be associated with betamimetic therapy, such as ritodrine or terbutaline (Cabaniss, 1993).

In general, SVT has very little baseline FHR variability, especially in rates greater than 240 bpm; stops and starts abruptly when initiated by

ectopy; responds to conventional transplacental treatment with digoxin at least 50% of the time and has one-to-one AV concordance (Allan, 1984; Allan et al., 1983; Chao, Ho & Hsieh, 1992; Gembruch, Redel, Bald & Hansmann, 1993; Kleinman et al., 1999; Shaffer & Wiggins, 1998; Strasburger, 2000).

Different mechanisms are responsible for SVT; SVT may be 1) reentrant or reciprocating (related to the circus movement of the electrical activity), 2) automatic (as result of irritable ectopic focus in the bundle of His) or 3) the result of atrial flutter or fibrillation (Gillette, 1976; Kleinman et al.,

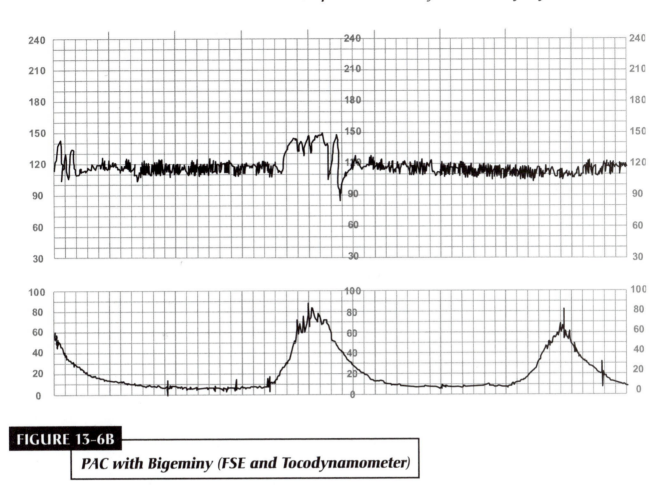

FIGURE 13-6B

PAC with Bigeminy (FSE and Tocodynamometer)

1999; Moak, 1990; Perry & Garson, 1990; Shaffer & Wiggins, 1998; Strasburger, 2000). However, most fetal SVTs are reentrant in nature (Kleinman et al., 1999; Shaffer & Wiggins, 1998; Simpson & Marx, 1994; Strasburger, 2000). Essentially, more than one pathway conducts the impulse, with the primary pathway being blocked. Because of the blockage, the electrical impulse is carried over the secondary pathway, but the reentry of the impulse occurs over the primary pathway, hence the circus movement. In 5–10% of patients, SVT has been associated with structural congenital heart disease (Beall & Paul, 1986; Reed, 1989); it is also associated with poor prognosis (Bergmans, Jonker & Kock 1985).

The rapid heart rate that occurs with SVT increases the workload of the fetal heart and, therefore, increases the cardiac oxygen demand. As a result, the stroke volume is decreased because of the decreased filling time that causes the cardiac output to decrease. The fetal body can no

longer meet the oxygen demand, causing congestive heart failure and increased breakdown, or hemolysis, of red blood cells (Strasburger, 2000; Tanel & Rhodes, 2001). The prolonged hemolysis then progresses to nonimmunologic hydrops fetalis—which is the development of generalized edema in the abdomen, scalp, liver and spleen—and fetal death (Murray, 2001; Strasburger, 2000). The rate and progression of the hydrops depend on the severity of the hemodynamic compromise, as well as gestational age (Strasburger, 2000). The undelivered or untreated fetus may develop cardiac failure and ischemic cerebral disease. Often, the fetus will demonstrate evidence of pericardial or pleural effusion, cardiomegaly, polyhydramnios, scalp edema or ascites, all of which are suggestive of congestive heart failure (Shaffer & Wiggins, 1998; Strasburger, 2000).

On occasion, an SVT can come directly from the atria without relying on the ventricles to sustain the tachycardic rate. This type of SVT is

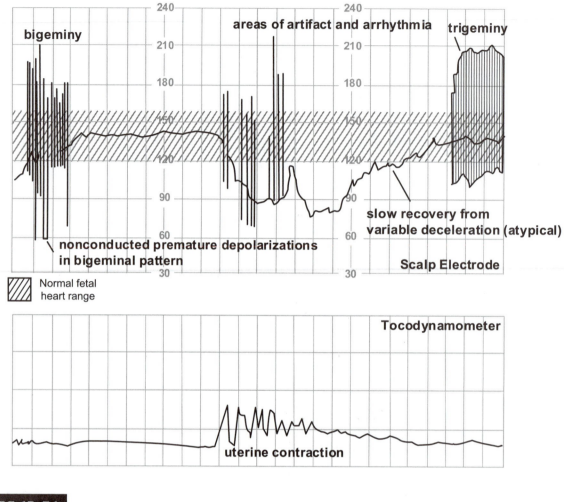

FIGURE 13-7A

PAC with Trigeminy (FSE and Tocodynamometer)
Note: From *Fetal Monitoring Interpretation*, by M. L. Cabaniss, 1993, p. 475.
Copyright © 1993 Lippincott-Raven. Reprinted with permission.

referred to as primary atrial tachycardia. The Doppler reading will show a fixed one-to-one AV relationship; i.e., the impulses are generated by the atria, not the ventricles, and the atrial rate is faster than the ventricular rate (Murray, 2001; Strasburger, 2000; Tanel & Rhodes, 2001). When this occurs, the fetus often manifests Wolff-Parkinson-White (WPW) syndrome, which is the most common type of fetal tachycardia, accounting for two thirds of all fetal tachycardias (Crosson & Brenner, 1999). Wolff-Parkinson-White syndrome is difficult to diagnose in utero and, when present, it is far more likely to be diagnosed at birth

rather than in utero. It has been reported to be present in about 8–15% of neonates at birth (Ferrer, 1998; Murray, 2001; Strasburger, 2000).

Atrial Flutter

If persistent, SVT can lead to more devastating, yet unusual, dysrhythmic patterns known as atrial flutter (Figure 13-10) and atrial fibrillation (Kleinman et al., 1999; Shaffer & Wiggins, 1998; Strasburger, 2000). Although their incidence is low, these patterns are associated with a high fetal mortality rate, often as a result of the difficulty

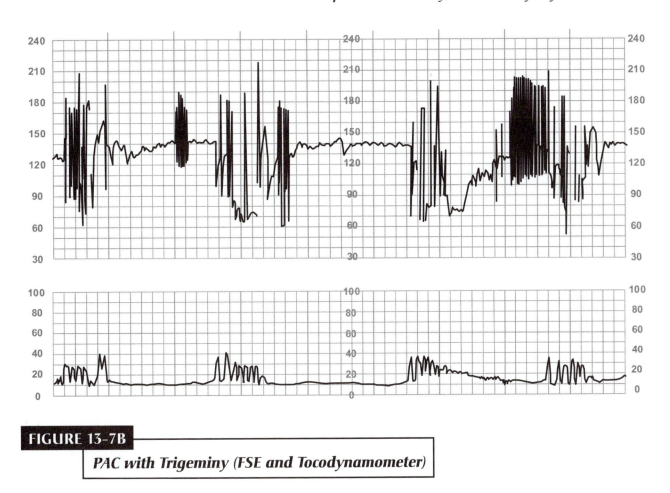

PAC with Trigeminy (FSE and Tocodynamometer)

controlling the dysrhythmic pattern and its high association with congenital cardiac anomalies (Kleinman et al., 1999; Shaffer & Wiggins, 1998; Strasburger, 2000). Like SVT, atrial flutter is also a reentry dysrhythmia. In atrial flutter, the AV node is not part of the circus movement and is responsible only for the transmission of the atrial flutter waves to the ventricles (Kleinman et al., 1999; Strasburger, 2000). Typically, the atrial rate in atrial flutter and atrial fibrillation varies from 400–500 bpm for the fetus and 300–360 bpm for the neonate. Because of the significantly increased FHR, the ventricular response varies, resulting in the rate being either fixed (2:1 or 3:1 AV block) and regular or variable and irregular (i.e., varying degrees of AV block) (Case & Fyfe, 1990; Shaffer & Wiggins, 1998). The ECG reading will usually display regularly recurring saw-toothed atrial activity instead of the normal P wave. The monitor tracing also may show half counting of the FHR, as with SVT (Cabaniss, 1993).

Atrial flutter has been associated with reentrant SVT, atrial septal defect, hypoplastic left heart syndrome, Ebstein's malformation of the tricuspid valve, cardiomyopathy and, more rarely, with familial rickets and dislocated hip (Ferrer, 1998; Kleinman et al., 1983; Shenker, 1979).

Atrial Fibrillation

Atrial fibrillation is even more rare than atrial flutter (Kleinman et al., 1999; Strasburger, 2000). Atrial fibrillation may be associated with fetomaternal hemorrhage, neonatal WPW syndrome and cardiac structural abnormalities, with the cardiac abnormalities contributing the most to the high mortality rate. When atrial fibrillation occurs in the antepartum period it is often accompanied by a variable degree of AV block that will cause the ventricular rate to vary from 60 to 200 bpm. The ECG reading will often show low-amplitude irreg-

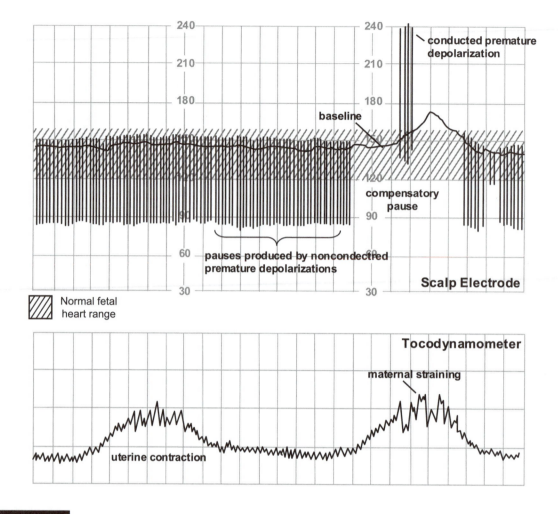

FIGURE 13-8A

Nonconducted PAC (FSE and Tocodynamometer)
Note: From *Fetal Monitoring Interpretation,* by M. L. Cabaniss, 1993, p. 483.
Copyright © 1993 Lippincott-Raven. Reprinted with permission.

ular atrial activity with complexes of various sizes (Cabaniss, 1993).

Ventricular Dysrhythmias

As the term implies, ventricular dysrhythmias are ventricular in origin and are the result of premature electrical discharge below the AV junction. Just as with PACs, these patterns are referred to as "premature beat" patterns, yet occur less frequently (3–8%) than supraventricular dysrhythmias (Cabaniss, 1993; Kleinman et al., 1999; Strasburger, 2000).

PVCs

Premature ventricular contractions in the fetus are extremely rare (Murray, 2001; Strasburger, 2000). They have been associated with cardiomyopathy, long QT syndrome, complete AV block with rates less than 55 bpm, hydrops fetalis, myocarditis, digitalis toxicity, cocaine use, hyperkalemia (although rare in pregnancy) due to hyperemesis, structural cardiac anomalies or unknown reasons (Allan et al., 1984; Cabaniss, 1993; Ferrer, 1998; Murray, 2001; Silverman, Kleinman, Copel, Weinstein, Santulli & Hobbins, 1985; Southall et al., 1979).

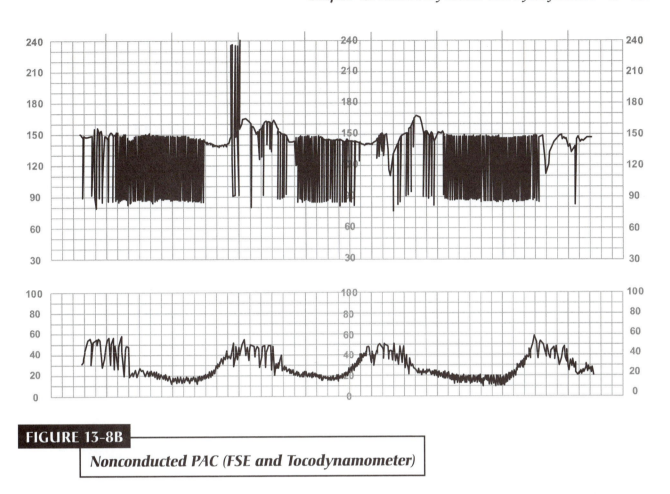

FIGURE 13-8B

Nonconducted PAC (FSE and Tocodynamometer)

The frequency may be increased by maternal use of caffeine, nicotine or alcohol, similar to PACs (Cabaniss, 1993).

On the fetal ECG, PVCs will show no P wave, and the premature QRS is bizarre and wide, with the T wave usually directed opposite to the polarity of the QRS complex. The full compensatory pause may or may not be present. The fetal monitor tracing for PVCs will show vertical spikes, usually of equal distance above and below the normal FHR baseline, and can resemble a "chimney" shape (Figure 13-11). The tracing may also appear as three parallel horizontal lines, with the upper line representing the rate produced by the premature beat, the lower line representing the compensatory pause and the middle line representing the rate produced by normal cardiac cycles. Because the middle line represents the rate produced by the cardiac cycles, it can give some semblance of variability, but it is not beat-to-beat. The tracing

may also show a long lower spike without the top spike (Cabaniss, 1993). Therefore, it cannot be assessed as short-term variability.

PVCs with Bigeminy, Trigeminy or Both

As with PACs, PVCs can occur with bigeminy, trigeminy or both (Cabaniss, 1993; Strasburger, 2000). Premature ventricular contractions with bigeminy will show no middle line; therefore, the FHR and variability are obscured (Figure 13-12) (Cabaniss, 1993; Murray, 2001).

Premature ventricular contractions with trigeminy show a FHR pattern in a regular pattern of vertical parallel lines (Figure 13-13). The rate represented by the top line is produced by the premature beat, whereas the rate represented by the bottom line is produced by the full compensatory pause. The middle line represents the FHR, but because it represents only every third beat, it does

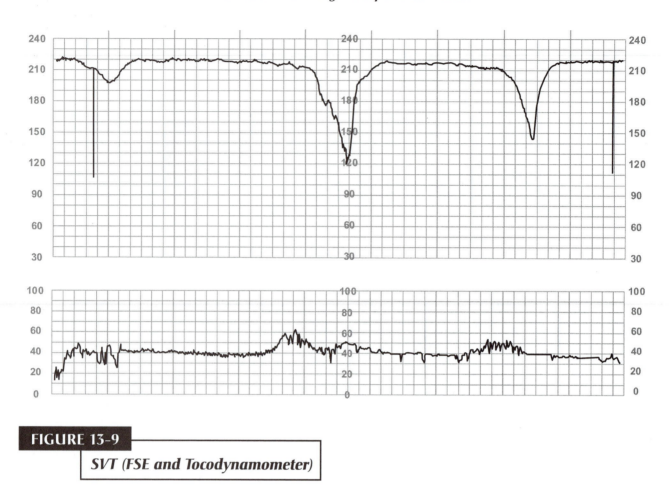

FIGURE 13-9

SVT (FSE and Tocodynamometer)

not represent true beat-to-beat variability (Cabaniss, 1993). If PVCs occur with bigeminy or trigeminy, the monitor tracing may appear as a vertical line downward and upward from the baseline, with the upward line appearing longer than the downward line. In this case, the unequal distance of the vertical line reflects the premature beat and the compensatory pause of the PVC (Cabaniss, 1993; Murray, 2001). In the FSE mode, as the electrical activity of the heart is displayed, a premature ventricular depolarization (or contraction) appears in the pattern as just described. Ultrasonography reflects the irregular motions of the heart wall or heart valve and displays the change. In a tracing showing a PVC with both bigeminy and trigeminy, the baseline FHR can appear as an interrupted line, giving the appearance of a dotted line between the PVCs (or spikes) (Figure 13-14 A, B).

As with atrial dysrhythmias, these patterns are considered benign events and tend to disappear in late labor, particularly during uterine contractions or soon after birth (Cabaniss, 1993; Strasburger, 2000). In general, they require no treatment in utero or postnatally (Strasburger, 2000). If PVCs are present, the mother should avoid cardiac stimulants (Strasburger, 2000). On occasion, pharmacological therapy is used to correct the patterns but is usually not warranted, as the fetus is seldom jeopardized, and these patterns are known to convert spontaneously.

Ventricular Tachycardia

Ventricular tachycardia is a rare fetal abnormality in which FHR varies between 170 and 400 bpm (Shaffer & Wiggins, 1998; Strasburger, 2000). Ventricular tachycardia in the fetus is usually an

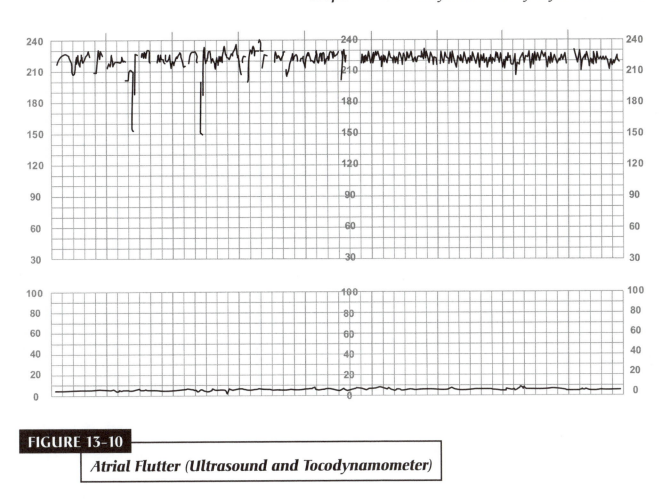

FIGURE 13-10

Atrial Flutter (Ultrasound and Tocodynamometer)

accelerated ventricular rhythm that competes with the normal sinus rhythm and AV dissociation, because the ventricular rate is faster than the atrial rate (Shaffer & Wiggins, 1998; Strasburger, 2000). Sustained rapid ventricular tachycardia has been reported rarely (Kleinman et al., 1999; Strasburger, 2000). A fetus with ventricular tachycardia may not be ill at all and may not require treatment (Kleinman et al., 1999; Shaffer & Wiggins, 1998; Strasburger, 2000). However, the dysrhythmic pattern should be distinguished from other types of tachycardia to avoid a negative impact on the fetus (Shaffer & Wiggins, 1998).

AV Dysrhythmias

Atrioventricular dysrhythmias consist of second- and third-degree AV block (Crosson & Brenner,

1999; Kleinman et al., 1999; Shaffer & Wiggins, 1998; Strasburger, 2000). These dysrhythmic patterns result from an AV conduction defect. First-degree AV block is difficult to recognize in the fetus and has no known pathophysiology (Cabaniss, 1993). Second-degree AV block, Mobitz type I, or Wenckebach, is not seen in the fetus (Cabaniss, 1993). However, second-degree AV block, Mobitz type II, occurs but is difficult to diagnose in the fetus because the atrial and ventricular rates may appear as the same rate.

Second-Degree AV Block

Second-degree AV block, Mobitz type II, is associated with rapid atrial rate due to SVT, atrial flutter or atrial fibrillation. Second-degree AV block is associated with maternal collagen vascular dis-

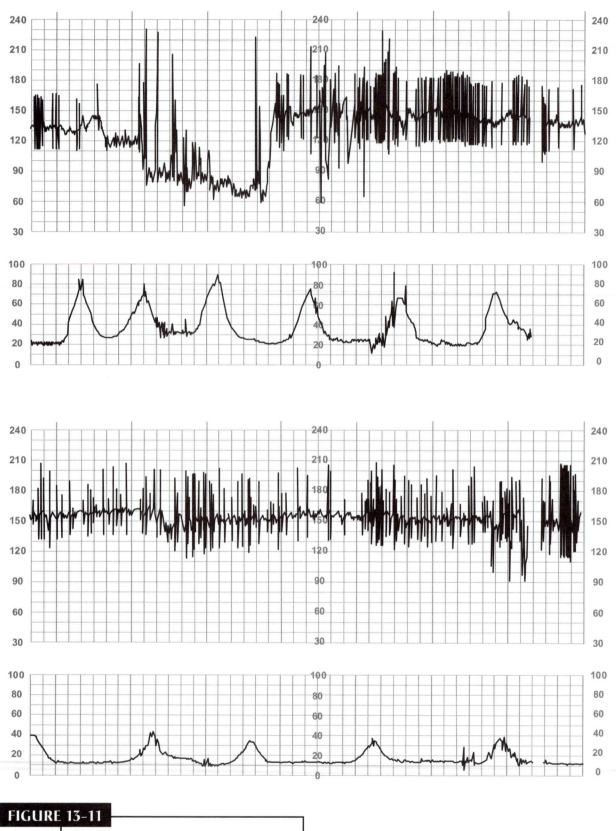

FIGURE 13-11

PVC (FSE and Tocodynamometer)

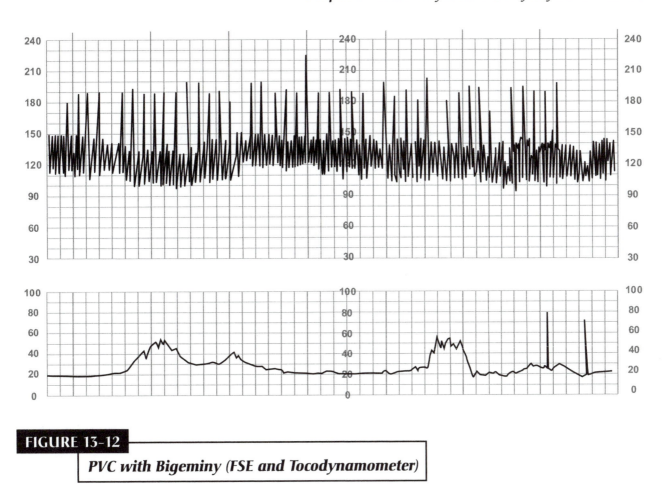

FIGURE 13-12

PVC with Bigeminy (FSE and Tocodynamometer)

ease and cardiac structural defects (Crosson & Brenner, 1999; Kleinman et al., 1999; Strasburger, 2000). The relationship between maternal collagen disease and AV block centers on the antibodies developed by the mother to a soluble tissue ribonucleotide antigen known as Ro. Ro antigens deposit themselves along the fetal cardiac tissue and involve the AV node and the atrial and ventricular myocardium of the fetus. An inflammatory reaction occurs, leading to fibrosis, calcification and, eventually, interruption of the fetal conduction pathway. Thus, AV block develops (Alexander, Buyon, Provost & Guarnieri, 1992; Esscher & Scott, 1979; Lanham, Walport & Hughes, 1983; Strasburger, 2000; Watson & Katz, 1991).

The block represents failure of some of the atrial pulses to be conducted. The hallmark of second-degree heart block is a regular atrial rhythm. Clinical deterioration, specifically fetal hydrops fetalis, is less with this pattern, and treatment is

often not needed unless fetal deterioration occurs (Strasburger, 2000).

Third-Degree AV Block

Third-degree, or complete, AV block may also be seen in the fetus (Figure 13-15 A, B). Complete AV block is caused by either maternal anti-SSA (B) antibodies or congenital heart disease. Whether treatment is beneficial in the fetus with AV block caused by antibodies is still under debate. If the mechanism thought to cause AV block is myocarditis, then corticosteroid treatment should be effective (Tulzer, 2000). Classically, fetuses with third-degree AV block fall into one of two categories: 1) congenital complete heart block (CCHB) associated with complex congenital heart disease or 2) complete heart block secondary to autoimmune disease-producing autoantibodies that destroy the fetal cardiac conductive

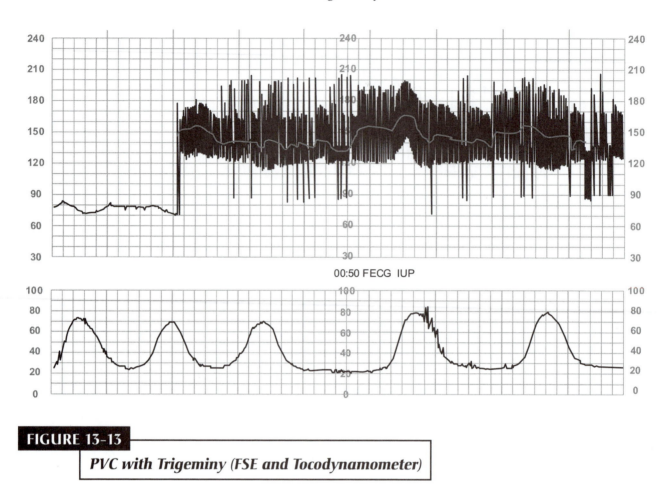

FIGURE 13-13

PVC with Trigeminy (FSE and Tocodynamometer)

tissue (Freidman, Zervoudakis & Buyon, 1998; Horsfall, Venables, Taylor & Maini, 1991; Litsey, Noonan, O'Connor, Cottrill & Mitchell, 1985; Moodley et al., 1986; Schmidt, Ulmer, Silverman, Kleinman & Copel, 1991; Tanel & Rhodes, 2001; Taylor, Scott, Gerlis, Esscher & Scott, 1986). The incidence of fetuses demonstrating third-degree heart block secondary to a variety of major congenital anomalies varies between 30% and 60% (Allan et al., 1984; Freidman et al., 1998; Shaffer & Wiggins, 1998; Strasburger, 2000). The most common presentation is regurgitation of the mitral or tricuspid valves, damage to the His-Purkinje tissues, inflammation of the AV node and the bundle of His or damage to fetal myocardium, all leading to congestive cardiomyopathy (Shaffer & Wiggins, 1998; Strasburger, 2000; Tulzer, 2000). In their research of autoimmune disease in pregnancy, Pinsky, Rayburn and Evans reported, "Subclinical and clinical autoimmune diseases

from mom were present in approximately one half of all affected fetuses" (1991; 306). Fetal hydrops may develop subsequent to cardiomyopathy. Steroid treatment is used to arrest the deposition of the immune complexes and halt further damage to the cardiac tissue.

Third-degree AV block has also been associated with fetal cytomegalovirus infection and antiphospholipid antibody syndrome (Kleinman et al., 1999; Strasburger, 2000).

Third-degree heart block represents the complete absence of conduction of P waves. The fetal tracing shows a 50–70 bpm rate unless the external Doppler is placed over the fetal atria, in which case a rapid rate will appear.

The overall prognosis for fetuses with AV block depends on the etiology, presence of hydrops fetalis and the atrial and ventricular rates. Fetuses with ventricular rates greater than 55 bpm and atrial rates greater than 120 bpm without evidence

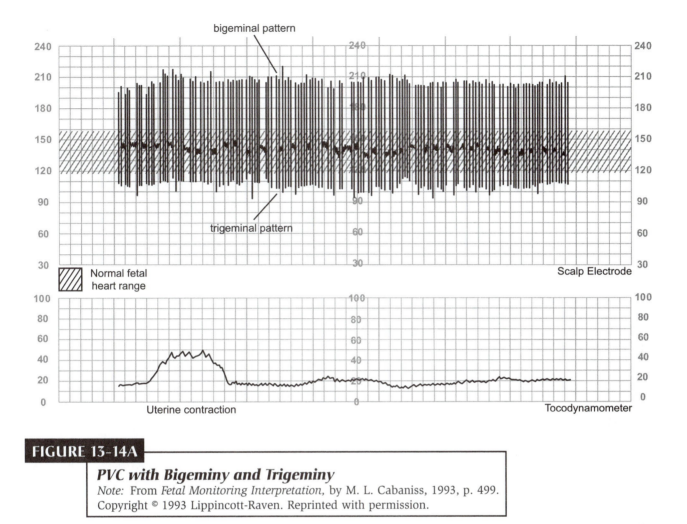

FIGURE 13-14A

PVC with Bigeminy and Trigeminy

Note: From *Fetal Monitoring Interpretation*, by M. L. Cabaniss, 1993, p. 499.
Copyright © 1993 Lippincott-Raven. Reprinted with permission.

of hydrops fetalis usually have positive prognoses (Shaffer & Wiggins, 1998; Strasburger, 2000).

Fifty to sixty-five percent of mothers whose fetuses demonstrate complete AV block will have laboratory or clinical evidence of connective tissue disease, such as systemic lupus erythematosus (Pinsky, Rayburn & Evans, 1991; Shaffer & Wiggins, 1998; Strasburger, 2000). However, third-degree AV block associated with maternal collagen disease, in general, has a better prognosis than heart block associated with structural lesions of the heart, which usually result in a poor fetal or neonatal prognosis. In approximately 53% of cases, complete AV block is associated with major cardiac malformation; in 25%, it is associated with chromosomal defects or a combination of both

malformation or chromosomal defects (Allan et al., 1984; Watson & Katz, 1991). Surprisingly, fetuses with third-degree AV block do well in utero and require intervention only at delivery. However, fetuses with hydrops, associated congenital cardiac malformations or ventricular rates below 50 bpm have poor outcomes, often resulting in death (Kleinman et al., 1999; Shaffer & Wiggins, 1998; Strasburger, 2000). When complex congenital heart disease is associated with complete AV block, the in utero fetal demise rate has been reported to be as high as 50%. If hydrops fetalis coexists, the death rate is 100% (Ferrer, 1998; Gudmundsson et al., 1991; Machado, Tynan, Curry & Allan, 1988).

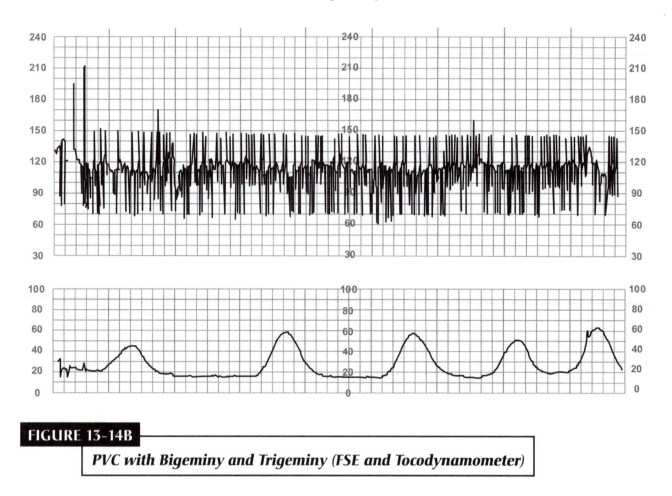

FIGURE 13-14B

PVC with Bigeminy and Trigeminy (FSE and Tocodynamometer)

Treatment

Treatment regimens have been established as a result of numerous research studies conducted over the past 10 years. Table 13-1 describes a selection of treatment recommendations.

Treating fetal dysrhythmias is a complex process. It requires a multidisciplinary team approach, an accurate diagnosis and an individualized treatment plan for both the woman and her fetus. Regardless of the situation, parents should be offered pretreatment counseling. Options range from conservative management to inutero treatment to pregnancy termination. Discussion of treatment options requires openness and cultural sensitivity on the part of the medical and nursing team. In mothers with maternal connective tissue disease and a previously affected fetus, prophylactic treatment may be warranted, as the risk of recurrent heart block in subsequent pregnancies

is as high as 33% (Buyon et al., 1988; Machado et al., 1988; Michaelsson & Engle, 1972; Rosenthal, Groves, Allan et al., 1996).

Treatment depends on the type of pattern. Medication should be avoided in the first trimester, if at all possible. Medications that have the longest record of safety should be considered as the first-line agents for treating dysrhythmic patterns (Joglar & Page, 2001). Simpson et al. support a conservative management scheme in which many cases of intermittent fetal tachycardia without evidence of fetal hemodynamic compromise are observed closely, possibly avoiding the need for potentially dangerous pharmacotherapy.

The risks inherent in antidysrhythmic therapy depend largely on the electrophysiologic mechanism of the dysrhythmia and the pattern observed. Once identified, the appropriate antidysrhythmic agents can be determined. Individual responses of the woman and her fetus to each agent should

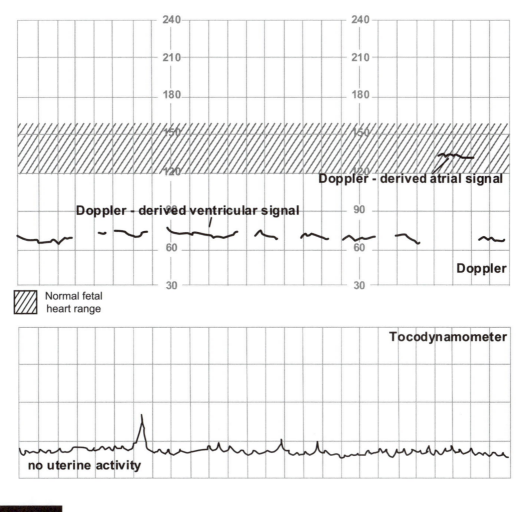

FIGURE 13-15A

Third-Degree (Complete) AV Block (Ultrasound and Tocodynamometer)
Note: From *Fetal Monitoring Interpretation,* by M. L. Cabaniss, 1993, p. 514. Copyright © 1993
Lippincott-Raven. Reprinted with permission.

be observed during treatment. The decision to treat fetal dysrhythmias should be based on an understanding of the natural history of the rhythm disturbances and cannot be predicated simply on the basis of presence of the dysrhythmia or on the frequency of episodes of fetal tachycardia.

Prior to antidysrhythmic therapy, a fetal EchoCG should be obtained. Once the EchoCG is obtained and drug treatment is initiated the woman should be monitored by means of a 12-lead continuous ECG during the drug loading-dose phase. In addition, the fetus should be monitored

either by ultrasonography or fetal EchoCG during the antidysrhythmic drug loading doses.

Treatment for alarming patterns, such as tachyarrhythmias, can be difficult and is often associated with significant morbidity and mortality. None of the antidysrhythmic agents are without significant risk to the fetus or the woman or both, and all have a variety of side effects. Use of these agents requires knowledge of pharmacology, underlying electrophysiologic mechanisms and the electrophysiologic and hemodynamic effect of the agents. The half-life of these agents also must

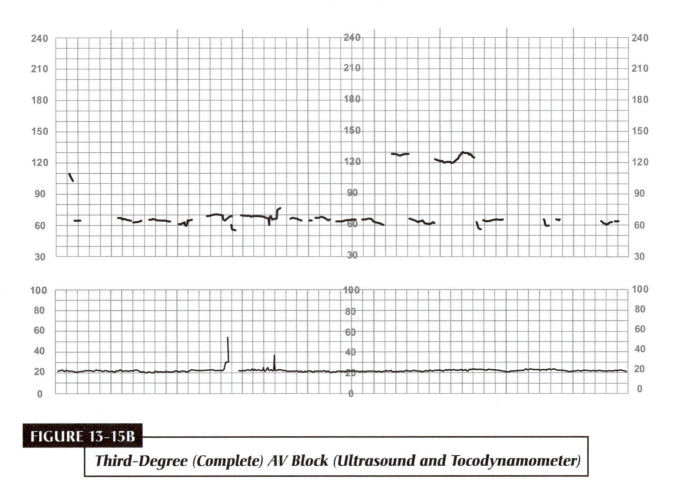

FIGURE 13-15B

Third-Degree (Complete) AV Block (Ultrasound and Tocodynamometer)

be considered when changing medications or using a combined regimen of antidysrhythmic agents. Regardless of the agent used, all antidysrhythmic therapy should be initiated on an inpatient basis with external fetal cardiac monitoring for 12–24 hours.

In the pharmacology arena, antidysrhythmic agents are also referred as antiarrhythmic agents. They are classified according to their predominant effects on the action potential of the agent. For example, a Class I agent would block the voltage-sensitive sodium channels in the same manner anesthetics would. Therefore, Class I agents generally cause a decrease in exciteability and conduction velocity within the heart. However, classification is not clear-cut, because these agents can demonstrate actions, or have active metabolites belonging to a different class of drugs. The classes of antidysrhythmic agents are Class IA, IB, IC, II, III, and IV. Class I is subdivided into three groups according to their effect on the duration of the action potential. (Table 13-2) (Mycek, Harvey, & Champe, 1997).

Patients taking medications with proarrhythmic effects—i.e., medications that can change a normal sinus rhythm pattern to arrhythmic/dysrhythmic pattern, the most common being beta-adrenergic sympathomimetics—should discontinue such medications. Patients should also be warned to avoid cocaine. Regardless of the pattern, all neonates will need care using a multidisciplinary team approach involving obstetric, pediatric cardiology and neonatology personnel until a definitive diagnosis and coordinated a plan of care can be established.

Treatment of sinus node variants is addressed in Chapter 7.

TABLE 13-1

Drug Therapy

DRUG	INDICATED USE	RECOMMENDED DOSAGE	SIDE EFFECTS	EFFECTIVENESS
Adenosine (Class IV, FDA Class C)	Supraventricular dysrhythmias	IV: 100–200 mcg/kg of EFW via rapid IV bolus into umbilical vein; fetal therapy via maternal IV not recommended PO: Not available	Bronchospasm (w/ asthmatic patients); dyspnea; transient arrhythmias (bradycardia) after cardioversion; known to ↑ AV block	Assists in identifying SVT (reentrant in nature); does not prevent recurrent SVT. First option for acute treatment of SVT (Joglar & Page, 2001).
Amiodarone (Class III, FDA Class D)	Supraventricular dysrhythmias; ventricular dysrhythmias	IV: 5 mg/kg over 20 min; 500–1,000 mg over 24 h, then oral administration PO: Loading dose: 1,200–1600 mg divided in two doses for 7–14 days; then 400–800 mg every day for 1–3 wk Maintenance: 200–400 mg/d	Can ↑ digoxin level; fetal hypothyroidism; maternal/fetal hyperthyroidism; corneal micro deposits; prematurity; low birthweight, congenital malformations; photosensitivity; life-threatening pulmonary alveolitis (not found to be dose-related); hepatitis; myopathy; neuropathy; nausea; rash; alopecia; tremors; insomnia; nightmares; fetal cretinism; hypotension	Considered "last-resort" drug; not recommended for use unless adequate doses of other antiarrhythmic drugs are unsuccessful or not tolerated. Adverse reactions require drug discontinuation in about 25% of patients. Can be found in breast milk for several weeks post drug administration.
Digoxin (Glycoside, FDA Class C)	Supraventricular dysrhythmias; atrial fibrillation (AF) rate control	IV: 1,200–1,500 mcg/24 h (loading only) Maintenance: 375–875 mcg/d PO: Divided BID	Toxicity = fetal arrhythmias; nausea & vomiting; anorexia; diarrhea; malaise; fatigue; confusion; facial pain; insomnia; depression. Vertigo and poor color vision may occur at low serum levels, especially if hypokalemia or hypomagnesemia is present. Interacts w/ other antiarrhythmic agents such as quinidine, verapamil, amiodarone and propafenone. Can also interact w/ erythromycin. Give lower dose if patient is in renal failure	Contraindicated in ventricular arrhythmias/WPW syndrome. May not be as effective in hydropic fetuses due to poor absorption. Requires frequent ECG monitoring to assess toxicity. Considered safe for breast feeding (Joglar & Page, 2001).

(table continues)

TABLE 13-1 (cont.)

Drug Therapy

DRUG	INDICATED USE	RECOMMENDED DOSAGE	SIDE EFFECTS	EFFECTIVENESS
Disopyramide (Class I-A, FDA Class C)	Supraventricular dysrhythmias; ventricular dysrhythmias	PO: Loading dose: 300 mg Maintenance: 100–200 mg q 6 h	Hypotension; negative inotropic effect; Torsades de Pointes; induction of uterine contractions; vagolytic effects; zero interaction with digoxin. Interacts w/ Class III cardiac agents	Rarely effective in children/adults; very limited experience in fetuses; other alternatives are available. May exacerbate CHF. May harm fetus. Compliance is often difficult because of side effects. Compatible w/ breastfeeding (Joglar & Page, 2001; Vautier-Rit et al., 2000).
Flecainide (Class I-C, FDA Class C)	Supraventricular dysrhythmias; ventricular arrhythmias	PO: 50–200 mg BID	Increased mortality/exacerbated CHF in patients w/ previous myocardial infarction/ dysfunction. Can provoke potentially lethal arrhythmias (reentrant V-tach). Can cause heart block in patients w/ abnormal conduction. ↓ FHR variability	Useful in fetal SVT w/o structural heart disease, especially those resistant to digoxin. First-line agent for treating fetal SVT w/ hydrops. Compatible w/ breastfeeding (Joglar & Page, 2001).
Ibultilide (Class III) (FDA Class C)	Acute AF/atrial flutter	0.1 mL/kg. If no effect, may give second dose of 0.1 mL/kg 10 minutes after first dose	Torsades de Pointes	No experience in pregnancy.
Lidocaine (Class I-B, FDA Class B)	Ventricular dysrhythmias; dysrhythmias due to digoxin toxicity	IV: 75–100 mg, then 2–4 mg/min Fetal IV: 1 mg (when used)	Dosage should be ↓ in patients w/ liver impairment. Toxicity can induce seizure activity. CNS adverse effects; bradycardia	Rare experience with fetal arrhythmias; not for chronic use or fetal indications. Avoid if fetal distress is present. Compatible w/ breastfeeding (Jogler & Page, 2001).

TABLE 13-1 (cont.)

Drug Therapy

DRUG	INDICATED USE	RECOMMENDED DOSAGE	SIDE EFFECTS	EFFECTIVENESS
Mexiletine (Class I-B, FDA Class C)	Ventricular dysrhythmias	IV: Not available in U.S. PO: Loading dose: 400 mg, then 100–400 mg q 8 h	Hypotension; bradycardia; GI side effects; CNS side effects. Interacts with beta-blockers and disopyramide. Low APGAR	Limited fetal use reported; not for use in fetal arrhythmias. Compatible w/ breastfeeding (Jogler & Page, 2001).
Phenytoin (Class I-B, FDA Class D)	Ventricular dysrhythmias; arrhythmias due to digoxin toxicity	IV: Not available in U.S. PO: 100–400 mg BID	Hypotension; vertigo; lethargy; dysarthria; mental retardation; gingivitis; macrocytic anemia; lupus; pulmonary infiltrates; growth restriction; fetal hydantion syndrome	Prolonged QT interval syndrome. Better alternative therapies are available. Caution advised w/ breastfeeding (Jogler & Page, 2001).
Procainamide (Class I-A, FDA Class C)	Supraventricular dysrhythmias; undiagnosed wide complex tachycardia	IV: 100 mg bolus over 2 min; up to 25 mg/min to 1 g over first hour Maintenance: 2–6 mg/min PO: 1 g; then up to 500 mg q 3 h	Hypotension with IV. Limit oral use to 3–6 mos. (especially in patients with lupus). Lupus-like syndrome w/ long-term use; ↑ digoxin level; GI symptoms; agranulocytosis. Interacts w/ Class III cardiac drugs, causing Torsades de Pointes. Known to accumulate in fetus if mother has high serum levels of drug in her system.	Long record of safety; oral dose frequency requirement may result in noncompliance. Compatible w/ breastfeeding; however, long-term use is not recommended (Jogler & Page, 2001).
Propafenone (Class I-C, FDA Class C)	Supraventricular dysrhythmias; ventricular dysrhythmias	IV: Not available in U.S. PO: 150–300 mg TID	Increases digoxin level; prolongs QRS complex; negative inotropic effects; proarrhythmia; GI side effects common. Avoid in patients w/ CAD or ventricular dysfunction.	Effective in treating dysrhythmias associated w/ WPW syndrome, ventricular premature complexes, and nonsustained V-tach. Unknown effect w/ breastfeeding.
Propranolol (Class II, FDA Class C/D)	Supraventricular dysrhythmias; ventricular dysrhythmias; AF rate control	IV: 1–6 mg slowly PO: 40–60 mg q 6 h	IUGR; bronchospasm; CNS depression. Interacts w/ other agents to ↑ heart block/↓ inotropic effect. May blunt hypoglycemia in patients w/ diabetes. May affect glucose tolerance in patients w/ non-insulin-dependent diabetes. Maternal hypotension. Contraindicated	Use of atenolol questionable. Has been successful in suppressing ectopy in fetuses w/ reentrant SVT (especially if ecurrent). May cause neonatal respiratory depression, rhypoglycemia or bradycardia. Has been associated with

(table continues)

TABLE 13-1 (cont.)

Drug Therapy

DRUG	INDICATED USE	RECOMMENDED DOSAGE	SIDE EFFECTS	EFFECTIVENESS
Propranolol (cont.)			in sick sinus syndrome and Raynaud's disease. Fetal apnea.	low birthweight infants. Compatible w/ breastfeeding (Joglar & Page, 2001).
Quinidine (Class I-A, FDA Class C)	Supraventricular dysrhythmias; ventricular dysrhythmias	PO: 200–300 mg q 6 h; 300–600 mg q 8–12 h if sustained dosage used	Hypotension; GI effects; Torsades de Pointes; ↑ digoxin levels. Monitor QRS/QTc intervals. Maternal/fetal thrombocytopenia. Idiosyncratic reactions (angioedema/vascular collapse) may occur more commonly. Eighth nerve toxicity	Does ↑ mortality; can result in increase in existing atrial dysrhythmias/V-tach resulting in sudden death. Caution advised w/ breastfeeding (Joglar & Page, 2001).
Sotalol (Class III, FDA Class B)	Supraventricular dysrhythmias; ventricular dysrhythmias; atrial tachycardias	IV: Not available in U.S. PO: 80–320 mg BID	Torsades de Pointes w/ hypokalemia; negative inotropic effect; sinus bradycardia; AV block	More successful experience w/ atrial flutter than w/ SVT.
Verapamil (Class IV, FDA Class C)	Supraventricular dysrhythmias; idiopathic V-tach; AF rate control	IV: 5–10 mg over 30–60 sec PO: 80–160 mg TID	Calcium channel blocker; negative inotropic agent; ↑ serum digoxin levels; ↓ SA/AV node function; maternal hypotension. Contraindicated in sick sinus syndrome, w/ MgSO₄ therapy, second- or third-degree heart block, shock, CHF, and w/ concomitant beta-blocker therapy. Fetal bradycardia; heart block. May cause V-fib if given to patient in V-tach. Fatigue; HA; dizziness; skin rash; peripheral edema	IV use for treatment of SVT w/ cardiac failure is contraindicated in neonates. Exercise caution w/ all patients. Compatible w/ breastfeeding (Joglar & Page, 2001).

Class I—Na⁺ (sodium) channel blockers; Class II—b-adrenoreceptor blockers; Class III—K⁺ (potassium) channel blockers; Class IV—Ca⁺⁺ (calcium) channel blockers (Mycek, M. J., Harvey, R. A. & Champe, P .C. (1997). *Lippincott's Illustrated Reviews: Pharmacology* (2nd ed.). Philadelphia: Lippincott-Raven (pp. 163–174).

Abbreviations: BID, twice daily; CAD, coronary artery disease; CHF, congestive heart failure; CNS, central nervous system; EFW, estimated fetal weight; GI, gastrointestinal; HA, headache; IV, intravenous; MgSO₄, magnesium sulfate; MI, myocardial infarction; PO, by mouth; q, every; TID, three times daily; V-fib, ventricular fibrillation; V-tach, ventricular tachycardia; w/, with; w/o, without.

Joglar, J. A., & Page, R. L. (2001). Antiarrhythmic drugs in pregnancy, *Current Opinion in Cardiology, 16,* 40–45.
Vautier-Rit S., Dufour, P., Vaksmann, G., Subtil, D., Vaast, P., Valat, A. S., Dubos, J. P., & Puech, F. (2000). Fetal arrhythmias: Diagnosis, prognosis, treatment; apropos of 33 cases. *Gynecologic & Obstetric Fertility, 28,* 729–737.

TABLE 13-2

Classification of Antidysrhythmic Drugs

CLASSIFICATION OF DRUG	MECHANISM OF ACTION	COMMENT
IA	β-Adrenoreceptor blocker	Blocks cells that are discharging at abnormally high rate (slows Phase 0 depolarization)
IB	Na⁺ channel blocker	Blocks cells that are depolarizing or firing rapidly shortening repolarization (shortens Phase 3 repolarization)
IC	Na⁺ channel blocker	Markedly slows conduction in all cardiac tissue (markedly slows Phase 0 depolarization)
II	β-Adrenoreceptor blocker	Depresses automaticity, prolongs AV conduction, and decreases heart rate and contractility. Used to treat supraventricular dysrhythmias caused by increased sympathetic nervous system activity; also used for atrial flutter, atrial fibrillation, and AV nodal reentrant tachycardia (suppresses Phase 4 depolarization).
III	K⁺ channel blocker	Block potassium channels diminishing outward potassium current during repolarization (prolongs Phase 3 repolarization)
IV	Ca⁺⁺ channel blocker	Blocks open or inactivated calcium channels slowing phase 4 spontaneous depolarization and slows conduction in tissues dependent on calcium currents, i.e., AV node (shortens action potential)

Adapted from: Mycek, M. J., Harvey, R. A. & Champe, P. C. (1997). *Lippincott's Illustrated Reviews: Pharmacology* (2nd ed.), Philadelphia: Lippincott-Raven (pp. 163–174).

Supraventricular Dysrhythmias

SVT

Treatment of SVT is highly effective and improves fetal outcome (Simpson & Sharland, 1998). Treatment recommendations range from observation only to early delivery of the affected fetus to prenatal drug therapy (Crosson & Brenner, 1999; Joglar & Page, 2001; Murray, 2001; Sharland, 2001; Strasburger, 2000; Tulzer, 2000). Observation is often used when the pregnancy is near term, the tachycardic episodes are short-lived, and fetal cardiac failure is not evident. Delivery prior to term depends on the gestational age and the presence of fetal cardiac failure. The risks of preterm delivery and its associated complications should be weighed against the risk of a continued cardiac dysrhythmic pattern and its associated complications. Prenatal drug therapy is advocated for a variety of patterns. Treatment depends on the gestational age, presence of cardiac failure, duration of the pattern and parental wishes. The most important prognostic indicator for a fetus is the presence or absence of hydrops fetalis (Sharland, 2001; Strasburger, 2000).

Supraventricular tachycardia can be converted with scalp stimulation, especially during the intrapartum period. Scalp stimulation stimulates the vagus nerve, thus stimulating the parasympathetic nervous system and lowering the FHR (Cabaniss, 1993; Murray, 2001).

In nonhydropic fetuses, digoxin monotherapy is very effective and safe, with conversion rates as high as 62%. However, the hydropic fetus with SVT remains a therapeutic challenge; in such cases, digoxin monotherapy is much less effective because of poor placental transfer and low fetal serum levels (20%) (Tulzer, 2000).

If found in the antepartum period, SVT often can be successfully converted pharmacologically using digoxin, adenosine, verapamil, procainamide, quinidine or propranolol via maternal route or percutaneous umbilical route. Digoxin is often considered to be the first-line agent for conversion of SVT found in the antepartum period (Joglar & Page, 2001; Kleinman et al., 1999; Strasburger, 2000). It is administered to the mother intravenously until the SVT converts to a normal sinus rhythm. Direct fetal administration of digoxin may be more effective but it requires repetitive invasive procedures, potentially exposing both the woman and her fetus to subsequent problems, such as infection and hemorrhage. As a result, direct fetal administration with digoxin is not recommended. Once the SVT is converted, the intravenous digoxin is converted to the oral route, and the woman is maintained on the drug until delivery. Cuneo and Strasburger (2000) found that fetuses also benefited from fetal intramuscular injections of antidysrhythmic agents coupled with transplacental antidysrhythmic therapy. In one United Kingdom study, flecainide was found to be the most effective and most rapidly acting drug, with a 59% conversion rate (Tulzer, 2000).

Because of their negative inotropic effects (i.e., weakening the force of cardiac contractions), verapamil and propranolol can cause maternal hypotension and can compromise the function of the fetal heart. Additionally, propranolol has also been associated with IUGR and is not as effective for treatment of SVT as other antidysrhythmic drugs. New to the armamentarium for SVT is sotalol, a Class III cardiac drug that has beta-blocker effects normally seen in Class II agents, as well as a potassium channel-blocker effect of the Class III cardiac drugs. In addition to the successful conversion of SVT, sotalol has also been effective in converting atrial tachycardias, such as atrial flutter or atrial fibrillation (Beaufort-Krol & Bink-Boelkens, 1997; Pinsky et al., 1991; Schmolling et al., 2000; Vautier-Rit et al., 2000). When directly injected into the umbilical cord, amiodarone successfully converts SVT in a hydropic fetus and resolves the hydrops (Mangione et al., 1999).

Medical management decision-making should weigh the risks of prematurity against the risks of cardiac failure and poor oxygen delivery in utero. The obstetric staff manages the route and timing of delivery of the fetus. Generally, delivery is recommended for term fetuses without hydrops. However, if a term fetus has hydrops, the fetus should be treated in utero; once the SVT has converted, delivery should proceed. If the fetus is preterm, intrauterine conversion therapy should be initiated along with assessment of fetal lung maturity. If the lungs are deemed mature and conversion of the SVT has been achieved, delivery should proceed. However, if the lungs are immature, intrauterine conversion therapy is recommended along with steroid therapy. Once the lungs are mature and conversion is achieved, delivery should proceed (Sharland, 2001; Strasburger, 2000; Tanel & Rhodes, 2001).

Atrial Flutter and Fibrillation

As with SVT, atrial flutter can be treated with scalp stimulation in the intrapartum period. However, if scalp stimulation does not result in conversion, definitive diagnosis with EchoCG or ECG in utero may alter the prognosis, and the plan of care may include more progressive medical management.

As with SVT, the administration of digoxin or propranolol is recommended initially in the antepartum period to control the ventricular response of the fetal heart (Kleinman et al., 1999; Pinsky et al., 1991; Schmolling et al., 2000; Shaffer & Wiggins, 1998; Strasburger, 2000; Vautier-Rit et al., 2000; Vlagsma, Hallensleben & Meijboom, 2001). If digoxin does not convert the heart rate pattern or the fetus continues to deteriorate, digoxin should be withdrawn and another drug therapy started (Kleinman et al., 1999; Pinsky et al., 1991; Schmolling et al., 2000; Shaffer & Wiggins, 1998; Vautier-Rit et al., 2000; Vlagsma et al., 2001). Class I cardiac drugs, such as flecainide, quinidine or procainamide, or Class III cardiac drugs, such as sotalol, amiodarone, or diltiazem, can also be used to convert atrial flutter (Kleinman et al., 1999; Pinsky et al., 1991; Schmolling et al., 2000; Shaffer & Wiggins, 1998; Strasburger, 2000; Tanel & Rhodes, 2001; Vautier-Rit et al., 2000; Vlagsma et al., 2001).

Class I agents are recommended because they slow AV conduction, thus slowing the flutter rate (Joglar & Page, 2001; Kleinman et al., 1999; Tanel & Rhodes, 2001). Verapamil is not recommended because it relies on an immature myocardium to allow for passage of calcium to the fetal heart (Joglar & Page, 2001; Kleinman et al., 1999).

Atrial flutter has been treated successfully with sotalol (Oudijk et al., 2000), quinidine (Ko, Deal, Strasburger & Benson, 1992) and amiodarone (Cuneo & Strasburger, 2000). However, although amiodarone has a long half-life, it has been associated with fetal cretinism and, as a result, is often not recommended (Crosson & Benner, 1999; Pinsky et al., 1991; Schmolling et al., 2000; Vautier-Rit et al., 2000; Vlagsma et al., 2001). Some studies have suggested sotalol should be the first-line agent for fetuses with atrial flutter (Beaufort-Krol & Bink-Boelkens, 1997; Oudijk et al., 2000). Meijboom et al. reported an 80% conversion rate for atrial flutter using sotalol (Meijboom, 1994).

Prior to the administration of antidysrhythmic agents, the fetus needs to be assessed for hydrops. If the fetus has hydrops, digoxin and propranolol are not recommended unless conversion to a normal sinus rhythm is considered urgent (Kleinman et al., 1999; Pinsky et al., 1991; Schmolling et al., 2000; Vautier-Rit et al., 2000; Vlagsma et al., 2001).

Treatment for atrial fibrillation is similar to that for atrial flutter. However, because of the difficulty to convert this pattern to a normal sinus rhythm using digoxin alone, other more potent cardiac drugs, as noted above, may be needed in place of digoxin.

Ventricular Tachycardia

As noted earlier, it is important to distinguish between accelerated ventricular tachycardia and sustained rapid ventricular tachycardia (Shaffer & Wiggins, 1998; Strasburger, 2000). The drug of choice for transplacental treatment of tachyarrhythmias with one-to-one AV conduction is usually digoxin; however, digoxin has little use in ventricular tachycardia (Strasburger, 2000). For ventricular tachycardia, amiodarone or sotalol, administered transplacentally, is recommended (Strasburger, 2000). If ventricular tachycardia is suspected and the fetus also as congestive cardiac failure, or in acute situations of rapid ventricular tachycardia, lidocaine can be given intracordally. (Cuneo & Strasburger, 2000; Ferrer, 1998; Kleinman et al., 1999). The intracordal administration of lidocaine can then be followed with maternal oral therapy with propranolol, mexiletine, quinidine, procainamide, amiodarone or sotalol (Kleinman et al., 1999).

AV Block

Effective management of a bradycardic pattern, regardless of the type, requires an accurate assessment of the etiology of the displayed pattern, validated presence of cardiac structural damage, evaluation of fetal well-being and fetal cardiac function needs.

Treatment of second-degree and third-degree AV block is essentially the same and is often directed towards increasing the FHR with atropine, isoproterenol or terbutaline. Digoxin has also been used to improve left ventricular function in fetuses demonstrating irregularities in left ventricular activity. Diuretics have also been studied and have shown some benefit to decreasing fluid overload (Buyon, Swersky, Fox, Bierman & Winchester, 1987; Buyon, Waltuck, Kleinman & Copel, 1995; Carreira, Gutierrez-Larraya & Gomez-Reino, 1993; Copel, et al., 1995; Groves, Allan & Rosenthal, 1996; Pinsky et al., 1991; Polin & Fox, 1999).

If the mother has high anti-Ro or anti-La titers, the use of steroids that cross the placenta, i.e., dexamethasone or betamethasone, should be considered. Early pacing of the fetus in utero is not recommended as there have been no successful outcomes to date (Copel, et al., 1995; Schmolling et al., 2000; Vautier-Rit et al., 2000; Vlagsma et al., 2001). Fetuses that do not have hydrops and have a ventricular heart rate above 55 bpm usually can be managed very much like normal pregnancies, with the addition of monitoring for hydrops and cardiac function, specifically ventricular function.

Hydropic fetuses are more difficult to manage, and current treatment modalities have not improved the outcome for these fetuses (Crosson & Brenner, 1999; Kleinman et al., 1999; Sharland, 2001). Successful conversion in such fetuses has been accomplished with maternal administration of isoproterenol, terbutaline or digoxin (Crosson & Brenner, 1999; Pinsky, Gillette, Garson & McNamara, 1982).

Intrauterine pacing of the fetal heart has also been tried in fetuses whose mothers were Ro/La negative; however, as of yet, it has been unsuccessful (Carpenter et al., 1986; Crosson & Brenner, 1999; Walkinshaw, Welch, McCormick & Walsh, 1994). After birth, fetal epicardial or endocardial leads can be placed temporarily (Weindling et al., 1994). Following temporary pacing, permanent pacemaker implantation should be investigated. Permanent pacemaker implantation is usually required in neonates with structural cardiac disease and in about 50% of patients with isolated AV block. The recommended criteria for pacemaker application in neonates with isolated block include 1) symptomatic fetus or neonate, 2) resting heart rate less than 60 bpm and 3) presence of wide complex escape rhythms (Crosson & Brenner, 1999). However, preterm delivery is not recommended, as it makes pacemaker implantation extremely difficult (Kleinman et al., 1999).

Monitoring in the labor and delivery arena requires no special accommodations. The bradycardic rate seen is usually not associated with a hypoxic fetus, and the rate will demonstrate normal FHR variations as seen in the normoxic fetus with a normal FHR baseline between 110 and 160 bpm (Cabaniss, 1993; Murray, 2001).

⌐▪ PROGNOSIS

The prognosis of a fetus with a dysrhythmic or arrhythmic pattern depends on a variety of issues, including the associated pathology, the type of pattern, the presence or absence of hydrops, the FHR and the adequacy of prescribed. Determin-ing these variables will help guide the multidisciplinary team to an individualized care plan for both the woman and her fetus. As noted earlier, all neonates demonstrating dysrhythmic patterns should be monitored by means of a 12-lead ECG to evaluate for ventricular function, especially preexcitation as seen in WPW syndrome, or for junctional reciprocating tachycardia. Should ectopy be found, an EchoCG is indicated to rule out cardiac structural defects. Neonates with controlled SVT should be given prophylactic treatment for 6–12 months. Neonates with atrial flutter alone and no evidence of WPW syndrome usually require short-term prophylaxis of less than 3–6 months (Beaufort-Krol & Bink-Boelkens, 1997; Groves, Allan & Rosenthal, 1995; Kleinman, Copel & Hobbins, 1987; Stevens, Schreiner, Hurwitz & Gresham, 1979).

A fetus with documented complete AV block should be delivered in a tertiary care center where emergency cardiac pacing can be achieved quickly if needed (Strasburger, 2000). For a fetus with isolated complete AV block complicated by hydrops fetalis, a heart rate below 50 bpm and a mother with a negative maternal anti-Ro antibody status, the prognosis is very poor (Machado et al., 1988; Schmidt et al., 1991). The same is true for fetuses with complete AV block that is associated with structural cardiac disease (Sharland, 2001).

⌐▪ CONCLUSION

Overall, the presumed mechanisms of cardiac failure associated with dysrhythmic patterns include the following: 1) decreased ventricular filling time (SVT, atrial fibrillation and atrial flutter), 2) dissociation between atrial and ventricular depolarization causing loss of atrial boost mechanism (supraventricular or ventricular dysrhythmias), 3) impairment of mild cardiac performance (ventricular dysrhythmias) and 4) decrease in cardiac output (third-degree heart block).

When a dysrhythmic pattern is identified, the clinician should identify the type of pattern, communicate the pattern to appropriate personnel and document the information appropriately. However, identification, diagnosis and treatment of fetuses with arrhythmic and dysrhythmic FHR patterns can be difficult. Multidisciplinary involvement is required throughout the pregnancy. Nurses caring for these patients should possess skills and knowledge of maternal–fetal physiology; fetal cardiac anatomy and physiology; pathophysiology of normal, arrhythmic and dysrhythmic patterns; assessment technology; treatment modalities and prognostic outcomes. This information will allow the nurse to assess the tracing, and participate in the multidisciplinary team that develops a comprehensive individualized care plan, and guide or assist with interventions necessary to obtain the best outcome possible for the fetus/neonate and the family.

REFERENCES

Alexander, E., Buyon, J. P., Provost, T. T., & Guarnieri, T. (1992). Anti Ro/SS-A antibodies in the pathophysiology of congenital heart block in neonatal lupus syndrome, an experimental model. In vitro electrophysiologic and immunocytochemical studies. *Arthritis & Rheumatology, 35,* 176–189.

Allan, L. D. (1984). Cardiac ultrasound of the fetus. *Archives of Disease in Childhood, 59,* 603–604.

Allan, L. D., Anderson, R. H., Sullivan, I. D., Campbell, S., Holt, D. W., & Tynan, M. (1983). Evaluation of fetal arrhythmias by echocardiography. *British Heart Journal, 50,* 240–245.

Allan, L. D., Crawford, D. C., Anderson, R. H., & Tynan, M. (1984). Evaluation and treatment of fetal arrhythmias. *Clinical Cardiology, 7,* 467–473.

Anderson, R. H., & Taylor, I. M. (1972). Development of atrioventricular specialized tissue in human heart. *British Heart Journal, 34,* 1205–1214.

Beall, M. H., & Paul, R. H. (1986). Artifacts, blocks, and arrhythmias: Confusing nonclassical heart rate tracings. *Clinical Obstetrics and Gynecology, 29*(1), 83–94.

Beaufort-Krol, G. C., & Bink-Boelkens, M. T. (1997). Effectiveness of sotalol for atrial flutter in children after surgery for congenital heart disease. *American Journal of Cardiology, 79,* 92–94.

Bergmans, M. G., Jonker, G. J., & Kock, H. C. (1985). Fetal supraventricular tachycardia: Review of the literature. *Obstetric and Gynecologic Survey, 40,* 61–68.

Bharti, S., & Lev, M. (1994). Embryology of the heart and great vessels. In C. Mavroudis & C. L. Backer, (Eds.), *Pediatric cardiac surgery* (pp. 1–13). St. Louis: CV Mosby.

Bianchi, D., Crobleholme, T., & D'Alton, M. (2000). *Fetology: Diagnosis and management of the fetal patient.* Philadelphia: McGraw-Hill.

Bruner, J. P., Gabbe, S. G., Levy, D. W., & Arger, P. H. (1993). Doppler ultrasonography of the umbilical cord in normal pregnancy. *Southern Medical Journal, Journal of the Southern Medical Association, 86*(1), 52-55.

Buyon, J., Roubey, R., Swersky, S., Pompeo, L., Parke. A., Baxi, L., & Winchester, R. (1988). Complete congenital heart block: Risk of occurrence and therapeutic approach to prevention. *Journal of Rheumatology, 15,* 1104–1108.

Buyon, J. P., Swersky, S. H., Fox, H. E., Bierman, F. Z., & Winchester, R. J. (1987). Intrauterine therapy for presumptive fetal myocarditis with acquired heart block due to systemic lupus erythematosus: Experience in a mother with predominance of SS-B (La) antibodies. *Arthritis & Rheumatology, 30*(1), 44–49.

Buyon, J. P., Waltuck, J., Kleinman, C., & Copel, J. (1995). In utero identification and therapy of congenital heart block. *Lupus, 4,* 116–121.

Cabaniss, M. L. (1993). *Fetal monitoring interpretation.* Philadelphia: Lippincott.

Cameron A., Nicholson, S., Nimrod, C., Harder, J., Davies, D., & Fritzler, M. (1988). Evaluation of fetal cardiac dysrhythmias with two-dimensional, M-mode & pulsed Doppler ultrasonography. *American Journal of Obstetrics and Gynecology, 158*(2), 286–290.

Carpenter, R. J., Strasburger, J. F., Garson, A., Smith, R. T., Deter, R. L., & Engelhardt, H. T. (1986). Fetal ventricular pacing for hydrops secondary to complete atrioventricular block. *Journal of the American College of Cardiology, 8,* 1434–1436.

Carreira, P. E., Gutierrez-Larraya, F., & Gomez-Reino, J. J. (1993). Successful intrauterine therapy with dexamethasone for fetal myocarditis and heart block in a woman with systemic lupus erythematosus. *Journal of Rheumatology, 20,* 1101–1104.

Case, D. L., & Fyfe, D. A. (1990). Fetal dysrhythmias. In P.C. Gillette & A. Garson, (Eds.), *Pediatric arrhythmias: Electrophysiology and pacing* (p. 637). Philadelphia: W.B. Saunders.

Chan, F. Y., Woo, S. K., Ghosh, A., Tang, M., & Lam, C. (1990). Prenatal diagnosis of congenital fetal arrhythmias by simultaneous pulsed Doppler velocimetry of the fetal abdominal aorta and inferior vena cava. *Obstetrics & Gynecology, 7,* 200–205.

Chao, R. C., Ho, E. S., & Hsieh, K. S. (1992). Fetal atrial flutter and fibrillation: Prenatal echocardiographic detection and management. *American Heart Journal, 124,* 1095–1098.

Copel, J. A., Buyon, J. P., & Kleinman, C. S. (1995). Successful in utero therapy of fetal heart block. *American Journal of Obstetrics and Gynecology, 173*(5), 1384–1390.

Copel, J. A., Morotti, R., Hobbins, J. C., & Kleinman, C. S. (1991). The antenatal diagnosis of congenital heart disease using fetal echocardiography: Is color flow mapping necessary? *Obstetrics and Gynecology, 78*(1), 1–8.

Crosson J. E., & Brenner, J. I. (1999). Fetal arrhythmias. In D. K. James, P. J. Steer, C. P. Weiner, & B. Gonik (Eds.), *High risk pregnancy: Management options* (2nd ed., pp. 371–378). London: W.B. Saunders.

Cuneo, B. F., & Strasburger, J. F. (2000). Management strategy for fetal tachycardia. *Obstetrics & Gynecology, 96,* 575–581.

DeVore, G. R., Siassi, B., & Platt, L. D. (1984). Fetal echocardiography. IV. M-mode assessment of ventricular size and contractility during the second and third trimesters of pregnancy in the normal fetus. *American Journal of Obstetrics and Gynecology, 150,* 981–988.

Drose, J. A. (1998). *Fetal echocardiography* (Chap 1, pp. 1–13). Philadelphia: W.B. Saunders.

Esscher, E., & Scott, J. S. (1979). Congenital heart block and maternal systemic lupus erythematosus. *British Medical Journal, 1*(6173), 1235–1238.

Feinstein, N. & McCartney, P. (1997). *Fetal Heart Monitoring Principles and Practices* (2nd ed.). Dubuque: Kendall/Hunt.

Feinstein, N. F., Sprague, A., & Trépanier, M. J. (2000). *Fetal heart rate auscultation.* Washington, D.C.: AWHONN.

Ferrer, P. L. (1998). Fetal arrhythmias. In B. J. Deal, G. S. Wolff, & H. Gelband (Eds.), *Current concepts in diagnosis and management of arrhythmias in infants and children* (pp. 17–63). Armonk, NY: Futura.

Fields, E. F. (1951). The development of the conducting system in the heart of sheep. *British Heart Journal, 13,* 129–147.

Freeman, R. K., Garite, T. J. & Nageotte, M. P. (1991). *Fetal Heart Rate Monitoring* (2nd ed.). Baltimore: Williams & Wilkins.

Freidman, D. M., Zervoudakis, I., & Buyon, J. P. (1998). Perinatal monitoring of fetal well-being in the presence of congenital heart block. *American Journal of Perinatology, 15,* 669–673.

Fyfe, D. A., Meyer, K. B., & Case, C. L. (1988). Sonographic assessment of fetal cardiac arrhythmias. *Journal of American College of Cardiology, 12,* 1292–1297.

Fyfe, D. A., Meyer, K. B., & Case C. L. (1993). Sonographic assessment of fetal cardiac arrhythmias. *Seminars in Ultrasound, CT and MRI, 14,* 286–297.

Gembruch, U., Redel, D. A., Bald, R., & Hansmann, M. (1993). Longitudinal study in 18 cases of fetal supraventricular tachycardia: Doppler echocardiographic findings and pathophysiologic implications. *American Heart Journal, 125,* 1290–1301.

Gewitz, M., & Philips, J. B. (1999). Fetal and neonatal cardiovascular physiology. In R. A. Polin & W. W. Fox (Eds.), *Fetal and neonatal physiology* (2nd ed., pp. 793–976). Philadelphia: W.B. Saunders.

Gillette, P. C. (1976). The mechanisms of supraventricular tachycardia in children. *Circulation, 54*(1), 133–139.

Gow, R. M., & Hamilton, R. M. (1992). Developmental biology of specialized conduction tissue. In R. M. Freedom, L. N. Benson, & J. F. Smallhorn (Eds.), *Neonatal heart disease* (pp. 65–81). London: Springer-Verlag.

Gow, R. M., & Walls, E. W. (1947). The development of specialized conducting tissue of the human heart. *Journal of Anatomy, 81,* 93–100.

Groves, A. M., Allan, L. D., & Rosenthal, E. (1995). Therapeutic trial of sympathomimetics in three cases of complete heart block in the fetus. *Circulation, 92,* 3394–3396.

Groves, A. M., Allan, L. D., & Rosenthal, E. (1996). Outcome of isolated congenital complete heart block diagnosed in utero. *Heart, 78,* 190–194.

Gudmundsson, S., Huhta, J. C., Wood, D. C., Tulzer, G., Cohen, A. W., & Weiner, S. (1991). Venous Doppler ultrasonography in the fetus with nonimmune hydrops. *American Journal of Obstetricians and Gynecologists, 164,* 33–37.

Ho, S., & Anderson, R. H. (1990). Embryology and anatomy of normal and abnormal conduction system. In P. C. Gillette & A. Carso (Eds.), *Pediatric arrhythmia: Electrophysiology and pacemaking* (p. 2) Philadelphia: W.B. Saunders.

Horsfall, A. C., Venables, P. J., Taylor, P. V., & Maini, R. N. (1991). Ro and La antigens and maternal anti-La idiotype on the surface of myocardial fibres in congenital heart block. *Journal of Autoimmunity, 4,* 165–176.

Joglar, J. A., & Page, R. L. (2001). Antiarrhythmic drugs in pregnancy, *Current Opinion in Cardiology, 16,* 40–45.

Kamino, K., Hirota, A., & Fujii, S. (1981). Localization of pacemaking activity in early embryonic heart monitored using voltage-sensitive dye. *Nature, 290,* 595–597.

King, T. L., & Simpson, K. R (2001). Fetal assessment during labor. In K. R. Simpson & P. A. Creehan (Eds.), *Perinatal nursing* (2nd ed., pp. 378–416). Philadelphia: Lippincott.

Kirby, M. L. (1998). Development of the fetal heart. In R. A. Polin & W. W. Fox (Eds.), *Fetal and neonatal physiology* (2nd ed., pp. 793–800). Philadelphia: W.B. Saunders.

Kleinman, C. S. (1986). Prenatal diagnosis and management of intrauterine arrhythmias. *Fetal Therapy, 1,* 92–95.

Kleinman, C. S., Copel, J. A., & Hobbins, J. C. (1987). Combined echocardiographic and Doppler assessment of fetal congenital atrioventricular block. *British Journal of Obstetrics and Gynaecology, 94,* 967–974.

Kleinman, C. S., Copel, J. A., Weinstein, E. M., Santulli, T. V., & Hobbins, J. C. (1985). In utero diagnosis and treatment of fetal supraventricular tachycardia. *Seminars in Perinatology, 9*, 113–129.

Kleinman, C. S., Donnerstein, R. L., Jaffe, C. C., DeVore, G. R., Weinstein, E. M., Lynch, D. C., Talner, N. S., Berkowitz, R. L., & Hobbins, J. C. (1983). Fetal echocardiography: A tool for evaluation of in utero cardiac arrhythmias and monitoring of in utero therapy: Analysis of 71 patients. *American Journal of Cardiology, 51*, 237–243.

Kleinman, C. S., Nehgme, R., & Copel, J. A. (1999). Fetal cardiac arrhythmias: Diagnosis and therapy. In R. K. Creasy & R. Resnik (Eds.), *Maternal-fetal medicine* (4th ed., pp. 301–318). Philadelphia: W.B. Saunders.

Ko, J. K., Deal, B. J., Strasburger, J. F., & Benson, D. W., Jr. (1992). Supraventricular tachycardia mechanisms and their age distribution in pediatric patients. *American Journal of Cardiology, 69*, 1028–1032.

Lanham, J. G., Walport, M. J., & Hughes, G. R. (1983). Congenital heart block and familial connective tissue disease. *Journal of Rheumatology, 10*, 823–825.

Litsey, S. E., Noonan, J. A., O'Connor, W. N., Cottrill, C. M., & Mitchell, B. (1985). Maternal connective tissue disease and congenital heart block: Demonstration of immunoglobulin in cardiac tissue. *New England Journal of Medicine, 312*, 93–100.

Machado, M. V., Tynan, M. J., Curry, P. V., & Allan, L. D. (1988). Fetal complete heart block. *British Heart Journal, 60*, 512–515.

Mangione, R., Guyon, F., Vergnaud, A., Jimenez, M., Saura, R., & Horovitz, J. (1999). Successful treatment of refractory supraventricular tachycardia by repeat intravascular injection of amiodarone in a fetus with hydrops. *European Journal of Obstetrics, Gynecology, and Reproductive Biology, 86*, 105–107.

Meijboom, E. J, van Engelen, A. D., van de Beek, E. W., Weijtens, O., Lautenschutz, J. M., & Benatar, A. A. (1994). Fetal arrhythmias. *Current Opinions in Cardiology, 9*, 97–102.

Michäelsson, M., & Engle, M. A. (1972). Congenital complete heart block: An international study of the natural history. *Cardiovascular Clinics, 4*, 85–101.

Moak, J. P. (1990). Basic electrophysiologic principles: Application to treatment of dysrhythmias. In: P .C. Gillette & A. Garson, Jr., (Eds.), *Pediatric cardiac dysrhythmias* (pp. 37–118). New York: Grune & Stratton.

Moodley, T. R., Vaughan, J. E., Chuntarpursat, I., Wood, D., Noddeboe, Y., & Schwarting, F. (1986). Congenital heart block detected in utero. A case report. *South African Medical Journal, 70*, 433–434.

Moore, K. L. (1988). *Essentials of human embryology,* Toronto: B.C. Deck.

Mucklow, J. C. (1986). The fate of drugs in pregnancy. *Clinics of Obstetrics and Gynaecology, 13*, 161–175.

Murray, M. L. (2001). *Antepartal and intrapartal fetal monitoring.* Albuquerque, NM: Learning Resources International, Inc.

Mycek, M. J., Harvey, R. A. & Champe, P. C. (1997). *Lippincott's Illustrated Reviews: Pharmacology* (2nd ed.), Philadelphia: Lippincott-Raven (pp. 163–174).

Nyberg, D. A., & Emerson, D. S. (1990). Cardiac malformations. In D. A Nyberg, B. S. Mahony, & D. H. Pretorius (Eds.), *Diagnostic ultrasound of fetal anomalies: Test and atlas* (pp. 300–341). Chicago: Yearbook Medical.

Oudijk, M. A., Michon, M. M., Kleinman, C. S., Kapusta, L., Stoutenbeek, P., Visser, G. H., & Meijboom, E. J. (2000). Sotalol to treat fetal dysrhythmias. *Circulation, 101*, 2721–2726.

Parer, J. T. (1997). *Handbook of fetal heart rate monitoring* (2nd ed.). Philadelphia: W.B. Saunders.

Perry, J. C., & Garson, A., Jr. (1990). Supraventricular tachycardia due to Wolff-Parkinson-White syndrome in children: Early disappearance and late recurrence. *Journal of the American College of Cardiologists, 16*(5), 1215–1220.

Pickoff, A. S. (1998). Developmental electrophysiology in the fetus and neonate. In R. A. Polin & W. W. Fox (Eds.), *Fetal and neonatal physiology* (2nd ed., pp. 891–913). Philadelphia: W.B. Saunders.

Pinsky, W. W., Gillette, P. C., Garson, A., & McNamara, D. G. (1982). Diagnosis, management, and long-term results of patients with congenital complete atrioventricular block. *Pediatrics, 69*, 728–733.

Pinsky, W. W., Rayburn, W. F., & Evans, M. L. (1991). Pharmacologic therapy for fetal arrhythmias. *Clinical Obstetrics and Gynecology, 34*, 304–309.

Reed, K. L. (1989). Fetal arrhythmias: Etiology, diagnosis, pathophysiology, and treatment. *Seminars in Perinatology, 13*, 294–304.

Reed, K. L. (1991). Introduction to fetal echocardiography. *Obstetrics and Gynecology Clinics of North America, 18*, 811–822.

Reed, K. L., Sahn, D. J., Marx, G. R, Anderson, C. F., & Shenker, L. (1987). Cardiac Doppler flows during fetal arrhythmias: Physiologic consequences. *Obstetrics and Gynecology, 70*, 1–6.

Reiss, R. E., Gabbe, S. G., & Petrie, R. H. (2001). Intrapartum fetal evaluation. In S. G. Gabbe, J. R. Niebyl, & J. L. Simpson (Eds.), *Obstetrics: Normal and problem pregnancies* (3rd ed., pp. 396–424). New York: Churchill-Livingstone.

Rosenthal, E, Groves, A., Allan, L. D., et al. (1996). Prognosis of an in utero congenital heart block. *Journal of the American College of Cardiology, 157*, 368–371.

Sadler, T. W. (1990). *Langman's medical embryology* (6th ed., pp. 179–227). Baltimore: Williams & Wilkins.

Schmidt, K. G., Ulmer, H. E., Silverman, N. H., Kleinman, C. S., & Copel, J. A. (1991). Perinatal outcome of fetal congenital complete atrioventricular block:

A multicenter experience. *Journal of American College of Cardiologists, 17,* 1360–1366.

Schmolling, J., Renke, K., Richter, O., Pfeiffer, K., Schlebusch, H., & Holler, T. (2000). Digoxin, flecainide, and amiodarone transfer across the placenta and the effects of an elevated umbilical venous pressure on the transfer rate. *Therapeutic Drug Monitor, 22,* 582–588.

Shaffer, E. M., & Wiggins, J. W. (1998). Fetal dysrhythmias. In J. A. Drose (Ed.), *Fetal echocardiography* (pp. 279–290). Philadelphia: W.B. Saunders.

Sharland, G. (2001). Fetal cardiology. *Seminars in Neonatology, 6*(1), 3–15.

Shenker, L. (1979). Fetal cardiac arrhythmias. *Obstetric and Gynecologic Survey, 34,* 561–572.

Shenker, L., Astle, C., Reed, K., & Anderson, C. (1986). Embryonic heart rates before the seventh week of pregnancy, *Journal of Reproductive Medicine, 31,* 333–335.

Silber, D. L., & Durnin, R. E. (1969). Intrauterine atrial tachycardia, associated with massive edema in a newborn. *American Journal of Diseases in Children, 117,* 722–726.

Silverman, N. H., Enderlein, M. A., Stranger, P., Teitel, D. F., Heymann, M. A., & Golbus, M. S. (1985). Recognition of fetal arrhythmias by echocardiography. *Journal of Clinical Ultrasound, 13,* 255–263.

Silverman, N. H., Kleinman, C. S., Rudolph, A. M., Copel, J. A., Weinstein, E. M., Enderlein, M. A., & Golbus, M. (1985). Fetal atrioventricular valve insufficiency associated with nonimmune hydrops: A two-dimensional echocardiographic and pulsed Doppler ultrasound study. *Circulation, 72,* 825–832.

Simpson, J. M., & Sharland, G. K. (1998). Fetal tachycardias: Management and outcome of 127 consecutive cases. *Heart, 79,* 576–581.

Simpson, L. L. (2000). Fetal supraventricular tachycardias: Diagnosis and management. *Seminars in Perinatology, 24,* 360–372.

Simpson, L. L., & Marx, G. R. (1994). Diagnosis and treatment of structural fetal cardiac abnormality and dysrhythmia. *Seminars in Perinatology, 18,* 215–227.

Southall, D. P., Arrowsmith, W. A., Oakley, J. R., McEnery, G., Anderson, R. H., & Shinebourne, E. A. (1979). Prolonged QT interval and cardiac arrhythmias in two neonates: Sudden infant death syndrome in one case. *Archives of Disease in Childhood, 54,* 776–779.

Southall, D. P, Richards, J., Hardwick, R. A, Shinebourne, E. A., Gibbens, G. L., Thelwall-Jones, H., de Swiet, M., & Johnston, P. G. (1980). Prospective study of fetal heart rate and rhythm patterns. *Archives of Disease in Childhood, 55,* 506–511.

Stevens, D. C., Schreiner, R. L., Hurwitz, R. A., & Gresham, E. L. (1979). Fetal and neonatal ventricular arrhythmia. *Pediatrics, 63*(5), 771–777.

Steward, P. A., & Wladimiroff, J. W. (1988). Fetal atrial arrhythmias associated with redundancy/aneurysm of the foramen ovale. *Journal of Clinical Ultrasound, 16,* 643–650.

Strasburger, J. F. (2000). Fetal arrhythmias. *Progress in Pediatric Cardiology, 11,* 1–17.

Tanel, R. E., & Rhodes, L. A. (2001). Fetal and neonatal arrhythmias. *Clinics in Perinatology, 28,* 187–207.

Taylor, P. V., Scott, J. S., Gerlis, L. M., Esscher, E., & Scott, O. (1986). Maternal antibodies against fetal cardiac antigens in congenital complete heart block. *New England Journal of Medicine, 315,* 667–672.

Tucker, S. M. (2000). *Pocket guide to fetal monitoring and assessment* (4th ed.). St. Louis: Mosby, Inc.

Tulzer, G. (2000). Fetal cardiology. *Current Opinion in Pediatrics, 12,* 492–496.

Uckan, E. M., & Townsend, N. S. (1999). Fetal adaptation. In L. K. Mandeville & N. K. Troiano (Eds.), *High-risk & critical care intrapartum nursing* (2nd ed., pp. 32–50). Philadelphia: Lippincott.

van Engelen, A. D., Weijtens, O., Brenner, J. I., Kleinman, C. S., Copel, J. A., Stoutenbeek, P., & Meijboom, E. J. (1994). Management outcome and follow-up of fetal tachycardia. *Journal of the American College of Cardiology, 24,* 1371–1375.

Vautier-Rit, S., Dufour, P., Vaksmann, G., Subtil, D., Vaast, P., Valat, A. S., Dubos, J. P., & Puech, F. (2000). Fetal arrhythmias: Diagnosis, prognosis, treatment, apropos of 33 cases. *Gynecologic & Obstetric Fertility, 28,* 729–737.

Vlagsma, R., Hallensleben, E., & Meijboom, E. J. (2001). Supraventricular tachycardia and premature atrial contractions in fetus. *Ned Tijdschr Geneeskd, 145*(7), 295–299.

Walkinshaw, S. A., Welch, C. R., McCormick, J., & Walsh, K. (1994). In utero pacing for fetal congenital heart block. *Fetal Diagnostic Therapy, 9,* 183–185.

Watson, W. J., & Katz, V. L. (1991). Steroid therapy for hydrops associated with antibody-mediated congenital heart block. *American Journal of Obstetrics and Gynecology, 165,* 553–554.

Weindling, S. N., Saul, J. P., Triedman, J. K., Burke, R. P., Jonas, R. A., Gamble, W. J., & Walsh, E. P. (1994). Staged pacing therapy for congenital complete heart block in premature infants. *American College of Cardiology, 74,* 412–413.

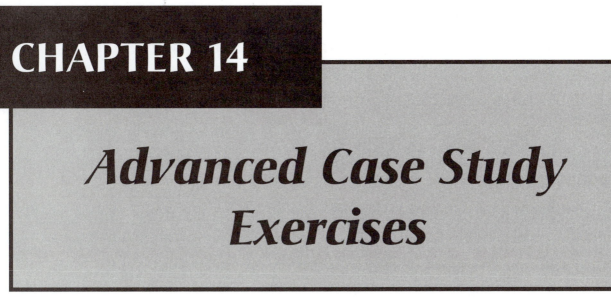

CHAPTER 14

Advanced Case Study Exercises

Rebecca L. Cypher

This chapter provides additional case study exercises as an adjunct to content presented in the Advanced FHMPP program. Included are a series of adaptations of actual case studies and electronic fetal monitoring (EFM) tracings from a variety of intrapartum clinical settings. This chapter is designed to promote and support critical thinking in the analysis of EFM tracings, in keeping with the framework used throughout the AWHONN Advanced FHMPP Workshop. The Systematic Approach to Interpretation Worksheet is provided to facilitate analysis of the case studies and EFM tracings.

For each case study exercise, readers are encouraged to a) review the brief history and data provided, b) analyze the EFM tracing and c) complete the Systematic Approach to Interpretation Worksheet. Answer keys for each exercise are provided at the end of each scenario. Readers should review their work and identify areas of strength and areas requiring more practice or review related to electronic fetal heart rate monitoring interpretation. In the clinical setting and in the FHMPP Workshop skill stations, longer EFM tracings may be available for interpretation and clinical decision-making purposes.

AWHONN Fetal Heart Monitoring Principles and Practices
Systematic Approach to Interpretation Worksheet

Case Study Exercise: _____

1. Contractions: *Frequency:* _____
   Duration: _____
   Intensity: _____
   Resting tone: _____

2. Baseline fetal heart rate: _____

3. Variability: Place a checkmark signifying the appropriate type of variability on the strip (LTV = long-term variability; STV = short-term variability).

   LTV Decreased (0–5 bpm) _____
   Average (6–25 bpm) _____
   Marked (> 25 bpm) _____
   Unable to assess _____

   STV Present _____
   Absent _____
   Unable to assess _____

4. Accelerations and decelerations. When present, circle P if periodic or NP if nonperiodic.

   Accelerations   P   NP
   Early decelerations   P
   Variable decelerations P   NP
   Late decelerations   P
   Prolonged decelerations   NP

5. List possible underlying physiologic mechanisms or rationales for observed patterns.

6. List in order of priority the physiologic goal(s) for observed patterns.

7. List interventions to achieve the physiologic goals and actions needed related to instrumentation or further assessment.

Case Study Exercise D: Brenda

Age:	35 years old
Gravida/Para:	2/1001
Gestational Age:	39 $^{1}/_{7}$ weeks
Medical History:	Unremarkable
Surgical History:	Unremarkable
Psychosocial History:	Depression: Took Fluoxetine (Prozac®) preconceptionally; however, self-discontinued medications during the first trimester when pregnancy was confirmed. Takes no medications for depression at present.
Past Obstetric History:	Low transverse cesarean delivery at 40 weeks of gestation for arrest of descent
Current Obstetric History:	Normal prenatal laboratory results
	2nd trimester ultrasound findings consistent with LMP
	Amniocentesis for advanced maternal age confirmed normal karyotype

Brenda presented to the obstetric triage unit because she fainted at a restaurant. She had been experiencing flu–like symptoms for 2 days. While in the obstetric triage unit she was treated for dehydration with intravenous fluids and given an antibiotic for her urinary tract infection. On admission, her vital signs were as follows: axillary temperature: 96.7°F (35.9°C); blood pressure: 101/52 mmHg; pulse: 85 bpm; respiration: 18 breaths/minute.

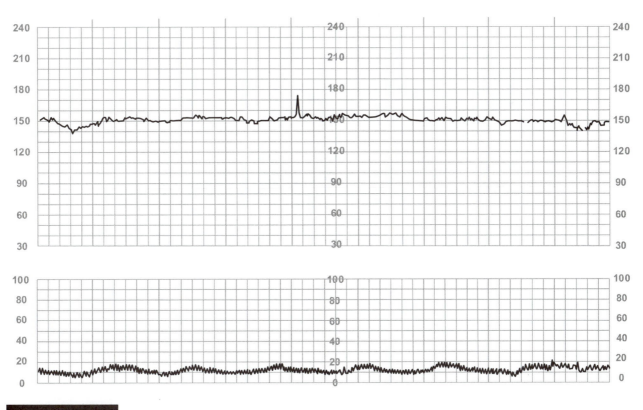

FIGURE 14-1

Tracing Segment D1: Obstetric Triage EFM Tracing at 7:45 P.M. Using External Monitoring

AWHONN Fetal Heart Monitoring Principles and Practices Systematic Approach to Interpretation Worksheet

Case Study Exercise: Brenda D1

1. Contractions: *Frequency:* **Uterine irritability**
   Duration: **30–40 sec.**
   Intensity: **Palpate**
   Resting tone: **Palpate**

2. Baseline fetal heart rate: **150–155 bpm**

3. Variability: Place a checkmark signifying the appropriate type of variability on the strip (LTV = long-term variability; STV = short-term variability).

LTV	**Decreased (0–5 bpm)**	✔
	Average (6–25 bpm)	
	Marked (> 25 bpm)	
	Unable to assess	
STV	Present	
	Absent	
	Unable to assess	✔

4. Accelerations and decelerations. When present, circle P if periodic or NP if nonperiodic.

Accelerations	P	NP
Early decelerations	P	
Variable decelerations	P	NP
Late decelerations	P	
Prolonged decelerations		NP

   None present

5. List possible underlying physiologic mechanisms or rationales for observed patterns.
   a. **Fetal sleep cycle**
   b. **Possible medication/narcotic intake prior to admission**
   c. **Possible loss of fetal reserves related to decreased LTV and possible absent STV**

6. List in order of priority the physiologic goal(s) for observed patterns.
   a. **Maximize oxygenation**
   b. **Maximize uterine blood flow**

7. List interventions to achieve the physiologic goals and actions needed related to instrumentation or further assessment.
   a. **Change maternal position to maximize uterine blood flow.**
   b. **Hydrate with intravenous fluids (IVF)**
   c. **Administer maternal supplemental oxygen via snug face mask if decreased LTV (variability) persists**
   d. **Notify the woman's obstetric health care provider if pattern persists**
   f. **Evaluate FHR responses to interventions**

Brenda was admitted to the labor and delivery unit at 3:00 A.M. because the fetal heart rate pattern continued to demonstrate decreased LTV, questionable late decelerations, and no accelerations in the obstetric triage unit. Oxytocin induction was ordered. An amniotomy was performed, and clear fluid was noted. A FSE and IUPC were placed. At 7:10 A.M., Brenda was progressing slowly, and the oxytocin was infusing at 20 mU/min. Vaginal examination revealed that her cervix was 2 cm dilated and 100% effaced, and the fetus was vertex and at –2 station. Epidural anesthesia was administered; however, Brenda continued to complain of experiencing the "worst pain she had ever felt."

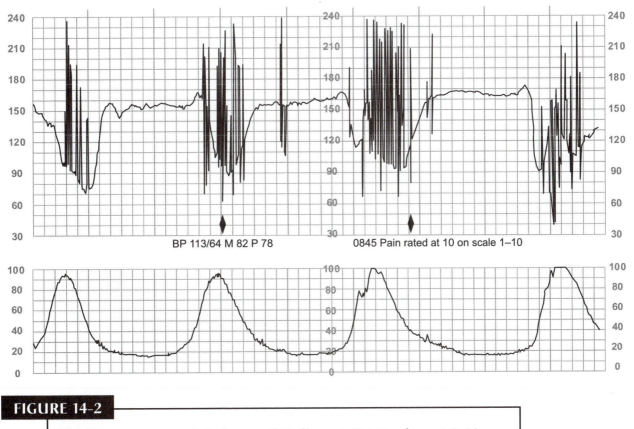

BP 113/64 M 82 P 78   0845 Pain rated at 10 on scale 1–10

FIGURE 14-2

Tracing Segment D2: Labor and Delivery EFM Tracing at 8:40 A.M. Using Internal Monitoring

AWHONN Fetal Heart Monitoring Principles and Practices
Systematic Approach to Interpretation Worksheet

Case Study Exercise: Brenda D2

1. Contractions: *Frequency:*   **q 2½–3 min.**
                             Duration: **90–100 sec.**
                             Intensity: **90–100 mmHg**
                             Resting tone: **15–18 mmHg**

2. Baseline fetal heart rate: **155–165 bpm, appears to be rising**

3. Variability: Place a checkmark signifying the appropriate type of variability on the strip (LTV = long-term variability; STV = short-term variability).

LTV	**Decreased (0–5 bpm)**	✔	*STV* **Present** ✔	
	Average (6–25 bpm)	✔	Absent	
	Marked (> 25 bpm)		Unable to assess	
	Unable to assess			

4. Accelerations and decelerations. When present, circle P if periodic or NP if nonperiodic.

         Accelerations
         Early decelerations
         Variable decelerations   (**P**)   NP
         Late decelerations
         Prolonged decelerations

5. List possible underlying physiologic mechanisms or rationales for observed patterns.
   a. **Baroreceptor and parasympathetic responses resulting in variable decelerations associated with umbilical cord compression or decreased amniotic fluid after artificial rupture of membranes (AROM)**
   b. **Fetal reserves present, resulting in presence of STV and recovery from the variable decelerations**
   c. **Artifact present on tracing**
   d. **Possible dysrhythmia present**

6. List in order of priority the physiologic goal(s) for observed patterns.
   a. **Maximize umbilical cord circulation**
   b. **Maximize uterine blood flow**
   c. **Maximize oxygenation**

7. List interventions to achieve the physiologic goals and actions needed related to instrumentation or further assessment.
   a. **Perform vaginal examination to assess for presence of prolapsed cord**
   b. **Change maternal position to maximize umbilical cord circulation and uterine blood flow**
   c. **Administer maternal supplemental oxygen via snug face mask**
   d. **Palpate uterus to confirm IUPC readings**
   e. **Notify the woman's obstetric primary care provider**
   f. **Notify the neonatal team of possible dysrhythmia in fetus**
   g. **Hydrate with IVF fluid bolus**
   h. **Consider amnioinfusion if pattern worsens**
   i. **Decrease oxytocin if pattern worsens**
   j. **Evaluate FHR response to interventions**

At 9:00 A.M., Brenda's vaginal examination revealed that her cervix was completely dilated, and the vertex fetus was at +1 station. She was instructed to push. The fetal heart rate tracing showed repetitive late decelerations and variable decelerations with late onset in timing. Brenda received three doses of ephedrine (10 mg, IV push) for blood pressures of 90/56, 73/50, 80/37, 67/36 and 69/42 mmHg. Her blood pressure did not respond to the ephedrine. Her pulse remained in the range of 89–107 bpm. The IUPC was no longer working despite being rezeroed.

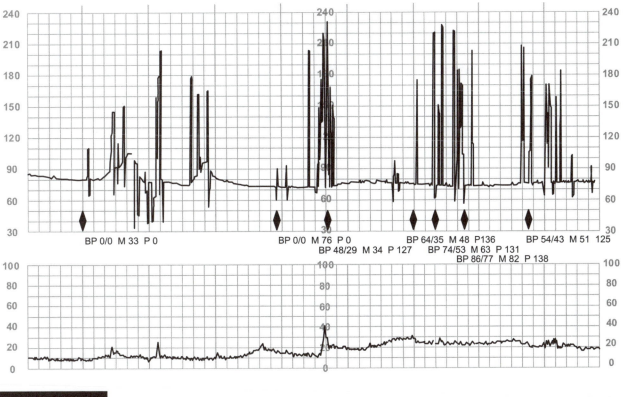

FIGURE 14-3

Tracing Segment D3: Labor and Delivery EFM Tracing at 9:30 A.M. Using Internal Monitoring

AWHONN Fetal Heart Monitoring Principles and Practices Systematic Approach to Interpretation Worksheet

Case Study Exercise: Brenda D3

1. Contractions:
   Frequency: **Unable to assess**
   Duration: **Unable to assess**
   Intensity: **Unable to assess; need to palpate**
   Resting tone: **Unable to assess; need to palpate**

2. Baseline fetal heart rate: **73–78 bpm (bradycardic rate)**

3. Variability: Place a checkmark signifying the appropriate type of variability on the strip (LTV = long-term variability; STV = short-term variability).

LTV		*STV*	
Decreased (0–5 bpm)	✔	Present	
Average (6–25 bpm)		**Absent**	✔
Marked (> 25 bpm)		Unable to assess	
Unable to assess			

4. Accelerations and decelerations. When present, circle P if periodic or NP if nonperiodic.

Accelerations	P	NP	Late decelerations	P	
Early decelerations	P		Prolonged decelerations		NP
Variable decelerations	P	NP	**None present**		

5. List possible underlying physiologic mechanisms or rationales for observed patterns.
   a. **Baroreceptor, chemoreceptor, autonomic nervous system and central nervous system responses associated with profound changes in fetal environment.**
   b. **Maternal hypotension**
   c. **Uterine rupture**
   d. **Dysrhythmic pattern**

6. List in order of priority the physiologic goal(s) for observed patterns.
   a. **Maximize umbilical circulation**
   b. **Maximize uterine blood flow**
   c. **Maximize oxygenation**

7. List interventions to achieve the physiologic goals and actions needed related to instrumentation or further assessment.
   a. **Continue to promote umbilical cord circulation and uterine blood flow through maternal position change and IV plasma expanders**
   b. **Quickly assess for possible causes while intervening (i.e., uterine rupture)**
   c. **Continue maternal supplemental oxygen via snug face mask**
   d. **Discontinue oxytocin**
   e. **Palpate uterus to confirm IUPC readings**
   f. **Notify the woman's obstetric primary care provider**
   g. **Notify the neonatal resuscitation team**
   h. **Prepare for emergent delivery**

Outcome:

An emergency cesarean delivery was performed. When the abdominal cavity was opened, the fetus and placenta were noted to be floating in the abdominal cavity. The patient continued to have uncontrolled bleeding, so an emergency hysterectomy and bilateral oophorectomy were performed. Estimated blood loss was 8,000 ml. A posterior uterine wall rupture was found.

Case Study Exercise E: Sakinah

Age:	28 years old
Gravida/Para:	2/0010
Gestational Age:	36 1/7 weeks
Medical History:	Sickle cell disease; most recent sickle crisis was 2 years ago
Surgical History:	Tonsillectomy at age 6 years
Psychosocial History:	Single; father of baby not involved, but family is supportive
Past Obstetric History:	Miscarriage at 8 weeks of gestation
Current Obstetric History:	Normal prenatal laboratory results
	Gestational diabetes controlled by diet
	Twin gestation (diamniotic/monochorionic)
	Monthly ultrasound examinations to monitor growth consistent with size and dates

Sakinah presented to antepartum testing for her biweekly nonstress test. Past testing was reassuring, showing reactive tracings and adequate amniotic fluid volume for a twin gestation. Sakinah stated both babies were moving well. She denied leaking fluid, bleeding, or regular/painful contractions. Her vital signs were as follows: temperature: 98.2°F (36.7°C); blood pressure: 104/60 mmHg; pulse: 78 bpm; and respiration: 20 breaths/minute.

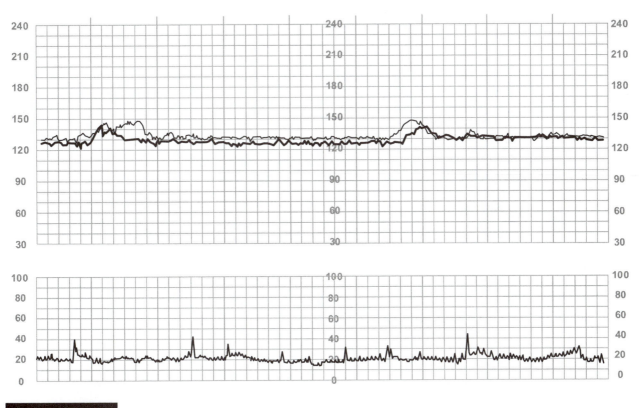

FIGURE 14-4

Tracing Segment E1: Antepartum Testing EFM Tracing at 2:00 P.M. Using External Monitoring. The Dark Line Represents Twin A, and the Light Line Represents Twin B.

AWHONN Fetal Heart Monitoring Principles and Practices
Systematic Approach to Interpretation Worksheet

Case Study Exercise: Sakinah E1

1. Contractions: *Frequency:*   **None**
                    Duration: **Not applicable**
                    Intensity: **Not applicable**
                    Resting tone: **Need to palpate**

2. Baseline fetal heart rate: **Twin A: 125–133 bpm, twin B: 130–137 bpm**

3. Variability: Place a checkmark signifying the appropriate type of variability on the strip (LTV = long-term variability; STV = short-term variability).

   LTV   Decreased (0–5 bpm)
          Average (6–25 bpm)   ✔ **(Twin A and twin B)**
          Marked (> 25 bpm)
          Unable to assess

   STV   Present
          Absent
          Unable to assess   ✔ **(Twin A and twin B)**

4. Accelerations and decelerations. When present, circle P if periodic or NP if nonperiodic.

   Accelerations   P   (NP) **(Twin A and twin B)**
   Early decelerations
   Variable decelerations
   Late decelerations
   Prolonged decelerations

5. List possible underlying physiologic mechanisms or rationales for observed patterns.
   a. **Fetal movement or response to environmental stimulus**
   b. **Direct sympathetic stimulation of the fetus**
   c. **Associated with nonacidotic, oxygenated fetus**

6. List in order of priority the physiologic goal(s) for observed patterns.
   a. **Maximize uterine blood flow**
   b. **Maximize umbilical circulation**
   c. **Maximize oxygenation**

7. List interventions to achieve the physiologic goals and actions needed related to instrumentation or further assessment.
   a. **Palpate contractions and adjust toco to monitor uterine activity more effectively**
   b. **Continue routine assessment and interventions for antepartum testing**

Case Study Exercise F: Hannah

Age: 16 years old

Gravida/Para: 1/0

Gestational Age: 39⁶/₇ weeks

Medical History: Unremarkable

Surgical History: Unremarkable

Psychosocial History: Attention deficit disorder; lives in foster care

Current Obstetric History: Normal prenatal laboratory results

Rh positive

Patient missed two scheduled ultrasound appointments

Hannah presented to the labor and delivery unit 4:00 P.M. with a complaint of spontaneous rupture of membranes 2 hours earlier that was green in color. Her contractions increased in frequency and intensity. Hannah stated the baby had not moved in the past 12 hours. Her vital signs were as follows: temperature: 98.6°F (37°C); blood pressure: 126/78 mmHg; pulse: 90 bpm; respiration: 24 breaths/minute. A fetal pulse oxygen saturation (FSpO₂) monitoring device had already been placed earlier due to earlier episodes of fetal tachycardia, decreased LTV and repetitive variable decelerations.

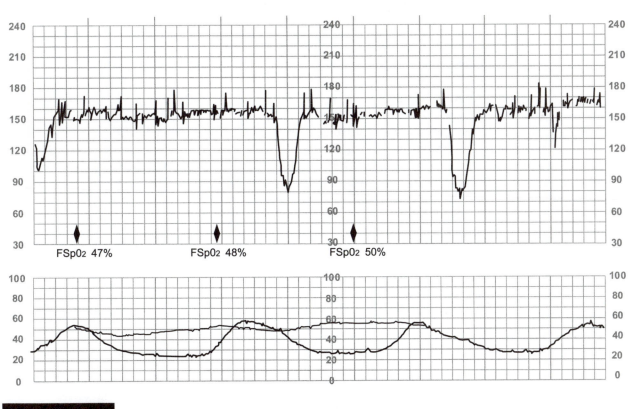

FIGURE 14-5

Tracing Segment F1: Labor and Delivery EFM Tracing at 5:20 A.M. Using Internal Monitoring and FSpO₂ Monitoring

AWHONN Fetal Heart Monitoring Principles and Practices
Systematic Approach to Interpretation Worksheet

Case Study Exercise: Hannah F1

1. Contractions: *Frequency:*   **q 2–3 min.**
                         Duration: **80–100 sec.**
                         Intensity: **50–55 mmHg**
                         Resting tone: **25 mmHg**

2. Baseline fetal heart rate: **155–160 bpm**

3. Variability: Place a checkmark signifying the appropriate type of variability on the strip (LTV = long-term variability; STV = short-term variability).

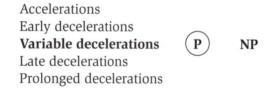

    LTV   **Decreased (0–5 bpm)**   ✔   *STV*   **Present**   ✔
               Average (6–25 bpm)   Absent
               Marked (> 25 bpm)   Unable to assess
               Unable to assess

4. Accelerations and decelerations. When present, circle P if periodic or NP if nonperiodic.

                  Accelerations
                  Early decelerations
                  Variable decelerations   Ⓟ   **NP**
                  Late decelerations
                  Prolonged decelerations

5. List possible underlying physiologic mechanisms or rationales for observed patterns.
   a. **Baroreceptor and parasympathetic responses resulting in variable decelerations and associated with umbilical cord compression or decreased amniotic fluid after rupture of membranes.**
   b. **Fetal reserves present, resulting in present STV and FSpO$_2$ reading of 47–50%**

6. List in order of priority the physiologic goal(s) for observed patterns.
   a. **Maximize umbilical cord circulation**
   b. **Maximize uterine blood flow**
   c. **Maximize oxygenation**

7. List interventions to achieve the physiologic goals and actions needed related to instrumentation or further assessment.
   a. **Perform vaginal examination to check for prolapsed cord**
   b. **Change maternal position to maximize umbilical cord circulation and uterine blood flow**
   c. **Administer maternal supplemental oxygen via snug face mask**
   d. **Palpate uterus to confirm IUPC readings**
   e. **Notify the woman's obstetric primary care provider**
   f. **Hydrate with IVFs**
   g. **Consider amnioinfusion if pattern continues or worsens.**
   h. **Continue to monitor FSpO$_2$ readings**
   i. **Continue to evaluate FHR response to interventions**

Glossary of Key Terms

Acceleration—A transitory increase in the fetal heart rate from the baseline rate; associated with sympathetic nervous stimulation.

Acidemia—An abnormal excess of hydrogen ion concentration in the blood that is due to increased acid build up or increased loss of base.

Acidosis—An abnormal excess hydrogen ion concentration in tissues that is due to increased acid buildup or increased loss of base.

Adrenergic response—Activated by, characteristic of, or secreting epinephrine or substances with similar activity. The term is applied to nerve fibers that transmit norepinephrine at a synapse when a nerve impulse passes (i.e., sympathetic fibers).

Aerobic metabolism—Biochemical and physiologic processes that take place in the presence of oxygen.

Alkalosis—An increase in pH value (decreased hydrogen ion concentration) above normal.

Amnioinfusion—Instillation of fluid into the uterus through an intrauterine catheter. Used to increase amniotic fluid volume in situations of oligohydramnios or umbilical cord compression with associated variable decelerations. Also used to dilute amniotic fluid in situations of meconium stained amniotic fluid.

Amniotic fluid index (AFI)—The amount of amniotic fluid measured by ultrasonography in centimeters. AFI is expressed as the sum of the measurements of the deepest amniotic fluid pockets in all four abdominal quadrants.

Amplitude—The distance between high and low points of FHR tracing oscillations. Also used in reference to long-term variability range in beats per minute.

Anaerobic metabolism—Biochemical and physiologic processes that take place in the absence of oxygen.

Antenatal—Occurring or formed before birth; used synonymously with prenatal.

Antepartum—The period of time that occurs before childbirth.

Antidysrhythmic therapy—Treatment regimens used to treat fetal dysrhythmias. Also referred to as antiarrhythmic therapy.

APT test—A diagnostic indicator that differentiates fetal from maternal red blood cells in a maternal or neonatal specimen (e.g., vaginal blood flow, meconium, or gastric aspirate).

Arrhythmia—A heart rate without rhythm. In EFM, describes sporadic, irregular fetal heart beats that may be heard or recorded on the FHR tracing. Arrhythmias are associated with variability of the R-R intervals but with normal P waves that occur in a regular fashion preceding each QRS complex. Term sometimes used interchangeably with dysrhythmia.

Artifact—Irregular variation or absence of FHR on the fetal monitor tracing that is due to mechanical limitations or electrical interference of the monitoring system.

Aspartate aminotransferase (AST)—An enzyme that contributes to protein metabolism. This enzyme is present in the liver and is important in the biosynthesis of amino acids as it catalyzes the reversible transfer of an amino group between glutamic and aspartic acid. The former term was SGOT (serum flutamic-oxaloacetic transaminase. When cell damage occurs, especially in the liver (as seen with severe preeclampsia, HELLP syndrome, or trauma), AST levels are increased and AST is released into the tissues and bloodstream.

Atrial flutter—A heart rhythm disturbance resulting in a tachycardiac FHR ranging from 400–500 bpm in the fetus and 300–360 bpm in the neonate. Due to the increased FHR, the ventricular response varies, resulting in the rate being either fixed (2:1 or 3:1 AV block) and regular or variable and irregular (e.g., varying degrees of AV block).

Atrial fibrillation—Tachycardiac atrial FHR rarely identified in the fetus. Often accompanied by a variable degree of AV block that will cause the ventricular rate to vary from 60 to 200 bpm.

Atrioventricular (AV) dysrhythmia—A heart rhythm disturbance resulting in a dysrhythmic patterns from a defect in the AV junction that disrupts or changes conduction of impulses through the AV node. AV dysrhythmias consist of second- and third-degree AV block.

Auscultation—An auditory assessment procedure or process of listening for sounds within the body, such as fetal heart sounds. Fetal heart sounds are auscultated to determine rate and rhythm. True auscultation is performed with a fetoscope, or stethoscope (e.g., Pinard), but this term frequently is used to include the use of a hand-held Doppler ultrasound device to detect FHR.

Autocorrelation—Microprocessor comparison of consecutive points of waveforms generated by the electronic fetal monitor. Comparison is based on ultrasound waves reflected from the moving fetal heart valves. Mechanism in second-generation fetal monitors.

Automaticity—The spontaneous, diastolic depolarization of normally specialized cells, e.g., the AV node, SA node, bundle of His or Purkinje fibers.

Baroreceptor—Pressure-sensitive stretch receptor in carotid sinus and aortic arch that responds to blood pressure changes by altering the FHR via the sympathetic (increase in rate) and parasympathetic (decrease in rate) nervous system.

Base deficit—Measures the amount of base buffer reserves below normal levels. A large positive base deficit (e.g., 10 mEq/liter) indicates that base buffers have been used to buffer acids, that sufficient base reserves are not present, and that metabolic acidosis is present.

Base excess—Measures the amount of base buffer reserves above normal levels. A large negative base excess (e.g., –10 mEq/liter) indicates that base buffers have been used to buffer acids, that sufficient base reserves are not present, and that metabolic acidosis is present.

Baseline fetal heart rate—Average FHR over 10 minutes, between uterine contractions, decelerations, or accelerations.

Beta-adrenergic receptors—Specific sites on smooth muscle cells (e.g., the myometrium of the uterus) where chemicals (agonists) can couple to produce a chemical reaction.

Beta-mimetic drugs—Chemical substances that are able to bind to beta-receptor sites on smooth muscle cells (i.e., myometrium of the uterus), causing a relaxing or depressant effect on the contractility of uterine myometrial cells. Beta-mimetic drugs belong to a group of chemicals called agonists.

Biophysical profile (BPP)—An antenatal assessment of fetal well-being that combines NST results with multiple physiologic parameters observed with real-time ultrasound. The BPP includes the assessment of the following five components: (a) fetal breathing movement, (b) gross body movement, (c) fetal tone, (d) amniotic fluid volume, and (e) fetal heart rate reactivity (NST).

Bishop Score—A method for determining cervical readiness for induction of labor by scoring 5 components: cervical dilation, effacement, consistency, position, and station of the presenting part. Higher scores are associated with successful induction of labor. Score also has been used as an assessment in preterm labor suppression.

Bradyarrhythmia—An irregular heart rate rhythm usually occurring when FHR is below 90 beats per minute (e.g., sinus bradycardia or heart block). Visualized by fetal echocardiography or ECG.

Bradycardia—Baseline FHR below 110 beats per minute for longer than 10 minutes.

Cardiotocography—The monitoring of the fetal heart rate and uterine contractions during labor and delivery. Also referred to as cardiotokography.

Certification—The process by which an accredited credentialing agency or organization documents an individual's knowledge in a nursing specialty.

Chemoreceptor—Sensory nerve endings or organs stimulated by a chemical response. Sensitive to change in oxygen, carbon dioxide, and pH levels in the blood. Chemoreceptors are located in the aortic and carotid bodies and in the medulla.

Combined deceleration patterns—Complex FHR patterns that cannot be classified as early, late or variable decelerations and that contain characteristics of more than one FHR pattern relative to shape and timing.

Compensatory response to hypoxemia—Describes the ability of the fetus to adjust to low blood oxygen levels by drawing from fetal reserves. The presence of STV implies fetal reserves.

Competence validation—Process of documenting the verification of individual's knowledge and skills according to predetermined criteria.

Conductivity—The capacity of the cardiac cells to conduct a current through the cells.

Conflict resolution—Process of resolving professional disagreements within the mechanisms of institutional policies, procedures, and protocols. Process may involve implementing the chain of command.

Contraction Stress Test (CST)—Antepartum assessment tool to assess fetal response to spontaneous or stimulated uterine contractions. Contractions may be produced via intravenous oxytocin administration or nipple stimulation. The uterine contractions should be 3 in 10 minutes of at least 40 seconds in length. The presence of late decelerations (a positive CST) could be an indicator of fetal compromise. Also referred to as Nipple Stimulation Test or Breast Stimulation Test (BST).

Deceleration—A transitory decrease in the FHR from the baseline rate.

Digyzotic—Pertaining to or derived from two separate zygotes (fertilized ovum), as in twin gestation occurring from two fertilized ovum. Results in fraternal twins.

Doppler—Generally refers to a hand-held instrument that emits ultrasound waves. It converts the waves reflected from the moving fetal heart into a fetal heart rate.

Doppler velocimetry—Use of specialized ultrasonography to measure the blood flow velocity in the uterine artery, umbilical arteries and fetal middle cerebral artery. Also referred to as Doppler flow.

Dysrhythmia—A disturbance in fetal heart rhythm associated with a disordered impulse formation, impulse conduction, or a combination of both. The pattern will demonstrate an abnormal P-QRS relationship evidenced by early P waves or bizarre-looking QRS complexes or both.

Early deceleration—A transitory decrease in the FHR from the baseline rate caused by compression of the fetal vertex during contractions and resultant vagal stimulation. Characterized by synchronous onset and offset with uterine contractions. Mirrors the contraction. Uniform in shape.

Electronic fetal monitoring—An auditory and visual assessment of the FHR and visual assessment of uterine activity with data generated by electronic technology. Generated data includes a digital and graphic display and a permanent record on paper or laser disk.

Excitability—The readiness of the cardiac cells to respond to a stimulus or irritation.

External fetal monitoring—A noninvasive auditory and visual assessment of the FHR with data generated by an ultrasonic transducer device to monitor the fetal heart rate and a tocodynamometer to monitor uterine contractions. Also referred to as an indirect method of monitoring.

Extrinsic influences—Factors in the fetal environment that affect the availability of oxygen to the fetus that may affect FHR characteristics (e.g., maternal, placental, or umbilical cord factors).

Favorable physiologic response—A reassuring FHR response associated with a fetus that is able to respond appropriately to the environment and maintain fetal reserves.

Fetal attitude—Assessment derived from Leopold's maneuvers that determines the relation of the fetal parts to each other. Fetal attitudes could be flexion or extension of the fetus.

Fetal lie—Assessment derived from Leopold's maneuvers that determines the relationship of the fetal body to the maternal body. Fetal lies would be longitudinal (fetal body is parallel to maternal spine), transverse (fetal body is at right angles (perpendicular) to maternal spine), or oblique (fetal body is at an angle between longitudinal and transverse lie).

Fetal pulse oximetry—A method of assessing fetal oxygen saturation during labor.

Fetal presentation—The lowest part of the fetus that comes out of the uterus first. Most often the presentation is vertex (head first), but it can also be breech (buttocks or feet first), shoulder (shoulder first), face or brow (face or brow first) or compound (hand with head or foot with buttocks).

Fetal scalp blood sampling—Invasive method of assessing pH level of the fetus. Requires ruptured membranes. Uses cone-shaped cylinder with a light source to permit scraping of the fetal scalp, collection of micro-sample of blood via capillary tube that is analyzed by a blood gas machine for the pH level.

Fetal scalp stimulation—An indirect method of assessing acid-base status of the fetus by vigorously rubbing the fetal head to elicit an acceleration. Can be performed with or without ruptured membranes. Is not used as a resuscitative measure.

Fetal surveillance—Assessment of fetal status via a variety of methods such as external or internal fetal monitoring, antenatal testing, fetal scalp stimulation, fetal scalp blood sampling, acoustical stimulation, pulse oximetry or ultrasound technology.

Fetal reserve—Additional amount of oxygen available to the fetus beyond the amount normally required by the fetus for metabolism.

Fetoscope—Stethoscope adapted for auscultation of the FHR (also known as DeLee fetoscope).

Funic souffle (bruit)—A soft "blowing" sound heard by auscultation over the umbilical cord. Synchronous with the FHR.

Heart block—An atrioventricular (AV) conduction defect in which the electrical impulses in the heart are not conducted normally from the atrium to the ventricles via the sinoatrial (SA) node, AV node, bundle of HIS, and Purkinje fibers. Results in bradycardia. May be fixed or intermittent.

Hydrostatic pressure—The pressure exerted by a fluid in a closed system, such as pressure created by amniotic fluid in the uterus. An intrauterine pressure catheter (IUPC) measures hydrostatic pressure in the uterus during and between uterine contractions.

Hyperglycemia—abnormally high levels of glucose in the blood.

Hypocalcemia—Abnormally low levels of calcium in the blood.

Hypoglycemia—Abnormally low levels of glucose in the blood.

Hypokalemia—Abnormally low levels of potassium in the blood.

Hypoxemia—Low levels of oxygen in the blood.

Hypoxia—Low levels of oxygen available in the tissue, inadequate to meet metabolic needs of the tissue.

Impending decompensation—The loss of fetal ability to respond physiologically to the feto-maternal environment; may include a loss of fetal reserves and inability to maintain the heart rate within normal range.

Intermittent auscultation—Listening to the FHR at periodic intervals either by fetoscope or hand-held Doppler.

Internal fetal monitoring—An electronic auditory and visual assessment of the FHR with data generated by a spiral electrode attached to the fetal presenting part to monitor the fetal heart rate and an intrauterine pressure catheter to monitor uterine contractions. Also referred to as a direct method of monitoring.

Intrapartum period—The period that includes labor and birth.

Intrauterine pressure catheter (IUPC)—A catheter used to directly measure intrauterine pressure during and between uterine contractions. The catheter may be fluid filled or sensor tipped.

Intrinsic influences—Internal fetal regulatory mechanisms that control the heart rate, including sympathetic, parasympathetic, and central nervous systems, baroreceptor, chemoreceptor, and hormonal responses.

Kleihauer-Betke test—A blood analysis used to detect the presence and relative amount of fetal hemoglobin in a maternal blood specimen. When blood specimen is stained on a slide, cells characterized with fetal hemoglobin can be viewed and counted to determine the ratio of fetal blood cells to maternal blood cells.

Late deceleration—A repetitive decrease in the FHR from the baseline rate typically caused by uteroplacental insufficiency. Deceleration is late in onset and in recovery in relationship to the uterine contraction and is uniform in shape.

Leopold's maneuvers—A systematic four step method of abdominal assessment used to determine fetal lie, presentation and position and identify the location for fetal heart rate auscultation.

Long-term variability (LTV)—Oscillatory changes in the FHR baseline. Most frequently described in terms of amplitude within the baseline range, but also includes frequency of oscillations (cycles) over 1 minute.

Medulla oblongata—The lower portion of the brain stem; the relay center for the parasympathetic and sympathetic nervous system.

Meta-analysis—A systematic approach to analyzing findings from multiple studies.

Metabolic acidosis—Decrease in blood pH associated with an increase in hydrogen ions, decrease in PO_2, and increase in base deficit (base excess). The PCO_2 may be normal.

Metabolic alkalosis—Increase in blood pH associated with a decrease in hydrogen ions and a decrease in PCO_2.

Mixed acidosis—Combination of metabolic and respiratory acidosis, associated with a decrease in pH, decrease in PO_2, an increase in PCO_2 levels, and an increase in base deficit.

Modified biophysical profile—Antepartal assessment that combines the NST and an ultrasound-obtained amniotic fluid index (AFI) in the third trimester.

Monozygotic—Pertaining to or derived from a single zygote (fertilized ovum), as in twin gesta-tion occurring from a single fertilized ovum. Results in identical twins.

Montevideo units—Total pressure in mm Hg for all uterine contractions within a 10-minute time frame. The baseline resting tone is subtracted from the peak uterine pressure for each contraction to determine the mm Hg.

Nadir—The lowest FHR value in a deceleration or depth of a deceleration. With electronic monitoring, it is visually the lowest point in the deceleration curve.

Neurohormonal response—Response that is both neural and hormonal mediated.

Nonimmunologic hydrops fetalis—The development of generalized edema in the abdomen, scalp, liver and spleen of the fetus.

Nonhypoxemic reflex response—A FHR response to an event not associated with de creased PO_2. Fetus quickly responds to change caused by an event (e.g., baroreceptor and vagal response affecting fetal blood pressure because of brief compression of the umbilical cord).

Nonperiodic pattern—Accelerations or decelerations of the FHR that occur independent of repetitive uterine contractions (e.g., deceleration or acceleration in response to vaginal exam, fetal movement, tetanic contraction, cord compression, or maternal vomiting).

Nonreassuring fetal heart rate pattern—A FHR pattern that may reflect an unfavorable physiologic fetal response to the feto-maternal environment. A descriptive term.

Nonstress Test (NST)—Antepartum assessment of fetal well-being. The FHR is monitored for 2 accelerations (15 bpm above the FHR baseline lasting for 15 seconds from the time the FHR leaves the baseline to the time it returns to the baseline) in 20 minutes. In the preterm infant before 32 weeks, two accelerations of 10 bpm lasting 10 seconds is considered a reactive test. The presence of accelerations indicates fetal well-being.

Overshoot—Exaggerated compensatory increase in the FHR after a variable deceleration. Usually at least 10 to 20 bpm increase with no variability, with no abruptness, and returns to the baseline gradually. Nonreassuring when repetitive and without baseline variability. Also referred to as rebound overshoot.

Oxytocin Challenge Test (OCT)—Antepartum assessment tool using exogenous (synthetic) oxytocin (pitocin) given via intravenous pump to produce uterine contractions. The uterine contractions should be 3 in 10 minutes of at least 40 seconds in duration.

Oxytocic—Having the effect of stimulating the uterus to contract.

Parasympathetic nervous system—Part of autonomic nervous system. Includes vagal nerves which decrease heart rate when stimulated.

Perinatal—The time between 20 weeks gestation and 28 days after birth.

Periodic pattern—Accelerations or decelerations of the FHR that occur in direct association with uterine contractions.

Periodic accelerations—Transitory increases in the FHR that occur repetitively and are associated with uterine contractions. May be attributed to fetal movement, mild partial umbilical cord compression, or sympathetic stimulation from fundal pressure on the fetal head in a breech presentation.

Phonocardiography—The graphic representation of heart sounds and murmurs, and includes pulse tracings (carotid, apex, and jugular pulse).

Piezoelectric effect—The crystals in the ultrasound transducer generate sound waves that are reflected back from moving structures. A shift in frequency of the waveforms reflected will identify the FHR.

Postterm pregnancy—Pregnancy lasting beyond 42 completed weeks of gestation.

Premature Atrial Contraction (PAC)—A heart rhythm alteration characterized by the early discharge of an atrial focus, as seen by a premature P wave followed by a narrow, normal-appearing QRS complex. Can be either conducted (i.e., PAC followed by a ventricular contraction, then a compensatory pause followed by normal sinus rhythm) or nonconducted (i.e., PAC followed by compensatory pause). Often followed by an incomplete compensatory pause, produced by the incomplete depolarization of the fetal heart. Etiologies include maternal ingestion of caffeine, alcohol or nicotine; maternal hyperthyroidism; trisomy 18 and drug exposure.

Premature Rupture of Membranes (PROM)—rupture of membranes that occurs after 37 com-pleted weeks of gestation, without signs and symptoms of labor.

Preterm PROM (PPROM)—rupture of membranes that occurs prior to 37 completed weeks of gestation, with or without signs and symptoms of labor.

Premature ventricular contraction (PVC)—Premature depolarization in the heart with resultant irregularity in the heart rate and rhythm. PVCs will show no P wave, and the premature QRS is bizarre and wide, with the T wave usually directed opposite to the polarity of the QRS complex. The full compensatory pause may or may not be present. Associated with cardiomyopathy, long QT syndrome, complete AV block with rates less than 55 bpm, hydrops fetalis, myocarditis, digitalis toxicity, cocaine use, hyperkalemia (although rare in pregnancy) due to hyperemesis, structural cardiac anomalies or unknown reasons.

Prolonged deceleration—Decrease in the fetal heart rate from the baseline for longer than 2 minutes but usually less than 10 minutes. Associated with stimuli, such as cord compression, uterine hypertonus, and response to medications.

Pseudosinusoidal pattern—A "sawtooth" undulating FHR pattern associated with periods of normal variability (STV and LTV) and accelerations. Less smooth, less constant than sinusoidal pattern and thought to be benign.

Reactivity—Presence of FHR accelerations meeting the criteria of 15 beats per minute increase over 15 seconds occurring at least twice in 20 minutes. Usually associated with normal variability.

Reassuring pattern—A FHR pattern that reflects a favorable physiologic response to the feto-maternal environment. A descriptive term.

Refractory window—An inhibitory period in which the electronic ultrasound transducer does not attempt to count the incoming signal. Mechanism in first-generation fetal monitors.

Respiratory acidosis—A decrease in pH associated with an increase in carbonic acid and increase in CO_2. The base deficit may be within normal range. If pulmonary or placental exchange is increased, the amount of CO_2 in the extracellular tissue may decrease.

Respiratory alkalosis—An increase in pH associated with a decrease in hydrogen ions and a decrease in PCO_2 often associated with hyperventilation.

Rhythm—Regularity or irregularity of the baseline FHR.

Saltatory—LTV that is greater than 25 bpm; also defined as marked LTV.

Short-term variability (STV)—Changes in the FHR from one beat to the next. Measures the R-to-R intervals of subsequent fetal cardiac cycles (QRS). Presence reflects fetal reserves. Measured only by direct spiral electrode.

Shoulders—Compensatory accelerations that may precede or follow variable decelerations. Generally of short duration (< 20 seconds) and < 20 bpm above the baseline.

Sinusoidal pattern—A persistent sine wave or recurrent undulating FHR pattern that is smooth (absent short-term variability), uniform, usually within the normal heart rate range, and without periods of normal FHR reactivity.

Solid sensor-tipped IUPC—An intrauterine pressure catheter that has a microprocessor transducer at the catheter tip which measures the intrauterine pressure directly.

Spiral electrode—An internal monitoring device applied directly to the fetal presenting part which receives signals from the electrocardiac impulses of the fetal heart. Used to directly determine FHR and STV based on changes in the R to R intervals in successive QRS complexes.

Strain gauge—A part of the IUPC that electronically converts uterine pressure changes into mmHg. Component of closed pressure system using a fluid-filled intrauterine catheter.

Supraventricular dysrhythmias—Patterns that originate above the ventricles, i.e., in the atria.

Supraventricular tachycardia—A sustained, rapid, regular dysrhythmia of atrial origin in excess of 180–210 bpm and may be paroxysmal (i.e., occurring suddenly or in waves/spasms) or continuous. At rates lower than 210 bpm, the FHR pattern may show some variability within the baseline rate at a rate of around 5–15 bpm. Supraventricular tachycardia is often characterized by a fixed R-R interval with P waves preceding each QRS complex, as identified by ECG.

Sympathetic nervous system—A part of the autonomic nervous system. Stimulation results in FHR increase.

Tachycardia—Baseline FHR above 160 beats per minute for longer than 10 minutes.

Tachysystole—Abnormally frequent uterine contractions.

Tocodynamometer (tocotransducer)—An external monitoring device that detects changes in uterine shape through the abdomen. Provides information about relative frequency and duration of contractions.

Tocolytic—A drug that has an effect of quieting or inhibiting smooth muscle activity (i.e., myometrium of the uterus).

Tonus—Intensity of uterine tone or intrauterine pressure between uterine contractions.

Ultrasound transducer—An external monitoring device that detects movement of the fetal heart valves open ing and closing through transmission of a sound wave and Doppler shift. Monitor processor converts reflected sound waves into a FHR.

Undulating pattern—A FHR pattern that has a characteristic repetitive sine wave shape. Includes sinusoidal and pseudosinusoidal patterns.

Unfavorable physiologic response—A FHR response associated with a fetus that is unable to respond appropriately to the feto-maternal environment and is demonstrating a loss of fetal-reserves.

Uterine bruit—The sound heard when listening to the blood flow in the maternal uterine vessels (also known as uterine souffle). Synchronous with maternal pulse.

Variable deceleration—An abrupt decrease in the FHR from the baseline rate most commonly in response to compression of the umbilical cord. Deceleration is irregular in shape, timing, and depth. May be associated with contractions (periodic) or not associated with contractions (nonperiodic).

Variability (baseline variability)—Variations or fluctuations of the FHR during a steady state (in the absence of contractions, decelerations, and accelerations). Changes are due to sympathetic and parasympathetic innervation. Generally used to describe beat-to-beat changes (STV) and oscillatory changes (LTV). Monitoring method determines which type of variability can be reliably described.

Ventricular dysrhythmia—Alterations in heart rhythm that is ventricular in origin and are the result of premature electrical discharge below the AV junction.

Ventricular tachycardia—An alteration in heart rate and a rare fetal abnormality in which FHR varies between 170 and 400 bpm.

Vibroacoustic stimulation (VAS)—Process of fetal stimulation using sound via an artificial larynx. The objective is to elicit a fetal startle or movement to evaluate fetal well-being. Also referred to as acoustic stimulation.

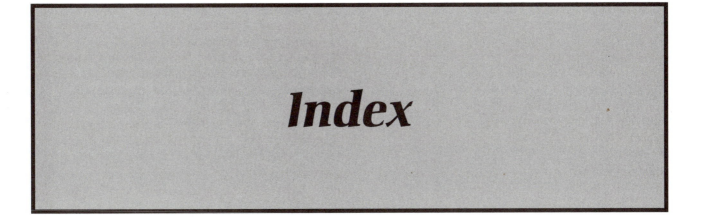

Index